CHILDREN *with* STARVING BRAINS

A MEDICAL TREATMENT GUIDE for AUTISM SPECTRUM DISORDER

4th Edition

JAQUELYN McCANDLESS, MD

With Contributions by
Teresa Binstock and
Jack Zimmerman, PhD

Also
J. Neubrander, MD, D. Lonsdale, MD,
Stan Kurtz, R. Deth, PhD, C. Schneider, MD
M. Elise, MD, S. Owens

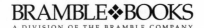

BRAMBLE❖BOOKS
A DIVISION OF THE BRAMBLE COMPANY

For information please contact:
Bramble Books
E-mail address: info@bramblebooks.com or visit our website, www.bramblebooks.com

The Library of Congress has cataloged the 2nd Edition as follows:

McCandless, Jaquelyn.
  Children with starving brains : a medical treatment guide for autism spectrum disorder / Jaquelyn McCandless ; with contributions by Teresa Binstock, and Jack Zimmerman.—2nd ed.
    p. ; cm.
Includes bibliographical references and index.
  ISBN 188364710X (alk. paper)
  1. Autism in children. 2. Autistic children—Rehabilitation. 3. Parent and child.
  [DNLM: 1. Autistic Disorder—therapy—Child—Popular Works. 2. Autistic Disorder—etiology—Child—Popular Works. 3. Complementary Therapies—Child—Popular Works. 4. Diet Therapy—Child—Popular Works. WM 203.5 M4775c 2003] I. Binstock, Teresa. II. Zimmerman, Jack, PhD. III. Title.

RJ506.A9M425 2003
618.92'898206—dc21

2003000311

3rd Edition ISBN: 978-1-883647-13-1
4th Edition ISBN: 978-1-883647-17-9

Cover art: Ken Bennett

First Printing 2002, 2nd Edition 2003, 3rd Edtion 2007, 4th Edition 2009

1   3   5   7   9   10   8   6   4   2
10 12 11 09

Printed in United States of America

The paper used in this publication meets the minimum requirements of
American National Standard for Information Sciences—
Permanence of Paper for Printed Library Materials, ANSI Z39.48-1984

CONTENTS

TWO

THREE

FOUR

FIVE

Gastrointestinal Healing...80

SIX

Feeding the Starving Brain 109

SEVEN

Removing the Heavy Metals 133

EIGHT

Immunity, Autoimmunity and Viruses 164

NINE

HBOT-HYPERBARIC OXYGEN THERAPY FOR AUTISM SPECTRUM DISORDERS 190

Written by James Neubrander, MD,
Reviewed and edited by Dan Rossignol, MD

TEN

ELEVEN

TWELVE

Starving Brains, Starving Hearts, What Does It All Mean?

Jack Zimmerman, PhD

APPENDICES

> **It is recommended that you check
> the Autism-Rx Guide Book website
> frequently for updates and new developments.**
>
> **www.starvingbrains.com**

ABOUT THE AUTHOR

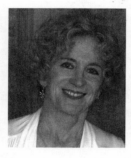**Jaquelyn McCandless** received her Doctorate in Medicine at the University of Illinois College of Medicine and is certified as a Diplomate of the American Board of Psychiatry and Neurology, beginning her practice of psychiatry in Southern California in 1966. Since the early 1990's, interest in women's issues and sexuality led more to an alternative medicine practice with a focus on anti-aging, brain nutrition and natural hormone therapy. In 1996 after her granddaughter Chelsey was diagnosed with autism when just 3 yrs of age, Dr. McCandless turned even more to basic medicine and began working with the complex biomedical aspects of developmentally delayed children. This has been her primary work for the last decade. She continues to search for effective treatments for those on the autistic spectrum and is currently expanding her interest and investigation of immune-enhancing agents toward helping those who struggle with the challenge of immune impairment, including persons affected by HIV+ AIDS and other autoimmune diseases.

DEDICATION

With love and gratitude to Bernard Rimland, PhD, 1928-2006, the "grand god-father of the movement for understanding and implementing the biomedical treatment of autism."

PREFACE TO 1ST & 2ND EDITIONS AND ACKNOWLEDGMENTS

In 1996, my beloved granddaughter Chelsey was diagnosed as having Autism Spectrum Disorder (ASD) at two years, nine months of age. Her diagnosis and unusually compelling nature inspired a reorientation of my professional life from the practice of psychiatry with a focus on alternative and anti-aging medicine to an immersion into the biomedical aspects of autism. Despite decades as a practicing physician, my embarrassing lack of knowledge about autism necessitated my going back into the basics of medicine. The heart of my journey which led to the writing of this book is actually a love story. Coming from a very large and loving family, having five biological children and three step-children plus thirteen grand-children certainly had already created a crucible of great love, wonder, and support for me. Yet something about Chelsey opened a part of my heart unbeknownst to me before. I discovered that all the children with this diagnosis touch that same place in me.

In my passion to understand the causes and therefore possible treatments for Chelsey, my medical brain became activated and information I didn't remember I had ever learned started becoming available to me in a new way I did not understand. The complexity of autism required me to put together a lot of medical information I hadn't connected before and led me into an entirely new approach to the practice of medicine which continues unabated today. For me, this transition has become a continuing and passionate adventure of mind-heart expansion, during which I have had enormous help. The ASD epidemic too well known now to families, teachers, and health care workers throughout this nation is opening up new paradigms in education and medicine, and I am excited to be a part of this movement. As my journey in these new directions continues, I want to recognize—in chronological order—individuals who have been particularly instrumental in helping me better understand and work with these children.

Dr. Bernard Rimland's ARI (Autism Research Institute) website and his studies about the treatment efficacy of vitamin B6 first started me on the path to seeing autism as a biochemical disorder. The B6 effect on Chelsey's hyperactivity was immediately noticeable. When the vitamin was skipped once for a few days, she managed to knock out her front teeth. Needless to say, we have never missed her daily dose since then. I consider Dr. Rimland the "grand god-father" of the movement for understanding biomedical treatment of autism. The organization Defeat Autism Now! that he co-founded is made up of the most generous, helpful, hopeful group of physicians, researchers, and parents as one could ever encounter. Many, including "Bernie" and myself, are parents or grandparents of a child with an autism-spectrum disorder. The group's willingness to share information about autism's biological nature and ways to help our children affected by autism merits respect and appreciation.

Though I have never had the privilege of personally meeting him, I saw a film portraying Dr. Ivar Lovaas at work with severely autistic children when Chelsey was three. His passionate dedication and effectiveness convinced me that many of these children are teachable, if you can get their attention, and inspired us to get Chelsey started on an intensive ABA program that has helped her immensely.

Karl Reichelt, MD, PhD, is an esteemed and caring researcher who helped me persuade Elizabeth, Chelsey's mother-of-four young children, to add the challenge of attempting a gluten-free, casein-free diet for Chelsey into her already very busy life. Dr. Reichelt patiently and generously e-mailed me from his research laboratory in Norway extensive and convincing information for implementing a dietary regime which in those days sounded like an impossible task. Within a week of starting this diet, Chelsey had her first formed bowel movement, leading not only to improvement in her health but finally to successful toilet training. That in itself was a more than adequate reward for the effort involved in enacting the diet.

Autism internet discussion boards have been and continue to be a resource not only for giving and sharing information but a way of being part of a passionate community of persons focused on autism as I am. Anytime of the day or night one can ask for and get help and encouragement from other parents and professionals all over the world. From the moment I ventured an e-post in 1998 to what was then the Secretin list (now called abmd) my professional life began changing course rapidly. The e-list groups have contributed greatly to my information base and strong desire to share what I've learned with as many parents and professionals as possible.

My friend and colleague Teresa Binstock told me she was formally diagnosed with Asperger's Syndrome in graduate school in 1997; she calls herself "aspergerian." Teresa's research and writings—both published and informal—first introduced me to the importance of investigating immune dysregulations, chronic viral infections, and other pathogenic aspects of subgroups within autism. She has assisted me in some of my most troubling cases and has "proof-read" and advised me on scientific aspects of this book, all of which has helped me immeasurably. She has tirelessly procured references and research papers for me to read during this writing project, especially for Chapter Eight on Immunity and Viruses. She is a fierce champion of the need for a change in the medical paradigm for autism. Teresa has helped me come to my operational dictum, "Heal the gut, feed the starving brain, treat for pathogens, remove the toxins, and help the immune system in every way possible," of course, all at the same time!! As a clinician, effective treatment is always my bottom line, and I and others (both parents and doctors) count on Teresa to lead us to the latest research, clarification of diagnosis, and optimal directions for healing.

I have Amy Holmes, MD to thank for inspiring me to work twice as hard as I ever have while making half the income. Prompted by Edelson et al, Bernard et al, and by the disciplined clinical protocols of Stephanie Cave, MD, Doctor Holmes became the beloved and respected "god-mother" of heavy-metal chelation for children with autism. As an inspired mother of an ASD child herself, she believed that doctors with children or grandchildren on the spectrum can be on the forefront of critically important changes in the prevailing medical model for diagnostic evaluation and treatment of these children.

I want to give a special acknowledgement to the person who helped me start writing this book. Just when I despaired of ever finding time to write because my autism patient waiting list was getting longer and longer, Dr. Maury Breecher contacted me and asked, "Do you want help in writing your book?" Maury is a medical writer and author with academic degrees in Mass Communications and Public Health. He told me that my passion for helping autistic kids attracted him to me. He shared my urgency about the importance of getting this material out to parents as quickly as possible. Maury helped me by a very productive series of interviews that got me in touch with how much I still needed to learn about autism. When no big publisher was interested in my book, Maury moved on, but those comprehensive, in-depth interviews and his early editorial guidance helped me get started on writing, and I will always be grateful to him.

Ironically, I must also credit the pediatricians and other doctors who dismiss autism spectrum children as having psychological problems, being products of bad parenting, or as hopeless genetic cases —and who make these judgments without biomedical testing while refusing to think "out of the box." My frustration with such physicians and their obsolete models has helped create a strong desire in me to provide information to parents so they can understand what their doctors may not yet realize: that whatever else it is, I believe most if not all children with autism have a complex medical illness and merit biomedical diagnostics and medical treatment. Although the epidemic of autism-spectrum disorders is forcing more doctors to contemplate this model, the field is so complex that evaluation and treatment must be specific to each individual child. Practitioners need to consider immune impairments, chronic infections, low-level accumulations of heavy-metals, special diets, and child-specific nutrient supplementation. Much of this new biochemistry of autism was not learned in their medical training.

It surely goes without saying that none of the experiences and explorations leading to this book would have happened for me if it had not been for Chelsey and all the other children with autism whose parents have entrusted me to help them in their efforts to heal their children. I especially want to thank my daughter Elizabeth for doing all the 24/7 hard work of all the biomedical treatments I've come up with in the seven (now ten) years Chelsey has been teaching us about autism. Liz has become a magnificent, wise, incredibly loving and understanding mother in this process, as is true for so many of the mothers (and fathers!). These special children are calling all of us to wake up; they are the messengers for what is happening in our toxic world and of what needs to happen in our institutions of medicine, education, and family life.

Last, first, and always: my husband of 33 years, Dr. Jack Zimmerman has helped me expand the love of our eight children and thirteen grandchildren to encompass all children. A PhD mathematician/poet turned visionary educator, author, and director of the Center for Council Training (an extension of the Ojai Foundation in Ojai CA), he has helped to develop a network of council facilitators that brings this process of authentic communication to tens of thousands of children in schools not only in Southern California but all over the country, with recently launched programs in Europe, Israel, and Hawaii. He is currently exploring with other concerned educators ways to introduce council to groups of special needs children in both private and public schools. His unstinting love and support in our healing work with Chelsey and his constant encouragement have helped me see the larger message that these hundreds of thousands of autism-spectrum children are bringing to the world. His role as editor has helped offset some of my limitations as a writer; our collaboration has deepened our love even more. His writing in Chapter Twelve and Appendix D and his poetry at the end of the book will give you the opportunity to experience his visionary mind and wonderful heart. Jack is a blessing and ever deepening source of strength and inspiration to me and to everyone who knows him.

Jaquelyn McCandless, MD

PREFACE TO THE 3RD (2007) & 4TH EDITION (2009)

The completion of the 3rd edition in early 2007 followed closely upon the death from prostate cancer of our beloved Dr. Bernie Rimland at the age of 78 in late November of 2006. He lived to see his most important message being heard resoundingly to a larger and larger number of parents and professionals worldwide: AUTISM IS TREATABLE, RECOVERY IS POSSIBLE. He is, was and will always be a giant in autism and left all of us a legacy of courage and dedication to which we will continue to aspire to help our autistic patients have as happy and fulfilling lives as possible.I explain more about ASD causation models in Chapter One to help parents understand the rationale behind the various biomedical treatments. Chapter Two discusses nutritional deficiency as a common denominator in almost all ASD children and emphasizes the importance of the gastrointestinal tract and its relationship with the immune system. Accumulation of toxins, especially heavy metals and the "autism/vaccination" controversy are discussed at length in Chapter Three on Impaired Detoxification, Toxic Accumulations, and Politics. Chapter Four is dedicated to diagnostic evaluations, including a description of laboratory tests that help guide treatment and monitor its progress.

Chapters Five to Eleven delineate the biomedical treatments for ASD that I use and have used in my practice for over eleven years. These include Gastrointestinal Healing, Feeding the Starving Brain, Detoxification Therapy, Methylation Strategies, new therapies including HBOT (subject of Chapter Nine by Dr. James Neubrander) and refinements of older treatments. Chapter Eight on Immunity, Autoimmunity and Viruses contains a contribution by parent Stan Kurtz on the recovery of his son from autism using anti-virals, anti-fungals, and a special diet. Chapter Ten discusses other newer developments besides HBOT; Chapter Eleven expounds on the nuances of mitochondrial dysfunction and treatment in ASD.

In Chapter Twelve, I have invited Jack Zimmerman, PhD, mathematician, author, and visionary educator (and my husband) to touch on the cultural significance of such large numbers of these special children coming into the world at this time. He looks at what the epidemic of ASD may say about family dynamics and medicine and the importance of hearing the message they bring as we learn ways to heal them and ourselves.

Appendix A allows researcher Teresa Binstock to bring her latest information gleaned from the research literature on the gastrointestinal tract in relation to the challenges in autism in this system. Appendix B also brought by Teresa presents her introduction and the alternative version of the now famous "autism/mercury paper" written by Sallie Bernard, Albert Enayati, Heidi Roger, Lyn Redwood, and Teresa Binstock. This was the paper that led to the removal of thimerosal from the Hepatitis B newborn vaccinations by late 2001, reproduced here by permission. Appendix C gives Teresa the opportunity to bring forth new and essential information on one of her favorite subjects, and one that should be important to everyone, the issue of the accelerating toxicity being brought into the world at this time. She discusses the implication of this increasing poisoning and its implication in human (and animal) disease. Appendix D is a summary of a great deal of literature research by Teresa Binstock on the importance of mitochondrial injury and contains many references for those who want to pursue the deeper scientific implications of these very critical structures that are so important to our health. Appendix E is a continuation of Jack Zimmerman's discussion of the cultural significance of the ASD epidemic in relation to education and the environment. We end the book with a compilation of Jack's poems relating to our work and life with our primary teacher in autism, called, "The Poetic Version of our Journey with Chelsey."

Jaquelyn McCandless, MD

INTRODUCTION

CHILDREN WITH REAL MEDICAL ILLNESSES

A Message of Hope

Children with Starving Brains is a message of hope to parents of children diagnosed with autism or any of the disorders associated with autistic spectrum disorder (ASD). This message is especially important if your child has recently been diagnosed and you are just embarking on the complicated journey of trying to find proper medical care. The book is also intended for parents who believe something is wrong with their child but do not know how to find qualified and knowledgeable medical help for diagnosis and treatment. If you do not already know, you will learn in Chapter One that we are in the midst of an epidemic of ASD. Many cases are as yet undiagnosed. Traditional treatment modalities encompass sensory integration, visual and auditory training, and behavioral modification; these are all important and are already well described in the current literature about autism. This book rather focuses on recently developed biomedical treatments that are showing great promise in improving the health and neurologic function of many children on the autism spectrum.

Autism is a condition often characterized by a failure to bond, lack of social interaction, avoidance of eye-to-eye contact, difficulties in language development, and repetitive behaviors known as "stimming" (self-stimulation). There are associated milder forms of this condition such as Asperger's Syndrome, PDD (Pervasive Developmental Disorders) and ADD/ADHD, or Attention Deficit/Hyperactivity Disorder. These are all known collectively as Autism Spectrum Disorder(s), or ASDs.

My main thesis in this book is that ASD is a complex syndrome based on physiological and bio-chemical disorders that have as a common end-point the cognitive and emotional impairment we associate with autism. In other words, these are medically ill children who can be greatly helped medically, behaviorally, and cognitively by proper diagnosis and treatment of their underlying medical conditions. This is a vital breakthrough in understanding and one that many old-line practitioners have had a hard time grasping. In the past, autism and other conditions in the autism spectrum were considered "psychiatric" or behavioral disorders, with only psychiatric or behavioral approaches considered as appropriate treatments. As we grow in our understanding that these are medical rather than mental disorders, we are exploring and learning new ways to use medical treatments tailored to meet each child's individual needs.

As a physician who is the grandparent of a child diagnosed with autism in 1996, I have come to realize that the traditional means of diagnosis and treatments for ASD leave much to be desired. By and large, the prevailing or mainstream treatment protocols are driven by the old-fashioned belief that ASDs are simply behavioral conditions caused by incurable genetic defects. For many years, the genetic-model represented progress, for at least it replaced the long-held psychoanalytic belief that autism was caused by "refrigerator mothers" who were unable to bond with and love their children properly. However, the current belief that autism is primarily or only genetic means that until very recently prevailing treatment protocols rarely advise anything other than behavior modification or educational therapy sometimes aided by mood-controlling drugs such as SSRI's (Prozac, Zoloft etc), stimulants (Ritalin, amphetamines etc), or behavior-controlling drugs such as Risperidone (Risperdal).

Since many mainstream physicians have been trained to accept that the basis for ASD is genetic, they routinely screen for genetic disorders such as Down syndrome or Fragile X and do not order appropriate laboratory tests for the gastrointestinal, immunological, and infection-related issues that beset ASD children. Often, parents are told there are no known treatments other than what behavior modification offers; some parents have even been informed emphatically that there is no evidence that vitamins or dietary changes would be of any benefit to their children. I intensely disagree with these judgments based on solid clinical experience. Increasingly, the old diagnostic and treatment models for ASD are being augmented by the biomedical approach. This significant paradigm shift is in part the result of the current epidemic of ASD, since now there are many health professionals who have a child, grandchild, nephew, niece, or someone close to them recently diagnosed with autism. Many of these physicians with "autism in the family" are contributing to the realization that the syndrome is actually a biomedical illness needing and responding to biomedical treatments.

After a long career in general psychiatry and alternative medicine, my own practice has shifted primarily to specializing in the treatment of developmentally delayed children, most of them on the ASD spectrum. Since I consider attention deficit disorder (ADD) and attention deficit hyperactivity disorder (ADHD) to be milder versions of the same problem, I also evaluate children with these disorders whose parents prefer to explore improvement through dietary, nutrient, and sometimes detoxification protocols before turning to stimulants or other prescription drugs. In trying to learn everything possible to help my granddaughter and the other children that have come into my practice, I have scoured the medical literature, attended medical conferences, participated in research-oriented internet groups, and surveyed alternative treatments being pioneered by an increasing number of physicians.

Defeat Autism Now!

It was a relief to learn that I was not alone in my search. I have been influenced by pioneering researchers including Bernard Rimland, PhD, William Shaw, PhD, Karl Reichelt, MD, PhD, Richard Deth, PhD, Jill James, PhD, James Adams, PhD, Ari Vojdani, PhD, and Andrew Wakefield, MD as well as pioneering physicians such as Sidney Baker, Michael Goldberg, Jim Neubrander, Derrick Lonsdale, Alan Goldblatt, John Green, Anju Usman, Marvin Boris, Amy

Holmes, Stephanie Cave, and Jeff Bradstreet. Significant contributions to my clinical practice have come from independent researchers Teresa Binstock and Susan Owens, as well as parent-researchers such as Victoria Beck, Sallie Bernard, and Allison Plant among many others.

These individuals and countless others I have met along my learning path have helped me realize that, when considered as a group, children on the autism spectrum have a multi-faceted disorder that may affect any and sometimes all of the major systems of the body. Inter-individual variation is their most consistent characteristic. In other words, each child is unique. The notion "one treatment size fits all" does not pertain to these children. Some of the factors that need to be considered in evaluating ASD children include:

- Were they autistic "from birth" or had they "regressed" after a period of normalcy?

- Are they low, medium, or high-functioning behaviorally and cognitively, including level of receptive and expressive speech and ability to learn?

- How are their biochemical profiles revealed by lab-tests correlated with symptoms?

- What is the familial history of autoimmune disorders, allergies, etc.?

- What is the child's personal developmental and medical history?

These categories help target diagnostic and treatment protocols. Most of the researchers and physicians just named, among many others, have joined together in a movement called Defeat Autism Now! that was started by Bernard Rimland, PhD, director of the Autism Research Institute in San Diego. I am proud to be associated with this movement. Members of Defeat Autism Now! are bonded by their belief that autism and associated ASD's are primarily medical disorders with behavioral and cognitive impairments that are by-products of the physical illnesses these children suffer. In other words, aside from rare genetic cases such as an autism derived from fragile X syndrome, these are physically ill children with real medical disorders. Since they are physically ill, they need biomedical intervention to maximize their healing potential. We have concluded there are many "autisms."

My clinical experience, when combined with the recent research and experience of dozens of Defeat Autism Now! practitioners, has led me to develop biomedical protocols for diagnostic evaluations and subsequent treatments. I think of this as a broad-spectrum approach. My patients and their parents have been my greatest teachers; some treatments that have become a mainstay of my practice were brought to me originally by parents seeking a doctor with an open mind to new tests and treatments they had heard about before I did. Nearly every child I have worked with has had immune irregularities, nutritional deficiencies, and gastrointestinal problems. Nevertheless, I have found each child to be remarkably different from each of his or her ASD "peers," not only in regard to biomedical profiles (as indicated by laboratory results) but also in response to various treatments. In an era when autism's primary model is changing, it is not surprising that parents also vary in their openness to a new medical model, in their willingness to do the indicated testing (assuming the financial means), and in their ability to follow through on the recommended treatments. The bottom line is that the protocol must be individualized for each child in the context of the family and circumstances in which he or she lives.

In 2003 I was invited to conduct a training for doctors and other health practitioners on my lab testing and biomedical protocols. 30 health personnel attended this first training, including registered nurse Maureen McDonnell, the coordinator of the large bi-coastal and bi-annual Defeat Autism Now! conferences. In her usual brilliant role as manifester and ultimate Defeat Autism Now! weaver, she recognized the need for this kind of endeavor, and suggested we create a series of "mini-Defeat Autism Now's" throughout the country in places distant from the coastal locations where we usually hold the larger meetings. Other doctors have joined the instructor division, and Maureen has started a coinciding nurses training along with the physicians' trainings. In this country, about 2000 doctors have now attended these training courses, and the instructors have taken the training to Europe, Australia, Israel, Scotland, Hong Kong and other locations to spread the biomedical teachings that Defeat Autism Now! researchers and physicians have pioneered.

What Can a Parent Expect From Biomedical Interventions?

From my experience and that of many Defeat Autism Now! physicians and caregivers, the behavioral and cognitive symptoms of most ASD children can be noticeably improved with proper biomedical treatments. Sometimes the improvement is dramatic enough for a child to lose his or her ASD diagnosis. That is a startling statement, so let me be clear so as not to raise false hopes. I am not promising that every child will get complete recovery. Nor am I promising that every child will show major improvement. My message of hope is that, if you try the treatments described in this book, your child is very likely to get better at least to some degree and, for some ASD children, perhaps even improve remarkably or recover from autism.

More specifically:

- A parent won't know how much his or her child will improve unless the various diagnostic methods and treatment protocols are tried.

- Not every child will enjoy profound improvements. Many, however, will. Most parents will see some improvement. Some parents may see no improvement or such improvements as occur may take much longer.

- Occasionally a child may get worse before he/she gets better. Lately, we're finding that many if not most of the regressions we see during treatment are being caused by gastrointestinal pathologies that we are learning more about as new research comes in. As these pathologies are identified and treated, improvement often resumes.

- Neutraceutical companies are working to find new immune enhancers, better enzymes, and better forms and mixtures of other vital nutrients to help in the various treatments.

- The earlier the evaluation is made and treatment started, the likelier it is that the child will improve.

Unfortunately, many pediatricians and other physicians are not experienced in diagnosing autism or any of the related ASD's. Some physicians may fear making the diagnosis because they were trained to believe that the autistic form of ASD is incurable. Also, although many of these children are actually quite ill, I sometimes hear a parent tell me, "But my child with autism never gets sick like my other kids do!" I have noticed that, although many children I see have a history of recurrent ear infections in their first year of life, this early pattern may be followed by a period of seemingly strong immunity. This may be because of a hyper-immune status in response to low-grade chronic infection. It also has been amazing to see an apparently healthy ASD child who has, nevertheless, had chronic diarrhea for years and has self-selected a daily diet limited to a few usually non-nutritious foods such as French fries, soda pop, and chips. Consequently, busy doctors after a quick physical may say the child looks fine, and parents may be told that their child's continuous loose stools are just "toddler diarrhea, a condition that will eventually be outgrown." In a neurotypical child, such pronouncements sometimes may be true. However, for an ASD child, intestinal treatment or change of diet may not only be warranted but essential for them to improve. Similarly, a pediatrician may counsel that a child who does not talk by 1-1/2 or 2 years of age is just a "late talker." In some instances this may also be true, but my advice is that any child who is not trying to talk by age 1-1/2 or at least by 2 ought to be evaluated for ASD, particularly if there are any other behavioral, gastrointestinal, or cognitive symptoms, however subtle they may seem.

This level of diagnostic sensitivity is important because effective treatment has a golden window of opportunity that unfortunately diminishes for most (but not all) as the child gets older. This is true for both educational and biomedical interventions. If your child has chronic diarrhea, frequently wakes up at night, self-selects a very restricted diet, has suffered repeated ear or other infections in the first year or at the cessation of breast feeding, isn't trying to say words by around 18 months, has a history of bad reactions to vaccinations, doesn't seem interested in other kids, and doesn't show the kind of curiosity and relatedness that most other kids do, find a physician to screen for ASD as soon as possible.

My personal experience and that of other Defeat Autism Now! physicians leads to an important principle for parents: Don't accept your doctor's advice if he or she counsels a "wait-and-see" attitude or promises that your child will "catch up." Especially hurry to seek help if your child had a period of normal development and then regressed. If your child has exhibited any of the traits described or has already been diagnosed with autism or ASD, this book will give you some guidelines for seeking interventions that may be of considerable help. Some of these interventions can be instituted by parents. However, diagnostics and treatments that include laboratory testing or prescription medications must, of course, be done with the cooperation of a health care professional. If you do not happen to live near a Defeat Autism Now! doctor or cannot get an appointment anytime soon, it is important to understand that a doctor these days with the availability of internet, faxing, and phone does not have to be seen very often to be able to give you excellent care for your child. An occasional trip once or twice a year to see someone experienced and competent may well be worth it rather than continue to waste time and money depending on professionals that have had no current training in the biomedical treatment of autistic children.

My Personal and Professional Involvement in the Bio-Medicine of Autism

My granddaughter Chelsey was diagnosed with autism in 1996 at 33 months of age. I had been working for many years in private practice in California as a physician certified by the American Board of Psychiatry and Neurology. I made it a point to keep abreast of all the new studies and medications pertaining to biological psychiatry as well as the psychotherapeutic approaches to emotional/mental illnesses. In the early nineties, I had begun an exploration of alternative medicine to learn how to use natural hormones, vitamins and other nutrients to help aging brains and bodies stay youthful and healthy. This research has helped me personally and in my current work with ASD children.

However, at the time Chelsey received her diagnosis, I knew almost nothing about autism. In 30 years of clinical practice I had seen but a few people with this diagnosis and had mainly been consulted for drug-based behavior control for these mysteriously impaired people. In retrospect, I realize I was woefully ignorant about autism. In my initial search to find help for Chelsey in 1996, I discovered to my dismay that my medical colleagues who practiced pediatric medicine knew little more than I. The prognosis they offered Chelsey was grim. As I regretfully look back on Chelsey's parents' as well as my own denial of the diagnosis and at the apparent scarcity of biomedical information available about autism, I now realize that we wasted precious time getting effective treatments started.

In fact, the importance of time is a prime reason for this book. It is designed to help parents get their children started on effective treatments faster. If you are a parent, this book will help you understand the rationale for the new treatments that are available now. If you are a physician, the book may help guide you through the process of deciding which testing and treatments to start first and in what order to initiate the others. This book should also provide information on where to go for additional knowledge about complicated, ASD-related conditions that are beyond the scope of the present discussion.

Another prime reason for documenting my broad-spectrum approach is that I and every autism specialist I know has a waiting list of anxious families who have heard about the new treatments and are having a hard time finding out how to get help for their children. I am hoping that this book will empower parents to put pressure on their doctors and their insurance companies to investigate the information becoming available that offers new hope for ASD children.

At the time we received Chelsey's diagnosis, it was thought—and unfortunately, in some quarters it is still believed—that autism is incurable and that it was caused by cold mothers who lacked nurturing and other parental skills. I have never accepted that my granddaughter and other ASD children are incurable. I also know without doubt that Chelsey's mother wasn't a *refrigerator mother, just as Dr. Bernie Rimland knew his beloved Gloria was not a refrigerator mother when their son Mark was diagnosed with autism.* Elizabeth has three other neurotypical thriving, happy children and is a dedicated loving parent to all of her children. Over the past ten years I have met hundreds of parents of ASD children and have been impressed by how the challenges of raising such a child often bring out the best in them. Their willingness and persistence to do everything possible to help their offspring proves that the parents of these developmentally challenged kids are among the most loving and capable of all caregivers.

Dr. Rimland's 1964 book *Infantile Autism: The Syndrome and Its Implications for a Neural Theory of Behavior*, demolished the generally held view at that time that autism was the psychological byproduct of "refrigerator mothers"—cold, unfeeling women who forced their children to withdraw into a protective shell of indifference. He concluded instead that the disorder, characterized by poor language skills and an inability to handle social relations, was the result of a fundamental biochemical defect underlain, perhaps, by defective genes but ultimately triggered by environmental assaults. Bernie Rimland was among the first to conclude that the United States was undergoing an epidemic of autism, one that increased the incidence of the disorder from a rare one case in several thousand births to the current government-accepted rate of one in every 166 children. In his usual pioneering and courageous way the originator and leader of the Defeat Autism Now! biomedical movement concluded that mercury in vaccines was the primary culprit in this increase and led a vociferous campaign among parents to have the heavy metal—used to kill contaminating bacteria—removed from the vaccines.

Dr. Rimland was also a forceful advocate for intensive behavioral therapy for autistic children, a therapy that many claim has restored their child to normality.

In late 2006, all of us suffered a tremendous loss in the death of Dr. Rimland from cancer at the age of 78. Tributes flowed in then and continue to flow in from all over the U.S. and the entire world for this incredibly dedicated, talented and courageous psychologist researcher to whom the autism world will forever owe an inestimable debt.

My Most Challenging Case

Over the years we have tried many different forms of therapy for Chelsey, some which seemed to help and many which did not. My beloved grandchild, the inspiration for this book, remains my first and most challenging case. At the time of her diagnosis, we only knew about various types of behavioral therapy, which we immediately instituted and continued full time for several years. Though early educational intervention and applied behavioral analysis did help her to focus and learn limited verbal skills, she remained quite impaired relationally, and suffered from chronic diarrhea and a severely restricted diet. I know now that chronic diarrhea is very common in these children and a sure tip-off that their biochemistry is abnormal. When she was almost five years old, we finally instituted a diet that removed certain common foods that we now know were toxic to her, even though the usual allergy testing did not reveal this. The results were dramatic; for the first time she started having normal bowel function. This lesson taught me the importance of food hypersensitivity awareness and testing for food allergies early in treatment.

Because many of the biomedical aspects of my current treatment protocol weren't developed until Chelsey was over five years of age, she didn't benefit from the early biomedical and detoxification therapies that are responsible for improvements, some quite dramatic, in my later crops of young patients. Unfortunately, biomedical improvement seems to take longer and may not be as complete with older children since biochemical abnormalities and toxic conditions have already become a part of their cellular functioning and are therefore harder to change. Though her recovery progresses at a slower pace than some of my younger patients, I will continue to remain open to new discoveries sure to come in this rapidly evolving field, while loving her with all my heart however she grows.

The "golden window" of opportunity I mentioned earlier is usually between 18 months to 5 years of age. Remember, however, that although that age range is an optimum period to begin treatment, it does not mean older children cannot improve. Older children and even adults can be helped, some remarkably so. It is never too late to provide every ASD person the benefits of the new diagnostics and therapies now available.

I and most other Defeat Autism Now! doctors have come to believe that early (even in some cases in utero or neonatal) injury to the immature immune systems of these children by toxins or pathogens starts a series of bio-chemical events that culminates eventually in neurocognitive deficits and behavioral challenges. Though there may be a genetic vulnerability in most if not all autism spectrum children, increasing evidence suggests that a toxic mercury-based preservative long used in vaccinations may have been the "trigger" for a susceptible subset of children, particularly since 1991 when Hepatitis B vaccinations were mandated for every newborn. I join many autism experts and parents who believe that the current epidemic of regressive autism began with this mandate. Statistics show a progressive rise in incidence beginning in 1988 when the MMR vaccination was mandated (although itself does not contain any mercury), and I and Teresa Binstock will be discussing the recent findings about MMR in other places in the book. However, the incredibly steep rise in incidence started in 1991, coinciding with the requirement for newborns to receive the HepB often within hours of birth. We believe that early injury by toxins—likely preceded by genetic predisposition and augmented by allergies, illnesses, and repeated antibiotic use—are among the factors that can initiate a cascade of problems starting with a weakened immune system and inflamed intestinal tract. A weakened immune system opens the door to bacterial and viral infections, overuse of antibiotics, intestinal yeast overgrowth, gut inflammation, and impaired nutritional status. The frequently noted "leaky gut" syndrome and its various effects enable toxins to spread throughout the body including the brain. Furthermore, in a transiently or chronically vulnerable child, immunizations with live viruses such as the MMR pose another challenge. In this complex scenario of possibilities, vaccine-associated mercury, viruses, or other toxins as well as the child's own overactive immune components (autoimmunity) can attack neurons and thereby interfere with synaptic development and nerve signaling. With much variation from child to child, these factors can combine to create brain malnutrition and the cognitive impairment characteristic of ASD children.

In summary, *Children With Starving Brains* will:

- **Help** parents understand why their child may have become chronically ill and how biomedical intervention may help

- **Identify** important diagnostic tools that can provide crucial information to help parents and physicians select the best treatment sequence

- **Explain** those therapies and identify safe and effective treatment options that can be started by parents or caregivers even before laboratory tests are ordered. This is important for parents having trouble finding a physician trained in treating children with ASD. Biomedical intervention for autism is new.

  Many physicians have not heard of or learned how to use these treatments as yet. However, a growing number are starting to take the time to learn these modalities because of the sheer numbers of children being diagnosed with ASD who need treatment now. Growing awareness in parents accelerates this process.

- **Encourage and inspire** parents to be their children's advocates in obtaining proper medical care (as they are doing in the field of education), and fight for insurance reform that will help them obtain the care they need. Joining support groups both locally and through the internet will provide a comforting and highly informative companionship with other parents who understand as no one else can what it means to love and care for a special needs child.

ONE

CAUSATION MODELS

*The Worldwide Autism
Spectrum Disorder (ASD) Epidemic*

C ould changes in diet calm your child and help him or her return to the world, pay attention. and behave better? Could
the addition of certain nutrients help your child make giant leaps
in developing vocabulary? Could the removal of mercury and heavy
metals from his or her body set the stage for outgrowing the Autism
Spectrum Disorder (ASD) diagnosis?

Yes. These treatments, sometimes individually but most often
in combination with one another, have enabled some children to
actually lose the diagnosis of autism or ASD. Many others, while remaining in the autistic spectrum, have made notable advancements
in cognition, behavior, and physical health.

This message of hope is needed now more than ever before. We
are in the midst of a worldwide ASD epidemic.[1] In one year alone
(from 1998 to 1999), there was a 26.01% increase in the numbers
of school age children classified as autistic, according to the U.S.
Department of Education.[2] In California, the number of school
age children diagnosed as autistic rose 210% in an 11-year period.[3]
There has been a sevenfold increase in ASD in the past decade.[4]
Similar increases in the incidence of autism and ASD have been
reported on the European continent. Included in the spectrum of

autistic disorders are Attention Deficit Disorder (ADD) and Attention Deficit Hyperactivity Disorder (ADHD). Six million children in the U.S. suffer from ADD or ADHD. Over two million children currently take Ritalin for either ADD or ADHD.

Definition of ASD and Incidence of Classic vs. Regressive Autism

The diagnostic criteria for autism agreed upon by most authorities are: severe abnormality of reciprocal social relatedness; severe abnormality of communication development (including language); restricted, repetitive behavior and patterns of behavior, interests, activities and imagination; and early onset (before age 3 to 5 years). Many authors would consider another criterion to be that of abnormal responses to sensory stimuli.[5]

Autistic Spectrum Disorder (ASD) is a group of developmental disorders ranging from full-fledged autism as described above to Attention Deficit Disorder (ADD), Attention Deficit Hyperactivity Disorder (ADHD) and Pervasive Developmental Disorder, (PDD). PDD is a catch-all diagnosis that children get when they do not meet developmental milestones and exhibit autistic symptoms, yet still retain at least some ability to speak and communicate. A child diagnosed with ADD has trouble maintaining focus. A hyperactive child with ADD is labeled ADHD. Both are considered milder forms of ASD. Typically, parents do not seek help for children with any of these conditions until they become aware that their child is not talking or developing as rapidly as other toddlers.

At the top end of the autistic spectrum is Asperger's Syndrome. It is the term used to describe an autistic child who functions at a high level. These children are often extremely intelligent. They use and understand a large vocabulary, but they have very narrow interests and exhibit many social deficits. An Asperger's Syndrome child may become the world's expert on washing machines, but washing machines may be the only thing he or she wants to talk about.

There are two basic types of autism: autism from birth (classic autism once known as Kanner's Syndrome) and regressive autism which generally occurs between 12 and 24 months of age after a period of normal development and behavior. The incidence of autism from birth remains an infrequent event—one or two out of 10,000 births. It is the incidence of regressive autism and associated autistic spectrum disorders that has soared, striking as many as one out of 150 children (in 2008) according to dozens of studies.

Some studies peg that estimate even higher. A recent one indicates that as many as one out of 150 California children may have regressive ASD.[6] A similar figure was reported by the Center for Disease Control (CDC) in a study of a township on the East Coast. That study identified 6.87 cases of ASD per 1,000 children, which is approximately one out of 150.[7] As far as the total number of ASD children, Dr. Jeff J. Bradstreet told a congressional committee that, "The government's own data indicate that there are as many as two million children in the U.S.A. with a significant developmental delay that can be categorized as ASD." *U.S. News & World Report* put it this way: "One out of every six children in America suffers from problems such as autism, aggression, dyslexia, and attention deficit hyperactivity disorder."[8]

It is considered by most of those now working with large numbers of ASD children that ADD, ADHD, PDD, and Asperger's Syndrome are the result of a milder version of the same pattern of genetic predisposition coupled with environmental triggers which we believe causes ASD. The environmental insults that trigger the damage can occur before birth while the fetus is still developing, during infancy, or while the child is a toddler. Whatever the timing, those environmental insults overburden undeveloped or just developing immune systems, often causing the children's immune systems to turn against their own bodies. When the immune system starts damaging its own body the process is called an autoimmune disease. Allergies, arthritis, and diabetes are other examples of autoimmune diseases. Many autistic/ASD children have families with histories of autoimmune diseases.

What Causes Autism and Other ASDs?

No one claims to understand everything about the causes of this epidemic, but there are theories that parents (and doctors) should be acquainted with because they are the basis for the treatments that will be described in later chapters. There is growing agreement that most cases of autism and ASD derive from a combination of genetic and environmental factors. Genetic factors may set the stage for ASD, yet in many individual cases, environmental factors appear to be the necessary trigger whereby genes then cause the disorder to be expressed.

There are many theories regarding the exact identity and mechanism of the environmental insults that trigger the cascade of physical, mental, and emotional dysfunctions which result in the starvation of a child's brain. No study, however, has definitively pinpointed a specific environmental toxin or contaminant as the one "smoking gun" behind autism, nor is it likely that just one toxin will be identified as the culprit. Instead, there is strong evidence incriminating not one, but several toxins and mechanisms of entry as primary villains behind the damage suffered by many of our children.

SIMPLY GENETIC?

Scientists have long thought that autism is a genetic disease. Yet gene research has been unable to identify a specific chromosome or location on a gene that is the site of a primary autism defect. These children rarely present facial and bodily dysmorphic features characteristic of the children with chromosomal defects that occur in very early gestation such as Down, Williams', and Fragile X children. Although a specific understanding of how genetics contributes to autism is still lacking, it is clear that there is likely to be a genetic "predisposition" or vulnerability in many ASD children. We know this from studies by Reed P. Warren and also because autism tends to show up more in twins than in the normal population. Furthermore, autism is nearly four times more prevalent in boys than in girls. These several findings suggest an association between autism and various genetic factors but do not mandate a clear role for genetics in every case of autism. In any one child, a clustering of environmental triggers may have been etiologically crucial for the onset of ASD. In many such children—with or without genetic predispositions—one or several of the environmental triggers may remain as a treatable pathology, such as a subclinical viral infection or heavy metal toxicity.

Aside from a few purely genetic syndromes that can induce autism, gene researchers have discovered an assortment of genetic markers common to many, but not all, autistic children. One of the genes that control the function and regulation of the immune system, the C4B gene, is involved in eliminating pathogens such as viruses and bacteria from the body. A deficient form of the C4B gene has been shown to have an increased frequency in autism, ADHD, and dyslexia.[9]

We talk about children with ASD as having "genetic susceptibility."—even as we realize that a "genetic susceptibility" may actually not exist in individual cases. At this time, however, acquired and genetic types of susceptibility are just beginning to be elucidated. Not surprisingly, studies about immune-related genes already appear in the autism literature.[10]

THE TOXIC CHEMICAL MODEL

It is shocking to realize that mothers-to-be may be drinking contaminated water, breathing air inside the home that is more dangerous than the air downwind of an industrial city, and absorbing toxic-chemicals from foods that may be acting as a time bomb within their bodies and those of their unborn children.

A recent report by a group of physicians in Boston states that millions of U.S. children exhibit learning disabilities, reduced IQ, and destructive, aggressive behavior because of exposure to toxic chemicals.[11] The report links pre- and post-natal toxic exposures to lifelong disabilities. In addition, a report from the National Academies of Science states that a combination of neurotoxicants and genetic factors may account for nearly 25% of developmental problems.[12] That includes Autism Spectrum Disorder. An important class of toxic chemicals are the polychlorinated biphenyls (PCBs) and organophosphate pesticides. The NAS report showed that babies who had significant amounts of PCBs performed poorer than unexposed babies in visual face recognition tests, ability to shut out distractions, and overall intelligence. The report went on to say that pesticides such as Dursban and Diazinon can cause brain damage. It was only in 2000 that the Environmental Protection Agency (EPA) banned Dursban from household use. It had been marketed to consumers in popular indoor roach and ant killers since 1956 to 2000.

THE HEAVY METAL CONTAMINATION MODEL

It is even more shocking to learn that the immune systems of genetically susceptible infants may have been attacked by heavy metals such as lead and mercury.

- **Lead:** The Boston Physicians' report referred to in the previous section states that one million American children currently have levels of lead in their bloodstreams above the threshold recognized by the (EPA) as adversely affecting behavior and cognition. Where does the lead come from? Many houses and apartments built before 1978 have paint that contains lead. Although the ban on lead paint has been in existence since the late 1970's, the presence of lead in older housing poses a serious hazard, especially to young children. Opening or closing a painted frame window can create small paint chips or lead dust that can be inhaled or which settles to the floor. Infants and very young crawling children often put their hands in their mouths and eat the dust and paint chips because they taste sweet. The CDC and the U.S. Public Health Service in a joint statement say: "Lead poisoning remains the most commonly and societally devastating environmental disease of young children." We now know that large numbers of children may suffer adverse health effects at blood levels that were once considered safe. Long-term exposure to low levels of lead may cause a buildup in the brain and other tissues resulting in neurological damage to children even before they are born, according to the EPA booklet that homesellers and landlords are required to give buyers or renters of dwellings that may still contain lead paint.[13] Consequently children's exposure to lead can retard and impair mental and physical development. "Lead exposure has already cut in half the number of U.S. children who might have had superior I.Q.'s (125 or higher)—some two million kids," says Herbert Needleman, MD, a professor of Psychiatry and Pediatrics at the University of Pittsburgh.[14] In a study released in June 2000, Dr. Needleman found that juvenile delinquents had significantly higher levels of lead in their bones than nondelinquent youths.[15]

- **Mercury:** Mercury, the substance found in old-fashioned thermometers, is ubiquitous in the environment. Fish are known to contain high levels of mercury. According to *U.S. News & World Report,* a toxicologist by the name of David Brown helped prepare a study of the mercury levels in the lakes of eight Northeastern states and three Canadian provinces. He found much higher levels of mercury in fish from supposedly pristine lakes than had been expected. Brown concluded that a "pregnant woman who ate a single fish from one of those lakes could, in theory, consume enough mercury to harm her unborn child."[16]

  Another source of prenatal exposure might be the mercury contained in the amalgam dental fillings of their pregnant mothers. No one realized the potential danger at the time, but Elizabeth, my own daughter, had dental repairs including fillings containing mercury when she was four months pregnant with Chelsey. Other countries such as Sweden and Canada have more stringent limits on amalgams for women of child-bearing age. Because of what we have learned about mercury, we now believe it is possible that those amalgams may have been a trigger for Chelsey's autism. No matter what the route or the combination of routes, it is my belief that a large portion of the current epidemic of regressive autism and ASD generally is a direct result of the mercury or other heavy metals that have entered the bodies of our kids. An important part of my practice at the present time is focused on evaluating and treating for toxic heavy metals in these children, as I describe in Chapter Seven.

VACCINATIONS

In infants and toddlers with increased susceptibility, vaccination with live viruses may have contributed to the child's autistic regression. Another contributor to the problem preceding the live virus injection was almost certainly the ethylmercury (in the form of thimerosal) which until recently was used as a preservative in multi-dose vials of some vaccines mandated for newborns. The correspondence between autistic traits and those that occur from mercury poisoning is highly significant and includes varying degrees of autoimmunity. In fact, all traits that define or are associated with autism have been described previously in mercury-poisoning literature (see Appendices B and C).

Mercury was for years used as an anti-fungal in paint but, due to toxicity, was taken out of indoor paint in 1991. Similarly, FDA hearings led, in 1982, to merthiolate's discontinuance because it contained ethyl-mercury. Unfortunately, no one thought to remove ethylmercury from the many vaccines mandated to protect our children from childhood illnesses. The mercury in those vaccines is a component of Thimerosal,[a] which is 49.6% ethylmercury by weight and which was used as a preservative to retard spoilage of vaccines in multi-use vials. Vaccinal ethylmercury may have "spoiled" the lives of thousands upon thousands of children and their families.

Indeed, the current cohort of kids being diagnosed with ASD has had more exposure to mercury from vaccines than the EPA thinks is safe for adults. That's because kids today have more total vaccinations (22 before two years of age) and have them closer together and earlier in life than ever before in history.

Prior to 1991, babies just learning to crawl were exposed to mercury fumes from commercial indoor paint. As we have just mentioned, in that year the FDA pressured paint manufacturers to remove mercury from their indoor house paint. The paint manufacturers complied. It is tragically ironic that in the same year the federal government, for public health reasons, mandated the unprecedented practice of inoculating newborn infants with the Hepatitis B vaccination on the very day of birth. Until 2001, that vaccine contained Thimerosal. So, while one part of the government was mandating that mercury be taken out of indoor paints, another was mandating that newborn infants be injected with the mercury-containing Hepatitis B vaccine. According to the CDC recommended immunization schedule, infants who get all their shots were exposed to 12.5 micrograms of mercury at birth, 62.4 micrograms at two months, 50 micrograms at four months, 62.5 micrograms at six months, and 50 micrograms at approximately 18 months. It is my belief that the mercury-containing Hep B vaccination given at birth when the immune system and liver are immature acted as a "trigger" that set into motion the cascade of events that have resulted in the gastrointestinal and neurological deficits we see in the current epidemic of autism. While a causal link between thimerosal and the current epidemic of autism has not yet been definitively proven, epidemiologic data support the connection. More recently the Institute of Medicine's staff has concluded that, indeed, the hypothesis is plausible. I feel it is only a matter of time before thimerosal's adverse effects are acknowledged; I might even use the term "admitted."

When British physician Andrew Wakefield first suggested the possible link between the MMR vaccine, acquired gut pathology, and autism, his work was belittled in a flurry of hastily assembled rebuttals. Nonetheless, special studies of inflamed intestinal tissue in a subgroup of ASD children demonstrated that measles virus (MV) was present in their biopsied intestinal tissue and that the measles virus found there was indeed the vaccine strain.[17] Other research has linked ASD with measles virus gut infestation. Recently, Harvard gastroenterologist Timothy Buie, MD described a cohort of nearly 400 children and reported that a subgroup indeed had the ileal-lymphoid hyperplasia first described by Wakefield and colleagues.[18] Importantly, Japanese researchers Kawashima et al reported that the vaccine-strain of MV was also present in the peripheral blood mononuclear cells in an ASD subgroup,[19] which may contribute to blood-brain-barrier inflammation and to low levels of viral infiltration into the central nervous system (CNS).

Most vaccinated children have been injected with a weakened form of the measles virus. The measles virus infects 40 million people and kills one million per year by suppressing the immune system and affecting the CNS. Most individuals who become seriously affected by wild-type measles virus live in under-developed nations. Overall, the measles vaccine has saved millions of lives. However, the measles vaccine is now given in a combination three-in-one shot that also contains mumps and rubella vaccines. The combined vaccine is called the MMR. The MMR is described as continuing to save millions of lives, but—given the intestinal-pathology data linked to vaccine strains of measles virus—the MMR may also have induced or contributed to regressive autism in thousands of children. That is the belief of Dr. Andrew Wakefield, who for years worked as a gastroenterologist/researcher at the Royal Free Hospital in London, England. He has relocated to the U.S. and is now based at Thoughtful House in Austin, TX.

This highly regarded clinician-researcher discovered a possible connection between autism and the specific measles viral strain associated with the MMR vaccination. As mentioned earlier, Dr. Wakefield found vaccine-derived viral genomes within intestinal tissue and peripheral blood mononuclear cells of a subgroup of autistic children. Those findings prompted an autism model in which the MMR can trigger the body's autoimmune reactions against the myelin basic protein (MBP) for a certain group of susceptible children. This model is consistent with data reported by long-time autism researcher VK Singh, whose articles describe that a high percentage of ASD children have elevated titers for antibodies against MBP and that these titers often co-occur with elevated titers against measles virus or human herpesvirus 6 (HHV-6).

Many experts including Bernard Rimland believe Dr. Wakefield's findings shed light on etiologically significant processes for a subgroup of ASD children. Despite medical officials' protests to the contrary, many parents, physicians, and researchers believe (a) that the MMR vaccine may be a real cause contributing to the rising incidence of autism, and (b) that adverse consequences may be more likely if the vaccinations occur as additional multiples (e.g., the MMR plus the DPT, all on the same day), and if the infant or toddler has increased susceptibility—whether acquired and/or genetic—at the time of vaccination.

THE AUTO-IMMUNITY/ALLERGY MODEL

As biomedical profiling increases, it is becoming clear that autism-spectrum children break down into defined "subgroups." For instance, a good number of autism spectrum children have elevated titers against various brain proteins. Similarly, many also have familial autoimmune or allergic diseases; many autistic children themselves have signs or symptoms of autoimmunity or allergy.[20]

An allergy results when the body's immune system overreacts to what it perceives to be a foreign invader. When a substance causes the body's immune system to respond, the substance is referred to as an "allergen." When an allergen such as dust or a plant pollen is inhaled, it is soon identified by the immune system as an intruder. The immune system then creates an antibody (a defender) to combat the perceived intruder. For example, in response to a plant pollen such as ragweed, an antibody called "immunoglobulin E," or simply IgE, is formed. The IgE antibodies attach themselves to tissue cells called mast cells and to other cells in the bloodstream called basophils. The mast cells and basophils (generally white blood cells) target the allergen and cruise through the blood stream, transporting the IgE to its target. When the allergen is reached, the IgE attaches to it and the mast cells and basophils release histamine. That chemical causes swelling in the lining of the nose and causes extra mucus to form. The afflicted person suffers congestion, sneezing, inflamed and irritated itching eyes and perhaps itching on skin areas exposed to the allergen. We take anti-histamines to combat those symptoms, but it is those symptoms that cause trapped allergens to be expelled along with the mucus.

Many autism spectrum children at least initially appear to have an immune dysregulation, in some ways overactive, in other ways suboptimal. Some researchers and physicians have theorized that when a particularly susceptible child suffers an environmental insult such as exposure to mercury or even to the weakened viruses in vaccines, the child's immune system responds by attacking not only the actual antigens but also look-alike antigens that are actually molecular structures within the child's brain.

A tip-off that an autoimmune process is at work is that the blood tests on many autistic children have been found to contain autoantibodies to a central nervous system protein known as myelin basic protein (MBP).[21] In a controlled study[22] that compared 33 autistic children with 18 normal children, 20 mentally retarded children, and 12 children with Down syndrome, anti-MBP antibodies were found in 19 of 33 (58%) of the autistic children, but in only in 8 of 88 (9%) of all the other subjects. This is an intriguing finding because myelination is an essential part of human brain development. Nerves can only conduct pulses of energy efficiently when properly sheathed with myelin. Like insulation on an electric wire, the fatty coating of myelin helps keep the electrical pulses confined, thus maintaining the integrity of the nerve's electrical signal. When the insulation on a wire is damaged or destroyed, the flow of electrical current may be interrupted and short-circuits occur. When the immune system attacks the body's own myelin, "short-circuits" can occur within the brain. Nerve axons cease to function properly.

The autoimmune findings in autism provide support for other subgroups and their causal models. As mentioned earlier, vaccinations that included ethylmercury or that contained live viruses may have affected children with dysregulated immunity, impaired nutritional status, and increased susceptibility.[23] In addition, a growing amount of clinical data suggest that some autistic children have chronic, *seemingly* subclinical infections which are etiologically significant to the child's negative traits.

THE VIRAL MODEL

The etiological significance of viral infections in ASD is well established by clinical data. Sidney Baker, MD, and Michael Goldberg, MD are physicians who have directed two major autism practices. Both Baker and Goldberg have reported that approximately 30% of their autistic patients respond favorably to acyclovir or Valtrex (an acyclovir variant). Efficacy studies have shown that, with descending usefulness, acyclovir is effective against herpes simplex virus, varicella, Epstein-Barr virus, and human herpesvirus 6 (HSV, VZV, EBV, HHV-6). My own clinical experience parallels what Baker and Goldberg have reported. When I first started seeing autistic patients I prescribed acyclovir or Valtrex for any of them that had elevated viral titers and found a positive response in about one-third of those treated. I was just learning, and may not have given a high enough dose for a long enough time for some of the children. This was my main treatment approach after diet, nutrients, and gut healing prior to starting to remove the heavy metals through chelation.

As we will see in Chapter Eight, these clinical findings have profound implications for the treatment of ASD children. First of all, acyclovir is benign for most children and adults. Thus a trial with acyclovir is easily enacted. Secondly, various herpes viruses are associated with verbal impairment, seizures, demyelination, and other autism-spectrum traits. All of this must be seen in the context of a child's overall medical portrait. Gut pathology must be minimized, nutritional status maximized, and heavy metals removed by physician-supervised chelation. A net effect of these treatments is that the child's immune status may improve to the point that his or her subclinical infection can be more successfully immunosuppressed. Generally, with notable exceptions based on a particular child's medical picture and lab findings, I will always heal the gut and start optimizing the nutrient intake first, chelate if there is evidence of heavy metal toxicity, and treat the viruses later in the treatment plan. However, my clinical experience has taught me that some children need a pharmaceutical antiviral like acyclovir or the plant alternative anti-virals right away along with or even preceding the chelation process. There is no doubt in my mind that viruses are a big player in many of our children's clinical pictures and further evidence of the immune dysregulation they endure. Since these infections are difficult to treat, I prefer to get the toxic load down and get the child's body into optimum health hoping their own immune system can start doing its job of viral immunosuppression.

THE GLUTEN/CASEIN, ENZYME DEFICIENCY, AND YEAST OVERGROWTH MODEL

Most autistic children have an inability to digest gluten and/or casein. Gluten refers to a mixture of proteins contained in wheat, rye, oats and barley and found in numerous other products. Casein is a milk protein. Alan Friedman, PhD, and fellow researchers theorize that an enzyme vital for the digestion of those substances ("DPP-IV") is missing (probably for genetic reasons) or is inactivated, possibly due to an autoimmune mechanism. Friedman's model posits that the absence or inactivation of the missing DPP-IV enzyme allows the accumulation in the body of opioid or morphine-like substances known as dermorphins. The buildup and accumulation of those substances may be one reason that autistic children frequently appear "spaced out." A common characteristic of autism is that the children generally ignore other people and seem to be living in their own inner worlds. Regardless of Friedman's hypothesis, many autistic spectrum children have one or several food hypersensitivities as determined by food-allergy tests and by elimination diets. Most ASD children studied have been shown to have inflamed gastrointestinal tracts, and it is believed that certain foods that the child is sensitive to such as gluten and casein irritate their intestines. Studies have shown that antibiotics also irritate the gut lining as well as impair the immune system. An initial and primary treatment for the inability to digest gluten and casein is a Gluten Free/Casein Free (GF/CF) diet. Chapter Five describes how to start and maintain your child on such a diet.

Children with impaired immune systems and inflamed intestines are particularly vulnerable to invasions by fungi, especially yeast of the Candida species. Fecal cultures and other lab-tests often identify overgrowths with *Candida albicans*. Indeed, some research indicates that Candida species and other fungi may be a significant cause of many of the untoward behaviors and health problems we see in autistic patients. Many of the children's medical histories document numerous episodes of ear infections and repeated use of antibiotics. As a result, the beneficial or "probiotic" flora in such children are likely to have been destroyed, thereby setting the stage for adverse fungal as well as bacterial colonizations. Similarly, organic mercury compounds can adversely affect intestinal flora. Thus vaccinal ethylmercury—which exits the body primarily via the intestinal tract—may also injure intestinal flora. When vaccinal ethylmercury poisoning is accompanied by antibiotic overuse, probiotic flora may decrease, resulting in an adverse intestinal colonization and the flourishing of intestinal yeast.

As these species of yeast multiply they excrete toxins. William Shaw, PhD, who conducted groundbreaking research on yeast and its effects on autistic children, points out that these toxins are capable of impairing the central nervous and immune systems.[24] An additional possible adverse connection with mercury is that it and other heavy metals destroy leukocytes and neutrophils, the specialized white blood cells that normally protect against fungi and bacteria.

Some of the health problems known to be caused by *Candida* overgrowth include diarrhea, stomachache, gas pains, constipation, headache, fatigue, and depression. Behavior problems include concentration difficulties, hyperactivity, short attention span, irritability, and aggression.

There are many safe ways to treat yeast overgrowth. These include taking "probiotics" (nutritional supplements which repopulate the intestinal tract with "good" microbes) and the use of anti-fungal nutraceuticals or mild prescription drugs to combat stubborn *Can-*

dida. Some children need to be put on special diets, low in sugar and other foods that cause yeasts to thrive. After treating their yeast infections, I have seen improvements in afflicted patients ranging from decreased hyperactivity and "stimming" to increased eye contact, better concentration, and increased speech.

THE METALLOTHIONEIN THEORY

This section discusses the work of William Walsh, PhD, a noted biochemist who works at the Pfeiffer Treatment Center in Naperville, IL. Based upon findings in thousands of individuals and nearly a thousand autism spectrum children, Dr. Walsh theorizes that a small peptide called metallothionein is the "missing link" in this disorder. Metallothionein (MT) is a protein with many roles in the body.[25] It is involved in the:

- Regulation of zinc and copper levels in the blood

- Detoxification of mercury and other toxic metals

- Development and functioning of the immune system and brain neurons

- Production of enzymes that break down casein and gluten

- Response to intestinal inflammation

MT also participates in the hippocampus region of the brain that modulates behavior control, emotional memory, and socialization. MT is such a vital substance that Dr. Walsh concludes that dysregulations of MT may be one of the primary causes of autism. He theorizes that autism results from the combination of a genetic defect involving marginal or defective MT functioning and an environmental insult during early development which disables MT.

In chemical profiles of 503 ASD patients Walsh and fellow researchers at the Pfeiffer Treatment Center, Naperville, IL discovered that 99% of those patients exhibited abnormal metal metabolism and showed evidence of MT dysfunction. He stated at the October 2001 Defeat Autism Now! conference in San Diego that environmental insults during gestation, infancy or early childhood may disable the metallothionein protein system, resulting in halted neuronal development and provoking the onset of autism.

In recent years, research studies and clinical lab-data have revealed that many children with ASD have abnormal copper and zinc levels in their blood. Since MT has an important role in regulating the balance of copper and zinc in healthy individuals, the fact that the majority of the patients in the Pfeiffer Treatment Center study had copper/zinc inbalances supports MT dysfunction as an important part of ASD pathology. Walsh's MT findings and supportive clinical lab-data have important treatment implications. Dr. Walsh and colleagues point out that MT functioning can be greatly improved through a two-step process that involves the removal of excess copper and other toxic metals in conjunction with nutrient therapies using zinc and other supplements known to encourage MT production and effectiveness. The Pfeiffer Center continues to actively research alternatives for autism prevention and treatment.

How Models of Causation Lead to Treatments That Work

The experts agree that autism spectrum disorder is a multi-factorial disorder. That means, for example, that very few believe mercury is the sole environmental insult or trigger for this disorder. Indeed, while many children get better when mercury and other heavy metals are removed from their bodies and brains, not all do. That fact alone implicates other causes in various subgroups and necessitates that we remain aware of other causation models in autism. In medical schools and universities, professors often tell their students, "There is nothing so practical as a good theory." That is because a theory is an attempt to explain a group of facts or phenomena. Once we have a model about what might be causing a disease, diagnostics and treatments can be designed in ways that address patterns of biomedical pathology.

Historically, valid medical theories often took decades before acceptance was commonplace. For instance, in the 19th century, Hungarian physician Ignaz Philipp Semmelweiss theorized that Childbirth Fever, that was killing huge numbers of women who had just given birth, somehow was transmitted by the hands of their doctors. In that era, doctors did not wash their hands very often and the germ theory of disease had not yet been accepted. Many doctors at that time actually performed autopsies on deceased childbirth fever victims and then assisted in live births without washing their hands! Semmelweiss was ridiculed by other physicians for his beliefs. It took years and the deaths of thousands of women before his theory was accepted. Now, thanks to the work of researchers such as Louis Pasteur, the germ theory of disease is accepted.

In my work I have come to believe that many autism spectrum children do not need drugs such as Ritalin or anti-psychotic medications. If possible, I want to correct the root of the problem and not just control behavior or other symptoms. In my opinion, the common denominator underlying the developmental disorders of almost all of these children regardless of the etiology is that proper nourishment does not reach their brain cells. I and many other clinicians are finding that almost all children begin improving when we (1) heal their inflamed digestive systems, (2) strengthen their immune systems by providing needed supplemental vitamins, minerals, and other nutrients; and (3) remove the toxins from their diets and the heavy metals from their bodies.

It was Dr. Bernard Rimland's pioneering work on the importance of Vitamin B6 for proper brain functioning and his publicizing of the benefits of DMG (dimethylglycine) for a certain subset of autistic children that started me on my search for information on the biochemical imbalances that underlie autism spectrum disorder. Because so many of these children self-restrict their diets to only a few, usually non-nutritious foods, it is easy to see that they need those nutrients as well as the replacement of other vitamins and minerals. It was clear to me that immune impairment was also a factor as shown by the history of high numbers of infections and antibiotic treatments in these children as well as immune deficiencies revealed by lab tests. I was avidly pursuing what role viruses might be playing in this disorder when I started hearing about the dangers of mercury toxicity from amalgams, mercury-laden fish, and vaccines. From e-mail communication with Amy Holmes, MD, of Baton Rouge, LA, the picture started getting clearer for me in a new way. Hearing about the use and benefit of oral chelation to reduce the heavy metal loads carried by these children, I began learning all I could about the harm mercury can inflict in a subset of susceptible children.

The presence of opportunistic viruses as shown by the high viral titers exhibited by many of these children went along with the mercury toxin idea, since mercury is a likely trigger to start this whole cascade of illness. Impaired immunity, gut inflammation, higher infection rate, increased use of antibiotics, impaired nutritional status, maldigestion/malabsorption, and decreased ability to handle toxins in the form of heavy metals or pathogens-—including viruses—is a sequence that fits most ASD children. I began to understand also that toxins in the brain, whether they are heavy metals, viruses or other pathogens, set up conditions that prevent nutrients from gaining entry into the brain cells even if the gut problems allow some nourishment to reach the brain. Autism spectrum disorder children's brain cells are starving for nutrients. An important part of my healing program is built around restoring healthful nutrition to their *starving brains*. One has to heal the gut, build up the child's immune system through a non-harmful diet and tailored supplementation, and block the intake of new toxins while lowering the load of those that have already accumulated. Only then is the brain enabled to take up needed nutrients.

Before parents and physicians can agree on the best treatment decisions, a good diagnosis is critical. Many treatment options are available and I have found that most of these children need many kinds of therapy, some applied simultaneously and some sequentially, to optimize the outcome. The different models of causation I have discussed in this chapter help me place children into subgroups so I can sequence the treatment optimally, starting with the most likely problem and working toward more esoteric treatments which are sometimes more expensive and require more invasive testing when the child is not making the improvement we had hoped for. The GF/CF/SF diet is a good example. Since I can say from direct experience and that of many others that almost all children benefit from removing casein and gluten from their diet, I do not have to advise an endoscopy and gut biopsy to prove the inflammation before suggesting this diet be adopted. Fortunately, dedicated researchers have already done the work for us.

History, family background, symptoms, and testing help me organize my treatment protocols based on which of the causation models are most likely operating. Like other Defeat Autism Now!

doctors I use lab testing to biomedically profile and specifically treat autism spectrum children. Patterns in these laboratory results and in treatment efficacy are prompting models of causation that may become the foundation for future autism protocols in mainstream medicine.

References

1 There is no general rule about the number of cases that must exist for an outbreak to be considered an epidemic. The classic definition of the term was stated by an epidemiologist by the name of Benenson in 1980. He defined an epidemic as "The occurrence in a community or region of a group of illnesses...of similar nature, clearly in excess of normal expectancy." In other words, an epidemic exists whenever the number of cases exceeds what is expected based on past experience for a given population.

2 22nd Annual Report to Congress on the Implementation of the Individuals with Disabilities Education Act, Table AA11, "Number and Change in Number of Children Ages, pp. 6-21, Served Under IDEA, Part B."

3 *U.S. News & World Report,* June 19, 2000, p. 47

4 Testimony on April 25, 2001 before the U.S. House of Representatives Committee on Governmental Reform by James J. Bradstreet, M.D., director of research for the International Autism Research Center.

5 Gillberg, C and Coleman, Mary, "The Biology of the Autistic Syndromes," 3rd Edition, 2000 Mac Keith Press, Chapter, Clinical Diagnosis

6 *Report on Autism to the California Legislature,* 1999.

7 Centers for Disease Control (CDC), April, 2000. "Prevalence of Autism in Brick Township, New Jersey, 1998: Community Report" available on the CDC website, http://www.cdc.gov/nceh/prograrams/cddh/dd/report.htm.

8 Shelia Kaplan and Jim Morris, "Kids At Risk," *U.S. News & world Report,* June 19, 2000, p. 47.

9 Warren, R.P., et al. (1996) 'Immunogenetic studies in autism and related disorders.' Molecular and Chemical Neuropathology, 28, pp. 77-81

10 Ibid

11 *In Harm's Way: Toxic Threats to Child Development* published in 2001 by the Greater Boston Physicians for Social Responsibility organization.

12 National Academies of Science Report, 2000.

13 "Protect Your Family from Lead in Your Home," EPA and United States Consumer Product Safety Commission pamphlet, 747-K-94-001, May, 1995.

14 Maury M. Breecher, PhD, M.P.H., *Healthy Homes in a Toxic World,* John Wiley & Sons, Inc.

15 *U.S. News & World Report,* June 19, 2000, p. 48.

16 Shelia Kaplan and Jim Morris, "Kids at Risk: Chemicals in the Environment Come Under Scrutiny as the Number of Childhood Learning Problems Soars, " *U.S. News & World Report,* June 19, 2000, p. 51.

[17] Wakefield, A.J. et al., "Ileal-lymphoid-nodular hyperplasia, non-specific colitis, and pervasive developmental disorder in children", Lancet 1998 Feb. 28;351(9103): 637-41

[18] www.feat.org/FEATnews: Report of Oasis 2001 Conference for Autism in Portland OR "Harvard Clinic Scientist Finds Gut/Autism Link, Like Wakefield Findings"

[19] Kawashima H. et al., "Detection and sequencing of measles virus from peripheral mononuclear cells from patients with inflammatory bowel disease." Dig. Dis. Sci. 2000 Apr;45(4): 723-9

[20] Comi, A.M. et al., "Familial clustering of autoimmune disorders and evaluation of medical risk factors in autism," Jour. Child. Neurol. 1999 Jun;14(6): 338-94

[21] Singh VK, Lin SX, Yang VC. Serological association of measles virus and human herpesvirus-6 with brain autoantibodies in autism. Clin Immunol Immunopathol 1998 Oct; 89 (1): pp. 105-8

[22] Brain, Behavior, and Immunity (Volume 7, pp. 97-103, 1993).

[23] Kawashima, H., et al., "Detection and sequencing of measles virus from peripheral mononuclear cells from patients with inflammatory bowel disease and autism." Dept. of Pediatrics, Tokyo Medical Univ., Japan, Dig. Dis. Sci. 2000 Apr;45(4): 723-9

[24] Shaw, William, Chapter 3, Biological Treatments for Autism and PDD, revised 2002 edition. Lenexa KS 66214

[25] Booklet, "Metallothionein and Autism." Pfeiffer Treatment Center, Naperville IL Oct 2001

TWO

GASTROINTESTINAL PATHOLOGY

Nutritional Deficiencies

Nutritional Deficiency as a Common Denominator

In this chapter, we will explain how medical researchers and Defeat Autism Now! clinicians are clarifying and solving pieces of the autism spectrum puzzle. Our discussion will broaden and deepen the understanding of some of the biomedical topics just touched on in Chapter One. The reader more interested in the treatment of autism than its biomedical origins can use this chapter as reference material for what comes later. Our recent progress in treatment is reflected in ever better understanding of the use of diagnostic testing and thus more effective treatments for individual children within subgroups of the underlying disease processes of this complex disorder. The shared symptom that integrates these seemingly disparate subgroups is the clinically substantiated fact that most autism-spectrum children have what I've come to call *starving brains*. Abnormalities shown in studies on these children compared to controls with neurotypical children reveal higher incidences of:

- Higher serum copper
- Zinc deficiency
- Magnesium deficiency
- Iron deficiency
- Higher copper/zinc ratios
- B12 deficiency
- Below normal glutamine
- Lower plasma sulphate
- Lower Vitamin B6
- Lower amino acids tyrosine, carnosine, lysine, hydroxylysine
- Lower methionine levels
- Higher glutamate
- Fatty acid deficiencies
- Calcium deficiency
- Inadequate levels of Vitamin D, E, and A

I cannot emphasize enough that the brain does not function in isolation. It is a team player; it needs vital nutrients as well as informational input. To fill these needs the brain depends heavily on complex interactions between the immune, endocrine, and gastrointestinal systems.

The early medical histories of many autism spectrum children indicate gastrointestinal challenges and/or recurrent otitis media (ear infections). When these findings are integrated with food-elimination results and studies of immune shifts and weaknesses, our attention is called to the significant interplay of gastointestinal health, nutritional status, and immune competence. This cluster of inter-relationships has relevance to diagnostics and treatments of ASD children, with many showing evidence of impaired immune systems and nutritionally deprived brains.

As the autistic child grows, parents, other physicians, and I are finding that the key to best outcome for many children is early bio-medical diagnostics followed by treatments which strengthen the immune system, heal the gut, and restore a healthful nutritional status. The proper combination of these treatments often succeeds in helping the brain receive the nourishment and neuronal input it needs to function properly. I call this series of treatments a "broad-spectrum approach;" some Defeat Autism Now! doctors simply refer to it as the Defeat Autism Now! protocol, with many variations per individual doctor.

This philosophy is based on years of laboratory experiments and trial-and-error clinical treatments involving thousands of patients. After sharing knowledge about several thousand cases, many Defeat Autism Now! doctors began to realize that, with much inter-individual variation, their autistic patients suffered from an interplay of immune dysregulations and gastrointestinal challenges with neurological ramifications. A primary clue toward developing a biomedical model of how to help ASD children was the oft-repeated observation that a great number of them have intractable diarrhea or constipation, abdominal pain, gaseousness and bloating, and—in many cases—foul smelling, light colored stools. In the historical context of a refrigerator-mother model that yielded to a "must be genetic" model, many pediatricians failed to connect these symptoms to the disease. In contrast, I and most, if not all Defeat Autism Now! practitioners believe we must treat the gastrointestinal problems to put these children on the road to recovery.

A second piece of the puzzle is that many children with autism, to the despair of their parents, have trouble sleeping through the night. In many cases, the first and second pieces of the puzzle are connected. Intestinal discomfort can impair sleep. Among Defeat Autism Now! doctors who recently participated in a well-attended physician training conference on autism in San Diego (October 2001), many agreed with Dr. Karl Reichelt's statement that many autistic children who awaken wailing and crying during the night suffer from reflux esophagitis.[1] That is, poor sleep habits occur because, during the night, stomach acid rises and burns the esophagus, the muscular membranous tube through which food passes to the stomach. No wonder these children wake up crying, often unable to tell us what is hurting them!

Causes of Gastrointestinal Problems in ASD Children

There can be many causes of gastrointestinal problems in children with autism. Multiple studies have shown malabsorption, maldigestion, gut pathogen overgrowth (fungal, bacterial and viral), and abnormal intestinal permeability in many ASD children. Many parents do not realize at first that there is a connection between their child's autism and their gastrointestinal abnormalities. Unfortunately, many doctors also have not yet learned about that connection. Constipation and diarrhea, and sometimes both at alternate times, are frequently reported by parents, as well as abnormal amounts of gas, belching, and foul smelling stools. Clinical biopsies reveal that many autistic children have an autism-specific ileal hyperplasia.[2][3][4] Many Defeat Autism Now! doctors and medical researchers believe that a primary factor in the children's chronic gastrointestinal disturbances is immune system impairment. However, since these two systems are so interrelated, it is often impossible to know whether the immune dysregulation or the gastrointestinal pathology came first. As we have already indicated in Chapter One, a history of food intolerances or allergies, inability to digest gluten and casein, and chronic fungal (yeast) infections are tip-offs that an immune impairment—whether acquired and/or genetic—contributes to the gastrointestinal pathology. An increasing amount of evidence supports the triggering role of external influences in starting the immune and gastrointestinal problems, such as vaccinations containing heavy metals and repeated antibiotics—environmental factors whose effects are magnified in children with increased susceptibility, be it transient or chronic, acquired or genetic.

The interplay of these complex domains—gastrointestinal, immune, infectious, and nutritional—makes it important to gather extensive information not only about the child's medical and vaccination history and symptoms, but also the family's medical history. In particular, we need to ascertain whether there is a family history of autoimmune, allergic, or infectious disease. I will provide more information about my philosophy of testing, the usefulness and costs of tests, and the sequence of testing I usually recommend in Chapter Four.

How the Immune and GI Systems Interact

To understand why we need to take a broad spectrum approach to treating ASD children, it may be helpful to understand some basics about how the immune and gastrointestinal systems interact. The immune system is our body's chief defense against pathogenic bacteria, fungi, and viruses. It distinguishes between self and foreign molecules inside the body and mobilizes armies of defensive cells and antibodies against those foreign molecules. However, it is supposed to kick into action only if something is wrong. Many and possibly most children with autism have some form of immune system malfunction. Often, such malfunction involves misidentifying cells as foreign that are actually part of *self.* In this type of immune dysfunction, the immune system is attacking its host's body. This is one type of process among others that can cause inflammation of the gastrointestinal tract. Examples include viral persistence within intestinal tissues[5] as well as adverse colonizations by fungal or bacterial pathogens. As we have indicated, gastrointestinal inflammation and its underlying causes contribute to a cascade of other difficulties that constitute a major part of the disease process in many autism spectrum children.

Because the intestinal tract represents an important barrier between external pathogens and our internal organs, nature has incorporated a number of immune mechanisms into the epithelium, the gut lining whose job it is to block outside pathogens from doing any damage. When the specialized immune cells lining the intestinal tract detect unknown or possibly harmful antigens, signals are generated and immune reinforcements are sent. Eventually, this response can include an "army" of cells to fight the invading antigens. This "army" has several types of specialized "soldiers." For instance, researchers have indentified Natural Killer cells (NK), cytotoxic T cells, helper T-cells, and B-cells. Some T-cells construct special molecules that aid in identifying and eliminating pathogens, while other cells produce and release antibodies that help only in the elimination process. A further distinction is that many T-cells can be categorized in accord with their primary role, with Thymus 1(Th1) cells participating in cell-mediated immunity and Th2 cells helping with antibody-mediated defenses. Recent studies demonstrate that an immune profile tending to have more Th2 cells is conducive to chronic fungal infections.[6] Autism-research studies have documented that many autistic children have immune-cell counts that demonstrate a Th2-like profile.[7] Not surprisingly, fecal-culture evaluations of many autistic children reveal intestinal colonization by Candida species.

Long-time autism-researcher Sudhir Gupta, MD, PhD—a professor of neurology, pathology, microbiology, and molecular genetics at the University of California, Irvine—has documented immune abnormalities in autism-spectrum children.[8] He found that a large group of autistic patients had relatively more Th2 cells than Th1 cells compared to neurotypical children. Dr. Gupta believes the decrease in Th1 cells may explain the susceptibility of autistic children to viral and fungal infections. In addition, the increase in their Th2 cells may also explain their increased autoimmune responses against brain tissue as indicated by Dr. Singh's findings of antibodies to the myelin basic protein (MBP) mentioned in Chapter One.

Dr. Gupta also points out that the immune system controls the release of various inflammatory mediators including Interleukin 1, Interleukin 8, and tumor necrosis factor (TNF)—all of which cause marked degrees of inflammation in the gut. His data and observations are helping identify at least a few of the immune dysfunctions and inflammatory bowel pathologies that cause so many autistic children to suffer. Furthermore, Dr. Gupta went on to say that the autopsied brains of autistic patients reveal alterations in neurotransmitters and neuropeptides, possibly even a loss of myelination (the protective covering) on nerve fibers similar to findings in the autopsied brains of multiple sclerosis patients. The brains of many autistic patients also showed increased levels of TNF, which creates inflammatory effects along the blood-brain barrier. Dr. Gupta stated that TNF increase causes inflammation leading to decreased blood flow and mitochondrial injury within the cells, decreased intracellular glutathione, and abnormal conduction or even cell death. Clearly, ischemic (oxygen deficient) brain cells would not be able to take in a full set of nutrients, even if provided by the diet.

HOW YEAST OVERGROWTH CAN INJURE
THE GASTROINTESTINAL SYSTEM

It is well known that a weakened immune system—whether through genetic predisposition or acquired as a result of intestinal problems—leaves children open to chronic infections. Therefore, it is not surprising that Canadian researchers found a strong relationship between the incidence of autism and the prevalence of ear infections. In fact, they found that the increased incidence of ear infections correlated with the most severe form of autism.[9] Similar studies of other symptoms that make up the autism spectrum follow a similar pattern. For example, studies on children with ADHD show that high rates of ear infections in a child's early years correlate with greater amounts of hyperactivity.[10]

Although in most affected individuals the infections are probably not the primary cause of autism or ADHD, they may be a first step because otitis media is generally presumed to have an infectious, bacterial origin and because bacterial infections are generally treated with antibiotics. Ironically, large, PCR-based (polymerase chain reaction) studies by Tasnee Chonmaitree and colleagues have demonstrated that approximately 35% of ear inflammations are not bacterial in origin. Furthermore, while antibiotics have saved millions of lives since World War II, many studies indicate that most medical doctors prescribe antibiotics far too often. One consequence of antibiotic overuse is that numerous bacteria are becoming resistant to antibiotics. Another ramification is that these "wonder drugs" kill protective (probiotic) bacteria in the gut as well as the pathogens. The destruction of beneficial gut-bacteria merits major concern. The process opens the door to overgrowth by fungi and bacteria. In many individual cases, the child's chronic diarrhea or constipation may be a symptom of yeast overgrowth.

How important are adverse intestinal colonizations by pathogenic fungi and/or bacteria? A noted researcher and clinical lab director—William Shaw, PhD—has written: "Abnormal byproducts of yeast and drug-resistant bacteria absorbed into the body from the intestine following the excessive use of antibiotics is the cause of these epidemics."[11] While I subscribe to the view that there are many factors and various causes for the current epidemic of autism,

I certainly agree that, in many autistic children, bacterial and fungal overgrowths are etiologically significant in the cascade of events that result in autism or one of the other autism spectrum disorders.

When we are healthy, Candida lives in an uneasy balance or truce with our mixtures of beneficial and potentially harmful bacteria. Furthermore, as can some species of bacteria such as Clostridia, Candida can survive without oxygen and does so by changing into an anaerobic (without oxygen) fungal form. Most antibiotics kill only oxygen-breathing bacteria. Candida survives antibiotics and can spread like wildfire following the sudden die-off of intestinal bacteria. If for any reason, an infant or toddler already has a weakened immune system, the resulting colonizations—whether fungal and/or bacterial—can be unhealthy for the intestine.

"LEAKY GUT", INCREASED PERMEABILITY OF THE INTESTINAL MUCOSA AND MALABSORPTION

Many yeast species excrete toxic by-products which cause a variety of digestive illnesses including irritable bowel syndrome, chronic constipation, or diarrhea. One of these toxic byproducts is an enzyme that allows the yeast to burrow into the intestinal wall which can contribute to what is termed the "leaky gut" syndrome. The yeast-generated toxins literally drill holes through the intestinal wall and seep into the child's bloodstream.[12] Ultimately, the toxic substances may inflame or cross the blood/brain barrier and, by interfering with the flow of nutrients to the brain, impair consciousness, cognition, speech, or behavior.

Another mechanism that may cause these children to have *starving brains* involves inadequate or inappropriate absorption of protein nutrients by the intestine. A healthy digestive system is able to take complex foods and break them down to forms that the cells of the body can absorb and metabolize into energy. As we have pointed out earlier, many children with autism have trouble digesting casein or gluten. Casein is a milk protein, and gluten is a plant protein found in wheat and related grains. Proteins are made of building blocks called amino acids; short strings or chains of amino acids are called peptides. During digestion, many proteins are broken down into single amino acids; others are transported as slightly larger chains. When ingested proteins are only partially digested, what remains are longer chain peptides. Some autism researchers have published articles in the scientific literature about malabsorption, maldigestion, and the related findings of unusual proteins and peptides in the urine of people with autism.[13] In many autistic children, those indigestible proteins and peptides come from casein and gluten; soy and corn can also be problematic.

Many peptide chains are flushed out in the urine. However, because many autistic children have leaky guts, an unacceptable amount of those substances can enter the bloodstream. The researchers we have already mentioned in Chapter One who found the unusual proteins and peptides in the urine of autistic patients discovered that those substances, when carried to the brain, have an opioid-like effect with a potency several times that of morphine, and named those unusual peptides *opioids*.

Paul Shattock, PhD, of the Autism Research Unit at the United Kingdom's University of Sunderland School of Health Sciences, says his studies indicate that there is "a rough correlation between the amount of opioids in the bodies of autistic children and the degree of severity of their impairments."[14] These natural morphine-like substances seem to drug the children and interfere with motivation, emotions, perception, response, and the normal development of their brains. Dr. Shattock says opioid peptides overstimulate nerve synapses and block normal signal transmissions to the brain.

In some children, the failure of the gut to properly digest the gluten and casein may, in part, be due to a low level of digestive enzymes. Such impairments can be acquired and, in some children, may be genetic. For children with impaired digestion, one treatment is to supplement their diet with certain digestive enzymes. However, a recent study found that although digestive enzymes helped, they were only half as effective as simply eliminating gluten and wheat from the diet. Furthermore, Dr. Shattock informs us that a two-year study found that many children with autism improve on the GF/CF diet, but that some regress if they return to eating wheat and milk products.

In my own practice, I have seen dramatic improvements in patients whose parents encourage or, let's be honest, require them to adhere to healthier diets. Even two-year-old ASD children are usually picky eaters. Regardless of age, it is often difficult, at least at the beginning of a new treatment plan, to encourage the child to discontinue sweet drinks and Chicken McNuggets. However, the potential benefits are worth it. As I will keep repeating, at present I strongly recommend that every parent of an autistic child totally eliminate gluten and casein from their children's diets for at least a four to six-month trial. In Chapter Five, I will tell you how to accomplish this.

FURTHER NOTES ON THE MERCURY/VACCINE CONNECTION

Many extensively researched papers and books have been written describing the toxic effects of mercury. Dr. Sudhir Gupta at the Fall 2001 Defeat Autism Now! Conference said, "Genes load the gun, environment pulls the trigger." He explained that sulfhydryl groups are present in cellular mitochondria, that mercury binds these groups, necrotizing DNA, altering cell membrane permeability, and affecting calcium transport. Mercury causes a shift from Th1 to Th2 immunity, dysregulates signaling mechanism, and induces autoimmunity. The noted researcher stated, "Thimerosal is a mitochondrial poison and autism is a disorder of mitochondria." This poison disturbs the ratio between death and rebirth of cells. Gupta produced a graph from his studies showing an increase in cell death rising in direct proportion to the amount of thimerosal present. Evidence is accruing that vaccinal mercury could have been a likely trigger for an entire generation of kids who, due to individual susceptibility, may have succumbed to this unanticipated form of mercury poisoning. I will be discussing the issue of impaired detoxification mechanisms and mercury more extensively in Chapter Three.

Putting the Puzzle Pieces Together

Which comes first, the "chicken" or the "egg?" This riddle can serve as an analogy for the controversy about which are the primary causative agents behind autism and other autism spectrum disorders. One can start from the proposition that abnormally large spaces present between the cell walls of the gut (possibly caused by genetics or by adverse pathogen colonizations) allow opioids and other toxic materials to enter the bloodstream. Since they are "out of place," the immune system recognizes these substances as foreign and makes antibodies against them. I didn't mention earlier that the immune system also has a "memory." When it sees what it perceives as an invader for the second, third, or subsequent time, it mobilizes even larger armies of antibodies to strike back. In our gastrointestinal tracts, the antibodies made to protect against those abnormal proteins and peptides get aimed at the foods that originated them. This appears to be one route by which food allergies and sensitivities arise.

Of course, those antibodies trigger inflammatory reactions in the gastrointestinal tract when the offending foods are consumed. Thus chronic inflammation, perhaps originally caused by yeast or perhaps by other invading microorganisms, keeps renewing itself. The constant inflammation weakens the protective coatings of another type of antibody (immunoglobulin A or IgA) that is normally present in healthy intestines. IgA is made in bone marrow and lymphoid tissue and protects us against bacterial and viral infections by facilitating phagocytosis (the absorption and destruction of pathogenic cells by the immune cells). IgA also inhibits the inflammatory effects of tumor necrosis factor, and is an important defense mechanism to prevent colonization of yeast and Clostridia. Patients with gastrointestinal pathology often have reduced levels of IgA. A child so affected would be less resistant to viruses, bacteria, parasites, and yeast.

Although some intestinal pathogens continue to pass through the permeable intestine into the bloodstream, they generally are destroyed by the immune reaction. Yet their cell-wall fragments can induce inflammation and, to some extent, may be transported to locations throughout the body including the liver, blood brain barrier, and the brain itself. In large enough amounts, those toxic substances can impair or even overwhelm the liver's ability to detoxify them. I believe that the buildup of this pathogenic debris can result in symptoms including brain fog, memory loss, and confusion. So you see, where we start the analytic process doesn't matter; autistic children's underlying pathologies are complex and remarkably interlinked. Nonetheless, of primary importance is what these various processes tell us about how we might intervene with healing treatments.

Clinical lab data from children with intestinal pathology, food hypersensitivities, or "leaky gut" often reveal a long list of vitamin and mineral deficiencies. In fact, I and many Defeat Autism Now! physicians believe that gastrointestinal pathology is why the majority of autistic children have abnormal nutritional profiles. Various tests and studies have documented deficiencies in many important vitamins and minerals including calcium, copper, magnesium, and zinc. Similarly, other studies have shown that ADHD children are deficient in vitamins B6 and B12; some have fatty acid deficiencies. All these deficiencies are physical manifestations of medical problems that can be treated. We will be discussing tests to diagnose these deficiencies in Chapter Four and nutrient-replacement treatments in Chapter Six.

Like the classic "chicken and egg" puzzler, what is cause and what is effect in the etiology or development of ASD in many individual cases may remain an unanswerable question. However, it is important that we are unraveling and understanding more and more about those complex processes. We don't need perfect understanding to begin effective treatments. Since research study data and clinical lab data increasingly point in similar directions, we now have sufficient evidence to try several common-sense treatment approaches.

In the present environment of increasingly hopeful understanding, the concept *subgroups* is vitally important. We know that some children respond to certain treatments and others respond to different ones. The variability of response may have to do with the initial trigger, the intensity of the injury, the length of time the condition has existed, and the amount of damage that has been done to the immune and gastrointestinal systems as well as to various body organs before treatment was initiated.

We cannot lose sight of the bottom line: even with variable responses to various treatments, most children improve with biomedical treatment. That is why several different treatment approaches have to be taken and possibly continued even if some of the treatments overlap. The earlier parents begin treatment, the greater the chances that the child will get better. Often, a synergistic effect occurs between treatments. That means a composite treatment approach may be more effective than implementing one treatment protocol at a time.

Note: the role of other toxins are set forth in Appendix C.

References

[1] Karl Reichelt, MD, PhD, at the DAN Fall, 2001 conference, Oct. 5-7, San Diego, CA.

[2] Wakefield A.J. et al., "Enterocolitis in children with developmental disorders." Amer Jour Gastroenterology 2000 Sep;95(9): 2285-95

[3] Furlano R.I. et al., "Colonic CD8 and gamma delta T-cell infiltration with epithelial damage in children with autism." Jour Pediatrics 2001 Mar;138(3): 366-72

[4] Buie, Tim, Pediatric Gastroenterologist, Mass Gen Hosp, Harvard Med School, Presentation Oasis II Conference 14 Oct 2001

[5] Wakefield A.J. et al., "Detection of herpesvirus DNA in the large intestine of patients with ulcerative colitis and Crohn's disease using nested polymerase chain reaction Jour. Med. Virology 1992 Nov;38(3): 183-90

[6] Gupta, Sudhir, MD, PhD, Professor of microbiology and molecular genetics at Univ CA at Irvine, Presentation at Defeat Autism Now! Conference, Oct 5, 2001, San Diego

[7] Ibid

[8] Ibid

[9] M. Kontstantareas and S. Homatidis, "Ear Infections in Autistic and Normal Children, *Journal of Autism and Developmental Diseases*, Vol. 17, p. 585, 1987.

[10] R. Hagerman and A. Falkenstein, "An Association Between Recurrent Otitis Media in Infancy and Later Hyperactivity," *Clinical Pediatrics, Vol. 26*, pp. 253-257, 1987.

[11] William Shaw, *Biological Treatments for Autism and PDD*, self-published, 1998.

[12] D'Eufemia P. et al. "Abnormal intestinal permeability in children with autism." Acta Paediatr 1996 Sep;85(9): 1076-9.

[13] *Malabsorption*
B. Walsh, "85% of 500 autistic patients meet criteria for malabsorption,"
J. Autism/Childhood Schizo, 1971 1(1): 48-62;
Maldigestion—elevated urinary peptides
P Shattock, *Brain Dysfunct* 1990; 3: 338-45 and 1991; 4: 323-4)
K. L. Reicheldt (*Develop Brain Dys* 1994; 7: 71-85, and others)
Z. Sun and R. Cade (*Autism* 1999; 3: pp. 85-96 and 1999; 3: 67-83)

[14] DAN Fall, 2001 conference, Oct. 5-7, San Diego, CA

THREE

IMPAIRED DETOXIFICATION, TOXIC ACCUMULATIONS, AND POLITICS

Toxic Threats to Child Development

An increasing body of clinical data indicates that many children with autism spectrum disorder cannot efficiently dispose of toxic substances that enter their bodies. For example, as metals accumulate, these children become ill with various forms of heavy metal poisoning. Laboratory tests documenting chelation induced metal outflow reveal that many ASD children have accumulated lead, tin, mercury, and/or some other heavy metals. Many of these children treated with physician supervised chelation (now called *detoxification)* preceded by gut-healing and nutritional support are showing major alleviation of autism-spectrum traits. Some children on this protocol have outgrown their diagnosis of autism.[1]

The reasons why natural detoxification is impaired for many ASD children remain to be determined. However, medical histories and medical literature are providing strong clues. The recent report by Greater Boston Physicians for Social Responsibility entitled *In Harm's Way: Toxic Threats to Child Development* [2] referred to in Chapter One links lifelong disabilities to toxic exposures of lead, mercury, other heavy metals, and pesticides prevalent in our environment during early childhood or even before birth. The Boston physicians' report states that "learning and behavioral disorders are increasing in frequency." They cite research that indicates toxic substances such as mercury, lead, and pesticides contribute to many neurobehavioral and cognitive disorders. The report further states: "Unlike an adult, the developing child exposed to neurotoxic chemicals during critical developmental windows of vulnerability may suffer from lifelong impacts on brain function."

Findings and news releases from the FDA and EPA have stressed that pregnant women should minimize fish consumption so as to reduce the intake of dietary mercury that can affect fetal development. In this context, it is not surprising that distinguished immunologist Hugh Fudenberg, MD, PhD, has long recommended the removal of metals for autistic children. In addition, Stephen Edelson, MD[3] and colleagues have published peer-reviewed studies wherein autism spectrum traits were significantly eliminated in response to chelation and related therapies. More recently, a revolutionary paper, first drafted by parents of autistic children and then published in 2000, called attention to the similarities between autism-spectrum traits and those induced by mercury poisoning.[4] That paper also drew upon FDA data regarding the presence of ethylmercury in some childhood vaccines and suggested that, at least in infants and toddlers with increased susceptibility, the ethylmercury injected during vaccinations may have induced intestinal and neurologic damage.

This seminal paper was pivotal in prompting an expanded interest in removing toxic metals from ASD children, which has led to encouraging clinical results thus far. In fact, pursuant to a vaccinal ethylmercury hearing on July 16, 2001, the Institute of Medicine (a division of the National Academy of Sciences) found the mercury/autism hypothesis to be plausible and subsequently funded two ongoing clinical studies wherein autism spectrum children are receiving chelation therapy in the context of gut healing and nutritional support. To say the least, all these developments were exciting and profoundly important to the treatment of ASD. To understand the impaired detoxification process more deeply, some background information about heavy metals will be helpful.

Heavy metals enter our bodies as a result of eating and breathing. Yes, food and air contain tiny quantities of toxic metals. They can even be absorbed through our skin. Furthermore, heavy metals are "bio-accumulative." That is, they can chemically bond to molecules within mammalian bodies, be difficult to excrete, and be passed up the food chain to humans. This is the reason we are warned of the dangers of mercury accumulation in fish, especially tuna and the large predator fish such as shark and swordfish. When heavy metals enter and accumulate in body tissues faster than the body can excrete them, a state of toxicity can develop that injures tissue and nerve cells. As we have stressed in previous chapters, a growing number of physicians, researchers, and parents now believe that impaired detoxification and excessive accumulation of toxic metals are primary etiological factors in many cases of autism and other autism spectrum disorders.

A recent study by James Adams, PhD, backs up that belief. In research financed by Arizona State University, he explored the question of whether "Mercury and other heavy metals contribute to the causes and/or symptoms of autism."[5] Dr. Adams and his colleagues studied 55 ASD children ages three to 24 and compared them to a control group of 30 "typical" children. Parents of both groups of children filled out a questionnaire designed to rate their known exposure to heavy metals. All the children also had hair analyses, dental exams, and underwent psychological testing including the Gilliam Autism Rating Scale, a commonly used test instrument to determine the severity of autism. The autistic children were found to have ten times the number of ear infections during the first three years of life compared to the normal children. Eighteen percent of the autism spectrum children also had experienced severe reactions to vaccines compared to zero percent of the "typical" children. The ASD children also had lower levels of mercury and lead in their hair than the "typical" children, indicating that excretion was not taking place as it did in the control group children. Dr. Adams points out that antibiotics which are often used to treat children's earaches, "greatly reduce mercury excretion." He stated that ASD children excrete "five times as much mercury" as typical children when given DMSA, an oral chelating agent used to remove heavy metals from the body.

"Together, our study suggests ASD children have inhibited ability to excrete heavy metals," Dr. Adams told scientists gathered at an international autism meeting in San Diego, CA in November of 2001. "Overall, mercury appears to be a major risk factor for ASD," he and his team of researchers concluded.[6]

Animal studies of lead and mercury have revealed that scientists previously had underestimated the levels of human exposure to these metals.[7] According to EPA guidelines, many neonates, infants, and toddlers have been injected with unsafe levels of ethylmercury through vaccinations. In retrospect, some of these children were certain to have become more susceptible to developing adverse effects as a consequence.[8] In short, our nation's children have experienced unprecedented exposure to heavy metals. This fact may be reflected in various epidemics whose increase cannot be due merely to "genetics." Our children's minds are at risk. The epidemics of autism, autism-spectrum disorders, and even Alzheimer's and other diseases may well be reflections of increased exposure to heavy metals.

The Mechanism of Heavy Metal Toxicity

As we have emphasized, mercury and other heavy metals can adversely affect the gastrointestinal, immune, nervous, and endocrine systems. Heavy metals alter cellular function and numerous metabolic processes in the body, including those related to the central and peripheral nervous systems.[9] Much of the damage produced by heavy metals comes from the proliferation of oxidative free radicals. A free radical is an energetically unbalanced molecule, composed of an unpaired electron that "steals" an electron from another molecule. Free radicals occur naturally when cell molecules react with oxygen (oxidize). However, excessive free-radical production occurs when a person is exposed to heavy metals or when an adult or child has genetic or acquired antioxidant deficiencies. Unchecked, the free radicals can cause tissue damage throughout the body including the brain. Fortunately, laboratory and clinical studies have shown that antioxidants such as vitamins A, C, E, and Co-Enzyme Q10 can protect against and, to some extent, repair free-radical damage.[10] Another substance important to proper detoxification is glutathione, which is considered elsewhere in this book.

Specific Heavy Metals: Lead and Mercury

LEAD

Lead is known as a neurotoxin—in plain English, a killer of brain cells. Excessive lead levels in children's blood have been linked to learning disabilities, to attention deficit disorder (ADD) and hyperactivity syndromes, and to reduced intelligence and school achievement scores. The greatest risk for harm, even with only minute or short-term exposure, occurs among infants, young children, and pregnant women and their fetuses. After a century of intensive study, the harm from lead "can now be characterized with fair certainty.[11]

Since childhood lead exposure has been ongoing since lead paint was first introduced in the 1890's, five generations of children have been injured while science has slowly advanced to where it is now capable of appreciating the magnitude of the problem. This same pattern of "after-the-fact" recognition of harm has been repeated for mercury.

In 1984, a federal study conducted by the Center for Disease Control (CDC) estimated that three to four million American children have unacceptably high levels of lead in their blood. This is an even higher figure than in the Boston Physicians' Report mentioned earlier. Dr. Suzanne Binder, a CDC official, stated, "Many people believed that when lead paint was banned from housing [in 1978], and lead was cut from gasoline [in the late 1970s], lead-poisoning problems disappeared, but they're wrong. We know that throughout the country children of all races, ethnic backgrounds, and income levels are being affected by lead already in the environment."[12]

In 1989, the U.S. Environmental Protection Agency (EPA) reported that more than one million elementary schools, high schools, and colleges are still using lead-lined water storage tanks or lead-containing components in their drinking fountains. The EPA estimates that drinking water accounts for approximately 20% of young children's lead exposure.[13] Other common sources are lead paint residue in older buildings (common in inner cities) and living in proximity to industrial areas or other sources of toxic chemical exposure, such as commercial agricultural land.

MERCURY

It is not as if the dangers of mercury had not already been understood by the chemical and pharmaceutical industries. No less a historic personality than Isaac Newton is said to have been affected by mercury poisoning. Historians note that Newton's personality changed dramatically at age 35, and again at age 51, after he conducted experiments involving heated mercury. In modern times, scientists who analyzed a lock of Newton's hair found unusually high levels of mercury probably from inhalation of the dangerous fumes.[14] Even 19th Century author Lewis Carroll knew that mercury is one of the most toxic substances on earth. Indeed, he indirectly referred to its dangers through the "Mad Hatter," his *Alice in Wonderland* character. When Lewis Carroll wrote that book, hat makers used mercury in the process of making hats. One of their occupational hazards was a type of mercury induced insanity called "Mad Hatter's" disease. Modern day manufacturers also have recognized the dangers of mercury.

As we have stated previously, concern about mercury stems from its effects on the brain, nervous system, and gastrointestinal system. Mercury poisoning induces cognitive and social deficits, including loss of speech or failure to develop it, memory impairment, poor concentration, word comprehension difficulties, and an assortment of autism-like behaviors including sleep difficulties, self-injurious behavior (e.g. head banging and self-biting,) agitation, unprovoked crying, and staring spells.[15]

Sources of mercury exposure include air and water pollution, amalgam dental fillings,[16] batteries, cosmetics, shampoos, mouthwashes, toothpaste, soaps, mercurial diuretics, electrical devices and relays, explosives, residues in foods (especially grains), fungicides, fluorescent lights, freshwater fish such as bass, pike, and trout, insecticides, pesticides, paints, petroleum products, saltwater fish such as halibut, shrimp, snapper, swordfish, shark, tuna, and shellfish. According to EPA estimates, about 1.16 million women in the U.S. of childbearing years eat sufficient amounts of mercury-contaminated fish to risk damaging the brain development of their children.[17]

Dental fillings are an important source of mercury contamination. Amalgam fillings release microscopic particles and vapors of mercury. This shedding of mercury is increased by chewing and by drinking hot liquids. Those vapors are absorbed by tooth roots, mucous membranes of the mouth and gums, and are inhaled and swallowed, thereby reaching the esophagus, stomach, and intestines. University of Calgary researchers report 10% of amalgam mercury eventually accumulates in body organs.[18]

Years after amalgam removal, some of my adult clients have shown high mercury urine output with a chelation challenge, with subsequent improvement in health after chelation.

Ingested mercury can be passed to the fetus in wombs of pregnant mothers from the mother's amalgams when she chews, and particularly when she has either placement or removal dental work involving amalgams. In March 2002 the parents of a five-year-old child brought suit against the American Dental Association, alleging mercury in the mother's nine dental fillings caused her son's autism. Also named as defendants were the California Dental Association and more than 20 corporations that deal in materials used to produce amalgam fillings, which are about 50% mercury by weight. The lawsuit accused them of fraud, negligence and illegal and deceptive business practices. Many lawsuits have been filed against drug companies alleging links between autism and vaccines containing mercury, but attorneys and scientists familiar with such litigation say this is believed to be the first to allege a connection between autism and amalgam fillings.

"I don't know that it's proven, but it's credible, very credible," said Dr. Boyd Haley, former chairman of the chemistry department at the University of Kentucky and an expert on mercury toxicity. "Mercury is one of the most neurotoxic compounds known to man." Dr. Haley said some studies show people with amalgam fillings have four to five times as much mercury in their blood and urine as people without such fillings.

Mercury in Vaccines

The insidious avenue of mercury poisoning through the ethylmercury preservative in several vaccines has already been mentioned in both Chapters One and Two. In this section I will summarize more of the terrifying details of how this came about.

Thimerosal is 49.6% ethylmercury by weight and, since the 1930's, has been used as a vaccine preservative intended to protect against bacterial contamination in multi-use containers.[19] The Manufacturers' Safety Data sheet for thimerosal states that the substance is "highly toxic," and warns about the danger of "cumulative effects" and "prolonged or repeated exposure" to mercury. That is because a danger point for mercury toxicity occurs when the rate of exposure exceeds the rate of elimination. This "threshold effect" then results in a neurotoxic shock to the immune system which can show itself months after exposure. As suggested earlier, this may be why children diagnosed with the "regressive" form of autism experience normal development from birth, then suddenly start regressing after further insults to their immune systems with other vaccines, notably the live viruses in the MMR.

As we have stated, a great deal of evidence implicates thimerosal as one of the primary etiologic triggers responsible for the current epidemic of "regressive autism," a trend that rapidly accelerated in the early 1990s. Furthermore, the historical record clearly shows that what were once considered "safe thresholds" for known neurotoxicants have continuously been "revised downward" as scientific knowledge advances."[20]

Ironically, as knowledge about the neurotoxicity of mercury accumulated during the 20th Century and as concerns were raised about mercury's ubiquitous and increasing environmental presence, no one thought to question its safety in vaccines—not even after an expert FDA panel had concluded in 1982 that thimerosal was unsafe and should be removed from all over-the-counter products! In fact, during the Institute of Medicine's (IOM) thimerosal/autism hearing on July 16, 2001, U.S. vaccine official Neal Halsey, MD, apologized for not having realized sooner that thimerosal-containing vaccines contained dangerously high levels of ethylmercury. It is a tragedy that this toxic substance in vaccines was overlooked.

The situation got out of hand in 1991 when the Hepatitis B vaccination was mandated for every newborn. This vaccine was loaded with thimerosal. Infants got not one, but three doses of Hepatitis B vaccine and three doses of the thimerosal-containing Hib or Human

Influenza B vaccine during the first six months of their lives. Not counting maternal exposures, for many infants the levels of mercury exceeded the EPA's guidelines for "safe" exposure *in adults*. The accumulation of mercury in their small bodies may have exceeded the threshold of their ability to excrete the toxin. Children who do not exhibit ASD symptoms may simply have had higher thresholds or stronger immune systems. Breast fed babies have been shown to be less susceptible to getting the disorder and some mothers have reported their child became autistic shortly after cessation of breast-feeding, which is known to convey many immunity benefits.

A reasonable person might assume that American health authorities would have learned from the experience of other countries. For example, over 15,000 lawsuits were filed against the mandatory Hep B vaccination program in France, which led to the French Minister of Health finally ending that program for all French school children in October of 1998.[21] However, it was not until late in 2001 that mercury was removed from the Hep B vaccine and most other vaccines in the U.S. By then an entire generation of kids had been put at risk. Yet this removal did not occur until after Bernard et al had sent their thimerosal/autism paper to officials at the CDC, FDA, AMA, and NIH. The long version of the paper contained more than 400 citations. It also contained the comparison table that described how mercury poisoning causes speech and hearing deficits, sensory disturbances including sensitivity to loud noises, aversion to touch, and cognitive and behavioral impairments. These same deficits are present in greater or lesser degrees in children with autism and autistic spectrum disorder. In brief, medical literature about mercury poisoning includes all the traits that define autism (DSM-IV) and other traits that are associated with ASD generally. The scientific justification was overwhelming. Ethylmercury should never have been injected into humans, regardless of age.

The Saga of Several Autism Parents and "Parent Power"

The role of vaccinal ethylmercury was first realized by several parents of autism spectrum children. Albert and Sima Enayati, Sallie

Bernard, Heidi Roger, and Lynn Redwood heard the FDA's 1999 announcement that some vaccines contained thimerosal, realized that mercury poisoning may have contributed to their children's autistic regression, and with Teresa Binstock began researching and writing the report that became known as the "Bernard et al mercury/autism paper." As the research materials accumulated and the paper took shape, this group began contacting officials at the CDC, FDA, AMA, and NIH. Surprisingly, officials at each of these agencies met with the co-authors and some of their supporters. The paper had called attention to a potentially important danger. Within the first year after the mercury/autism paper's long version was made available, vaccine manufacturers began removing thimerosal from most vaccines, vaccinating neonates with the hepatitis B vaccine was restricted, and thimerosal's adverse effects were reviewed by the Institute of Medicine and through a Congressional hearing led by Dan Burton of Indiana and the House Government Reform Committee.

The dedication and persistence of this small group of parents alerted the world to the autism epidemic's probable connection with vaccinal ethylmercury. When the Bernard et al co-authors calculated the amounts of mercury a child received for each of his or her recommended vaccines, they found that infants could be exposed to levels of mercury that exceeded the EPA's guideline of 0.1 micrograms of methylmercury per kilogram of infant body weight per day. Sally Bernard, Lyn Redwood, Albert Enayati and Heidi Roger then went on to create an advocacy group called "Safe Minds," which steadfastly lobbies against mercury-containing vaccines.

Since the distribution and publication of the "mercury/autism paper," thousands of parents have come to believe that their children's regression into autism was caused or augmented by vaccinations containing mercury. For many such parents, this belief was reinforced after chelation related lab tests confirmed high levels of mercury in their child. In 1999 the FDA issued a letter to vaccine manufacturers asking, *but not ordering,* that mercury-containing thimerosal be removed from vaccines. Finally, in 2000, the FDA cited a joint statement by the American Academy of Pediatrics and the U.S. Public Health Service that "called for the removal of thimerosal from vaccines as soon as possible."[22] Even after all that, the nation's physicians and hospitals were allowed until late in 2001 to use up already purchased stockpiles of mercury-containing vaccines, including the Hep B vaccine. In other words, despite the known toxicity of mercury and its organic compounds, more children may have been injured during the two-year period following the FDA's admission that many infant and toddler vaccines contained high levels of ethylmercury.

It is interesting to note that, pursuant to federal drug-safety laws, a coalition of more than 35 law firms in 25 states filed a lawsuit in October 2001 to force drug companies to study how the presence of mercury has affected children.[23] In Texas and Florida other groups of lawyers are suing vaccine and thimerosal manufacturers for damages, medical costs, and nursing care for what they believe to be the thimerosal-caused autism of young children. The threat of lawsuits may have been a factor in finally persuading vaccine makers to remove mercury from most vaccines given to children. However, despite this flurry of litigation, the most important fact is that many autism spectrum children show incredible improvement in response to physician-supervised chelation when combined with gut healing and nutritional support. The lawyers' ads on television asking, "Could your child have autism because of vaccines?" have raised awareness in many parents previously ignorant of the saga surrounding vaccines and autism. This awareness has also increased the need for more doctors who are willing to biomedically evaluate these children—including ordering laboratory tests for heavy metal accumulation. These tests and others will be discussed in Chapter Four and also Chapter Seven.

References

1   Amy Holmes, MD, Jane El-Dahr, MD, Stephanie Cave, MD, Defeat Autism Now! Conference Panel Presentation, San Diego CA, Oct. 2001

2   Greater Boston Physicians for Social Responsibility, May 2000, "In Harm's Way: Adverse Toxic Chemical Influences on Developmental Disabilities," 11 Garden St, Cambridge MA 02138, phone 617-497-7440

3   Edelson, S.B., Cantor, D.S. "Autism: xenobiotic influences." Toxicol Ind Health 1998;14: 553-563

4   Bernard, S., Enayati A., Redwood L., Roger H., Binstock T., "Autism: A Novel Form of Mercury Poisoning , Med Hypotheses 2001 Apr;56(4): 462-71. Original long version, online at http://www.autism.com/ari/mercury.html

[5]   Interview with Dr. Adams, 01-18-2002. Copy of handout about the study is available at http://eas.asu.edu/~autism/

[6]   Ibid

[7]   Greater Boston Physicians for Social Responsibility, May 2000, *In Harm's Way: Toxic Threats to Child Development*, p. 7.

[8]   Hattis D. et al. "Distributions of individual susceptibility among humans for toxic effects. How much protection does the traditional tenfold factor provide for what fraction of which kinds of chemicals and effects?" Ann NY Acad Sci 1999;104:s2: 381-90

[9]   Klassen C.D., editor. Casaret & Doull's Toxicology: the Basic Science of Poisons, 5th ed; McGraw-Hill, 1996

[10] James W. Anderson, MD and Maury M. Breecher, PhD, MPH, Dr. *Anderson's Antioxidant, Antiaging Health Program*, 1996, Carroll & Graf, Inc., NYC, p. 6

[11] Ibid, p. 119

[12] Breecher, M., Linde, S., 1992, *Healthy Homes in a Toxic World*, John Wiley and Sons, Inc.

[13] Ibid

[14] Maury M. Breecher, PhD, MPH and Shirley Linde, PhD, 1992, *Healthy Homes in a Toxic World*, John Wiley and Sons, Inc., p. 141.

[15] Bernard, S. et al., "Autism: a Novel Form of Mercury Poisoning," Med. Hypotheses 2001 Apr;56(4): pp. 462-71. Original long version, Jun 2000, http://www.autism.com/ari/mercury.html

[16] Eggleston, D. et al., "Correlation of dental amalgams with mercury in brain tissue," J. Pros. Dent. 58: 704-7, 1987

[17] Greater Boston Physicians for Social Responsibility, May 2000, *In Harm's Way: Toxic Threats to Child Development*, p. 4.

[18] Kupsinel, Roy MD, "Mercury amalgam toxicity," J. Orthomol. Psychiat, 13(4): pp. 140-57; 1984

[19] Vaccine Fact Sheets, National Vaccine Program Office, Centers for Disease Control website http://www.cdc.gov/od/nvpo/fs_tableVI_doc2.htm (This so-called "fact sheet" also contains the blunt statement that "There is no evidence that children have been harmed by the amount of mercury found in vaccines that contain thimerosal."

[20] Greater Boston Physicians for Social Responsibility, May 2000, *In Harm's Way: Toxic Threats to Child Development*, p. 14.

[21] http://www.909shot.com/hepfrance.htm

[22] Letter from Center for Biologics Evaluation and Research, a department within the U.S. Food and Drug Administration, July 4, 2000.

[23] Bob Wheaton, "Mom Says Mercury in Vaccine Harmed Child." *The Flint (Michigan) Journal*, Oct. 22, 2001.

[24] Westphal GA et al. Homozygous gene deletions of the glutathione S-transferases M1 and T1 are associated with thimerosal sensitization. Int Arch Occup Environ Health. 2000 Aug;73(6):384-8

[25] Cave, Stephanie (with Deborah Mitchell), "What Your Doctor May Not Tell You About Childhood Vaccinatiions," Warner Books Sept 2001

FOUR

CLINICAL AND DIAGNOSTIC EVALUATION

To briefly summarize the first three chapters: I have described how autism spectrum disorder is a complex multi-system medical illness with immunological, gastrointestinal, and neurological issues. The disorder is being increasingly recognized as having a variety of etiologies, and precise mechanisms are still being studied for both the genetic and environmental issues involved. The more scientists learn about autism, the more complex the disorder appears. Many of us have come to accept that a common etiology arises from a genetic susceptibility that gets triggered by one or more environmentally based injuries, pathogenic insults, and/or toxic exposures in the womb or early childhood. Since ASD can involve so many major systems of the body, I believe an affected child should receive an intensive clinical and diagnostic evaluation to identify the affected body systems and underlying pathologies as a basis for subsequent treatment. In this chapter I describe my current evaluation and testing procedures.

Biomedical Evaluation

Parents need to know at the outset that the complexity of ASD means that diagnostics and treatment are neither easy nor quick. A great deal of devotion, time, patience, and hard work is required;

the strains upon economic and emotional resources may be great. Prolonged treatment falls 24/7 on the shoulders of the parents, even when they have been fortunate enough to find a caring and knowledgeable health practitioner to guide their child's treatment.

A further challenge faces parents who are considering embarking upon the journey of biomedical approaches to ASD. That is, almost all but *not all* affected children improve. As of 2007, there is no clear way to determine whether a child will improve in a major way, or just a little, or not at all. However, the improvements that occur for many autistic children diagnosed and treated biomedically are likely *not* to occur if the parents and the child's primary physician fail to explore the possibilities available now.

When looking clinically at hundreds or even dozens of autism spectrum children, much variation is seen from child to child. These variations in medical history, health status, and biomedical profile call for a personalized evaluative approach for each child. The first step in my biomedical evaluation of a new patient consists of preparing a thorough family and child health history in the form of an extensive questionnaire followed by an interview, preferably in person but possibly by phone for those living at a distance. These histories often provide important clues in determining whether the child fits into one of the autism spectrum's biomedical subgroups. Does the family have a history of autoimmunity or allergies? Are there indications of viral presence, heavy metal toxicity, or other special categories? Is anyone else in the child's family affected by an autism-spectrum disorder? Answers to these questions often help us design a treatment likely to be effective.

FAMILY AND MEDICAL HISTORY

Family

An extensive questionnaire should detail family history, especially regarding relatives with autism spectrum disorder (ADD, ADHD, PDD, Asperger's, high-functioning autism), dyslexia, learning disorders, autoimmune disorders, Down Syndrome, Alzheimer's, mental retardation, mental illnesses such as recurrent depression, bi-polar disorders, and schizophrenia. Particular note should be taken of maternal health or toxic exposures, specifically:

Before conception: Mother's health (particularly autoimmune conditions and any indication of immune system impairment[1]), general nutritional status, genetic predispositions on either maternal or paternal sides of the family, maternal vaccinations near time of conception.

During gestation: Toxic exposures (e.g. mother's dental work done with amalgam placement or removal), ingestion of large amounts of mercury-contaminated fish, exposures to pesticides or other heavy metals such as lead, maternal malnutrition, Rh factors, viral or other maternal illnesses, pregnancy complications, medications.

During birthing and early infancy: Infant pre- or post-maturity, difficult labor, breast-feeding difficulty, milk or soy allergy in non-breast fed infants, feeding and digestive problems, vaccinations particularly with thimerosal, infections, antibiotic treatments.

Child

Delivery issues, labor and delivery problems, condition at birth, weight, APGAR score, and mother's age at delivery. Medical: breast-feeding experience, digestive problems, vaccination history with any noted reactions, infections, antibiotic use, seizures, other medications, allergies, surgeries, dental work. Further details are often extremely helpful. Specifically:

- **Development:** General: Eating patterns, toileting patterns, sleeping patterns. Size in relation to same age peers. Age walking began, speech began, speech delay, any regressions noted in language, peculiarities in speech, eye contact history.

- **Detailed vaccination history:** Dates given, number of shots given at one time, health status if known at time of vaccination, unusual reactions (excessive crying, fevers) noted. Many parents have documented the timings and amounts of ethyl-mercury injected during vaccinations, as well as incidents of multiple vaccinations per visit to their doctor.

- **Detailed dietary and stool history:** How long breast-fed, when milk/soy products introduced. Food likes and dislikes, allergies, need for and reaction to special diets. What kind of diet the rest of the family eats generally. History of diarrhea or constipation, reflux, presence of yeast infections, including treatments and results.

- **Personality:** Alertness, fears, phobias, repetitious activities, mood swings, hyper or hypoactive, temper tantrums, inconsolable crying spells. Attachment and relating issues: Closest bond, making and keeping friends, affection, reactions to other children, pets, baby-sitters, daycare, teacher reactions. Imagination pattern, motor development, handedness, eye contact, reaction to change, sense of humor, self-sufficiency. Need for special schooling, nature of any learning disabilities.

PRETESTING CONSIDERATIONS

Many parents usually go to a specialist in autism for a biomedical evaluation and treatment if they can find one. For these families, the primary pediatrician remains the person the child sees for general check-ups, routine vaccinations, and for treatment of infections, injuries, or chronic medical conditions. Many ASD children have already been tested to rule out the well-known genetic abnormalities before seeking help from an autism specialist.

For the autism biomedical consultation, it can be helpful for the specialist to see the child with his/her family, noting the relationships of the child with siblings and parents. General observation of health, skin color, general tone, motor development, alertness, eye contact, fearfulness, speech patterns, handedness, and attachment and relating behavior helps the physician have a base line for comparison with later stages in the child's treatment and development. Watching the child play with toys is instructive; asking the child to write or draw gives a lot of information about language receptiveness as well as fine motor development and level of conceptualizing. Extent and quality of verbalization should be noted for comparison as treatment progresses.

In cases where the pre-testing evaluation (and perhaps follow-up treatment as well) is done at a distance, serial candid photographs of the child and monthly status report forms filled out by the parents are very helpful in documenting progress. For me, e-mailing has often been convenient, saves time trying to return phone calls, and leaves a dated record for the patient's chart for both me and the parents. E-mail has become one of my favorite ways to get progress reports from the parents and give them feedback on testing results and further treatment considerations. Besides the telephone being more disruptive and intrusive and less efficient than e-mail (if there is anyone busier than a doctor it is the mother of a special needs child!), this method of communication helps to avoid misinterpretation of my treatment intentions and instructions by having them all down on paper and dated.

New Diagnostics in ASD Based on Screening

The medical history and interview are followed by diagnostic lab tests to determine what biomedical issues need to be addressed. The new diagnostics in autism are based upon *screening*. Many biomedical irregularities in an autistic child are subtle. The lab tests are not intended to confirm an obvious illness, but to reveal underlying pathologies. The use of lab-based screening provides data that often reveals an imbalanced or even etiologically significant pathology that provides the basis for subsequent treatments.

For example, heavy metal screening is particularly important for children who received the Hepatitis B vaccination as neonates or young infants, between the years 1991 (the year it was mandated), and late 2001, (the year the CDC finally ordered thimerosal removed from the newborn Hepatitis B vaccine). Heavy metal screening is also recommended for autism-spectrum children whose mothers received RhoGam treatment during pregnancy or had amalgam removal or placement during pregnancy. Children in these categories have a higher risk of overexposure to the neurotoxic effects of mercury. Proper diagnostic testing for heavy metals is essential for determining appropriate and effective chelation treatments (see Chapter Seven).

Data from thousands of autistic children reveal the existence of "subgroups" of similar biomedical profiles. Which subgroup best describes a child is virtually impossible to know without a thorough evaluation. It takes medical histories, responses to several simple treatments, and lab-test data combined to provide a portrait of a child's biomedical characteristics. Despite the existence of subgroups of ASD children, each one has a unique profile.

Initial Strategies in Test Evaluation

As I have emphasized already, many autism spectrum children have intestinal problems, and in my experience most of those children respond favorably to a gluten-free/casein-free/soy-free diet. This is one of my first recommendations to most parents. Food hypersensitivity can occur even in the absence of obvious intestinal symptoms that are not usually the immediate allergic reactions tested by mainstream doctors. Also, a child may be sensitive to foods other than wheat and milk products. A food hypersensitivity test should occur early in the diagnostic sequence. Because many ASD children have food hypersensitivity or an intestinal pathology, many of them show improvements when prescribed various nutritional supplements.

After several months of a gluten-free and casein-free diet reinforced with nutritional supplements, another test may be warranted to assess if hypersensitivities have changed. Many children I see are already on the GF/CF/SF diet when they come for their evaluation; a lot of time is saved when this is the case.

At the time of the child's first visit, I order a complete blood count and a metabolic panel so as to obtain a base-line for future reference. Because so many of these children have been found to have intestinal colonizations by pathogenic bacteria, fungi, or parasites, a urine test to check for fungal and bacterial metabolites and sometimes a fecal-culture evaluation is often ordered right away as well (see below).

MORE TESTS, A NEW PHILOSOPHY

Except for the basic routine screening tests that almost any local lab can do (CBC, Chemistry Panel, and Thyroid Panel), most insurance plans do not pay for all (or sometimes any, depending on the insurance plan) of the specialty tests needed for ASD children. A fairly complete lab-test panel can range in cost from $1,200 to $3,000 (depending upon which tests are ordered). It is important for parents to understand that even with all this medically useful data there is no absolute guarantee that it will always lead to a clear diagnosis and to treatments that invariably work.

In the long run, a certain percentage of children evaluated and treated biomedically make wonderful progress, and some have even lost their diagnosis as autistic. A larger percentage make major progress toward improvement but, to various degrees, remain somewhere "on the spectrum"; unfortunately another small group makes little or no progress. At this time, the only way by which parents can learn whether or not the biomedical approach "works" and was worth the investment is to have tried it.

After the medical histories are obtained, the GF/CF/SF diet started, and some basic nutritional supplementation initiated, many options arise. A fairly complete battery of tests can be ordered if the parents are willing, or further lab-tests can be done sequentially, a few at a time. This depends on the parents' medical philosophy, awareness and knowledge about the biomedical approach, as well as their health insurance coverage and economic situation.

In making this decision, parents should know that when data are obtained all at one time, their interrelationships are often easier to recognize. The interrelationships among all major systems are so complex that comprehensive information is useful, if only to rule out certain conditions. When lab-tests are too scattered across time, they are less helpful in obtaining a good portrait of current condition. Therefore, the ideal situation is to have a child receive all the major testing at the time of the evaluation, although I understand this is not always possible or affordable. Sometimes a child will have had some tests done fairly recently by another doctor and understandably parents will not want to repeat those. Historical perspective is helpful, but current testing is usually essential to guide optimal treatment.

PARENTS, DOCTORS AND TESTING PHILOSOPHY

Often, biological pathologies are subtle and the child's underlying disease processes are not obvious. For instance, children with inflamed gastrointestinal tracts can amazingly have few or no symptoms of this problem, and it will not be learned until testing that they have pathogen overgrowth often accompanied by markedly imbalanced amino acid patterns or vitamin, mineral, and fatty acid deficiencies.

Parents differ in regard to testing their affected child. Some parents are very desirous of having many tests done to get as much diagnostic information as possible. Others so dislike the idea of the child having a venipuncture ("needle stick") that they will actually delay seeking a biomedical evaluation for this reason. Insurance company variabilities complicate matters further. For many of these children, "autism" or ASD may not be the diagnosis appropriate for their insurance applications. There often are underlying disease processes that are etiologically significant and that can be identified, treated, and coded, such as immune deficiency, gastroenteritis, heavy metal poisoning, viral infections, etc.

Doctors too vary in regard to testing. Some still think in accord with the "must be genetic" model and believe that biomedical testing is frivolous and unnecessary. Obviously, I disagree. In contrast, the growing number of physicians who are moving towards biomedical models for ASD are allowing those models to modify their clinical approaches. Let us consider several general approaches a physician might take.

Some physicians feel that they do not need to test the child very much and suggest treatments according to an intuitive assessment of the child's past history and current problems. Other physicians, particularly if pressed for time, may diagnose and treat in accord with an established protocol that may not reflect the unique biomedical nature of a particular child. In contrast, some physicians order a thorough set of lab tests early in the diagnostic process as a general principle. The latter approach can be very useful when the physician is experienced in the biomedical aspects of ASD and is capable of interpreting a set of complex data. Sometimes physicians will cooperate with anxious parents who want extensive testing even if they don't feel it may be necessary.

I have noticed a trend that provides a practical perspective on testing. The longer a practitioner works with these children, the more "streamlined" his or her assessment becomes, and less testing is necessary—at least in early phases of the treatment regimen. Later, if the child develops further problems or is not making progress, then more extensive tests (along with more advanced treatment protocols) can and should be considered. Since each child is unique biomedically, parents should not be surprised if, for an exceptionally challenging situation, a consultation with a neurological, immunological, endocrine or gastrointestinal specialist is recommended. Examples of such complicated cases are the severe seizure disorders or highly allergic children who might have a negative reaction to certain treatment regimes. Often these specialists do not know much about autism in general (as yet!), but know a lot about a particular child's medical problems related to their specialty.

My philosophy as a clinician is to order those tests which will give me information useful in selecting and guiding treatment. However, since lab tests are expensive and not always reimbursed, a frank discussion with the child's parents is important. I try to find out their philosophy and economic situation as regards their child's medical care. I feel that timing is often quite important and some tests have higher priority than others. Furthermore, the physical act of holding an uncomprehending child down to obtain a blood test is traumatic to both the child and the parents. Thus, I sometimes order non-invasive (urine, hair, and stool) tests in the beginning and try to have most of the initial evaluation work requiring blood tests organized so that only one blood draw (with a "butterfly" needle so that all tubes can be obtained with one venipuncture) is necessary for the initial evaluation. A prescription for an anesthetic (lidocaine 2.5% and prilocaine 2.5%) cream to numb the venipuncture site helps some children. They still don't like to be held down but at least they learn that the "stick" doesn't hurt.

If the initial screening tests indicate the likelihood of heavy metal toxicity, assessment of the child's readiness for oral chelation treatment is very important. We have learned that gastrointestinal health and nutritional status must be maximized before starting chelation for optimal outcome. I want to stress that chelation therapy in my opinion should not be done without active participation of a physician. Several types of lab tests are virtually mandatory. One type monitors metals presence and metals outflow. Another type of lab test will monitor the child's health during chelation. The medications used during the oral chelation detoxification process can be stressful to the liver. Some children need to have chelation halted temporarily if the child's lab tests so indicate liver stress or excessive pathogen overgrowth. That is why this treatment should be done under the supervision of a knowledgeable health practitioner who knows how to monitor the progress of these children through the most up-to-date tests available. Medically developed chelation protocols are available from the Autism Research Institute website online and are described in Chapter Seven.

Descriptions of Specific Laboratory Tests

NECESSARY PRELIMINARY SCREENING TESTS

- **CBC (Complete Blood Count)with Differential and Platelets**
- **Comprehensive Metabolic Panel**
- **Thyroid panel (T3, T4, TSH)**

These tests can all be obtained with one draw at any local laboratory in your vicinity and are often covered by insurance. These tests help us to check the child's general health for such conditions as anemia, liver or kidney impairment, or thyroid imbalance, all of which are not uncommon in ASD children.

- **Urinalysis**

Small children may need to have a urine sample brought from home in a clean glass jar; very young children can be fitted with a plastic urine collector to get a specimen. A urinalysis will check for bleeding, bladder infections, or evidence of kidney disease by the presence or absence of bilirubin, protein, or casts from the kidneys.

- **Hair analysis**

By now, many parents have heard about the heavy metal toxicity problem, and are willing to do a hair analysis. In my opinion, this is an informative non-invasive and inexpensive screening test. I highly recommend Doctor's Data Laboratory for this test. This laboratory has probably the world's largest database regarding hair analysis. Hair is an excretory tissue rather than a functional tissue. Hair element analysis provides important information which, in conjunction with symptoms and other laboratory data, can assist the physician with a diagnosis of physiological disorders associated with abnormalities in essential and toxic element metabolism. Toxic elements may be up to several hundred times more highly concentrated in hair than in blood or urine. Therefore, hair is the tissue of choice for detection of cumulative body burden and recent exposure to elements such as arsenic, aluminum, cadmium, lead, and mercury. With experience reading these tests, hair analysis results can often ascertain mercury poisoning. For example, in many cases the test can determine the presence of mercury poisoning, even though (except for recent large exposure) it will seldom show up directly as a high level of mercury on the test. The special discernment here is knowing what mercury does to the essential minerals in the body. Dr. Andrew Cutler,[2] a chemist who suffered for many years and was finally treated for mercury poisoning from amalgams, has been very helpful to the chelating community in teaching us his system of "counting rules" on the hair analyses to help determine mercury toxicity.

Hair analysis is basically a preliminary screen, however, and often needs to be followed by more specific blood and urine testing to validate those results. Recent as yet unpublished studies indicate that hair in autistic children often displays lower levels of toxic metals than their siblings and parents. This may actually turn out to be further evidence of impaired detoxification in our ASD children.

Blood tests must be viewed carefully as well. Physicians who are not familiar with heavy metal poisoning will often order a blood test for mercury, and when it returns with negative results, assure the parents that their child does not have mercury poisoning and does not need chelation. Blood tests only reveal recent large exposures, and will show nothing of the mercury in the brain that is behind the blood-brain-barrier and no longer available for assessment in peripheral blood studies. I have had some disappointing experiences with colleagues who refused to participate in the investigation after ordering and receiving a negative blood test; parents need to know that the doctor who does this is not aware of the new biomedicine of mercury poisoning in ASD children.

Hair testing must be ordered by a health care professional. Doctor's Data Lab charges about $50 if you send in payment with the hair specimen. Since insurance will rarely if ever pay for this test, I advise parents to send their payment along with the hair, because if laboratories have to bill insurance and wait to get money they may never receive, they end up billing the patient for all the extra paperwork and phone costs. Explicitly, if the hair analysis is billed to insurance without advance payment, the lab charges a higher fee, which is billed to the client when insurance denies the claim. If insurance does pay, the patient is reimbursed. This is true for much of the testing and patients can often save a lot of money in lab testing by paying at the time they send in the samples. Though patients complain about this, it is understandable that the extra personnel and phone costs in handling insurance claims needs to be re-imbursed and creates a need for the lab to have differential charge policies. I personally feel parents should focus their efforts on insurance reform rather than anger at lab billing policies. (I do not receive anything from the labs I use, not even a discount for myself!)

Specialized Laboratory Tests as Individually Indicated

I recommend a basic blood count, metabolic chemistry, and thyroid panel be obtained as a base-line for all children. Special tests are ordered according to the symptoms and history of the child and often include immune system tests, tests for the presence and levels of viruses and fungi, and food hypersensitivity testing for wheat and milk tolerance. I do the peptide test now only for parents who are very resistant to going onto a gluten and milk-free diet, and want laboratory proof that their children are indeed intolerant of these large peptides. Extensive food tolerance and plasma amino acid panels are helpful to direct proper nutrition and nutrient protocols. These preliminary tests often indicate the need for treating Candida yeast or other pathogenic overgrowths in the gut and elimination of foods containing wheat, milk and often soy as well as one of the first steps. Treatments for these conditions are explained in Chapter Five. Blood, stool and urine studies can identify pathogens or pathogen metabolites and provide the basis for proper supportive and anti-pathogen treatments. Blood tests help target areas where the biochemistry can be improved by proper supplementation. Hair, urine and blood testing together can help determine whether heavy metal toxicity is present and then direct the removal and necessary mineral and nutrient support for chelation. Proper monitoring throughout the treatment process helps us fine-tune dosages of medications and nutrients and maintain optimal health of the children undergoing treatment.

There are multiple more refined tests for special cases as indicated by the clinical progress, but these listed below are the ones I most commonly find helpful in my practice during the initial evaluative phase. Some children who have a seizure issue may need to be referred to a pediatric neurologist to obtain 24-hour EEG studies if they have not already done so. Intractable infectious cases with major immunological derangement may need work with an immunologist or an infectious disease specialist. Some digestive problems are so severe that the child may need to be sent to a gastroenterologist for endoscopic studies. Rarely, a child may need to be referred to an endocrinologist for management of brittle diabetes or severe thyroid problems, or to an allergist for severe asthma treatment. Occasionally, such specialists may have been consulted even before the child is brought in for an autism-related biomedical evaluation. It is important for all the child's doctors to work as a team so that the treatments do not conflict, even though many mainstream doctors as yet know little about the biomedical approach to autism. Parents need to be prepared for some physicians to become threatened with information and treatments they do not as yet understand and so disparage the use of diet and nutrients in the treatment of their children.

URINARY PEPTIDE TESTS FOR CASEIN AND GLUTEN

This is a chromatographic test for the exorphin peptides, including the large peptides produced by wheat (gluten) and milk (casein). *Quantitatively accurate measurement of these peptides is still not yet in the realm of routine clinical testing, and results in terms of clinical application have been very confusing over the years.* Children with high values may show no gut symptoms or any benefit by removal of casein and gluten from their diets; many children with normal values may respond amazingly well to a GF/CF diet. I no longer routinely order this test for my clients unless the parents are extremely desirous of it, hoping it may free them from having to use the GF/CF diet. Still, no matter what the test shows, particularly if the child has a restricted diet and any bowel problems, I suggest that all of them undergo a trial of the diet if they are not already on it, since the great majority of children with autism benefit.

Parents are often surprised and pleased to see definite clinical improvements in most cases even before starting chelation. I have also found that the parents' willingness to adhere to the challenging task of keeping their children on this diet often indicates their willingness to go through the prolonged and grueling process entailed in healing their children. This includes getting their children to take multiple nutrients, observing strict chelation medication schedules, and procuring testing necessary to guide treatment.

ORGANIC ACID TEST (OAT-URINE)

The Organic Acid Test is one of the routine tests I order because of the ubiquitousness of the yeast problem and metabolic imbalances. The OAT test measures key components in the child's biochemical factory. Metabolic function testing by organic acid analysis provides indicators of how efficiently metabolism is functioning, how well it is converting food into usable products for health, and where problems may be occurring. It is especially important for revealing those microbial imbalances that cause the buildup of metabolic toxins that can be identified in overnight urine. As mentioned earlier, most cases of yeast infection result in symptoms of chronic diarrhea, constipation or an alternation of the two, as well as gas, bloating, abdominal discomfort, and foul-smelling stools. However, I have occasionally encountered children with yeast overgrowth as shown by lab tests who do not have any obvious bowel symptoms. Clinically, if children remain very picky about food, I suspect a chronic gut inflammation and pathogen colonization in spite of the lack of symptoms.

90-FOOD IgG ANTIBODIES TEST (SERUM)

Delayed or hidden food sensitivities are typically not noticeable for several hours or days after ingestion of a particular food.

Frequently, these reactions reflect chronic exposures to the commonly eaten derivatives of corn, wheat, milk and egg. This comprehensive panel is a valuable tool in the clinical management of food allergic patients. For those children who are not benefiting from the GF/CF diet or who benefited at first but then regress, I order this test to make sure some of the common foods they eat are not affecting them. IgG indicates delayed sensitivity (not the IgE, or immediate allergic reaction that most allergists obtain), which afflicts the children with autism more frequently. In that sense, it is more a food sensitivity test than a true allergy test, indicating that even without an obvious allergic reaction, these foods are stressing the gut and contributing to its continued inflamed state. When these offending foods are removed children often make another leap in their healing process.

AMINO ACIDS, (PLASMA)

Amino acids are the building blocks of protein and are essential for many bodily processes. The digestive tract breaks down protein from food into individual amino acids, which are then absorbed into the blood stream. These amino acids:

- Build the structural proteins of muscle and connective tissue
- Make enzymes which control every chemical reaction in the body
- Make a variety of brain neurotransmitters and hormones
- Generate energy
- Stabilize blood sugar
- Aid in detoxification and anti-oxidant protection.

Because of poor dietary habits or inadequate digestion and absorption of proteins, most ASD children have amino acid imbalances. The vast majority of these imbalances seem to be related to maldigestion or disorders in the metabolism of methionine and cysteine, and often will indicate an insufficiency of taurine. Low taurine can affect both detoxication and uptake of essential lipids from the diet and can cause a deficiency of vitamins A, E, D, and essential fatty acids. To get a baseline test, the first amino acid analysis should be done with the child eating his/her usual diet but without taking nutritional supplements for 3 days prior to the test. Later testing can be done with the child using their usual food and supplements for fine-tuning their regimen. More information can be provided with a 24-hour urine amino acid study, but the specter of trying to collect 24 hours of urine from most of these ASD children is daunting and I and others usually use the the fasting plasma analysis.

COMPREHENSIVE MICROBIAL/DIGESTIVE STOOL ANALYSIS

For children who continue to have bowel problems even though they are on the diet and use probiotics, this is a valuable test of the nature of the digestive tract to guide further treatment strategies. This analysis evaluates digestion, absorption, gut flora, immune status, and the colonic environment, and can evaluate for parasites using microscopic examination. A sensitivity panel for treating pathogenic flora is provided by some labs but must be specifically requested and costs extra, of course. However, the panel is invaluable in treating repeated bouts of pathogen infestation to make sure the proper anti-fungal or anti-biotic agent is being used.

FATTY ACID ANALYSIS (PLASMA)

ASD children typically have very poor diets and particularly diets that contain "good fats" found in vegetables, nuts, whole grains, and fish (which I now suggest not be eaten by the children in treatment with me because of mercury levels in most of the fish available.) The hydrogenation process used in modern food processing destroys important fatty acids and creates structurally altered fatty acids called trans fatty acids that may be harmful to the body. Please see more about fatty acids in Chapter Six on nutrients.

The plasma fatty acid test can measure over 30 different fatty acids in body stores——essentials and their derivatives, saturated, and trans fatty acids. This test is usually further along in my testing sequence unless malnutrition seems apparent at the outset of the evaluation; I always order it for ADD-ADHD or bi-polar children, as many studies are coming out showing the efficacy of treatment of these children (and adults) with fatty acids. This test helps me guide dietary modifications and supplements that can move the child toward a healthy balance of their fatty acid levels.

TESTS FOR METALLOTHIONEIN DYSFUNCTION

Dr. William Walsh at the Pfeiffer Treatment Center located in Naperville, IL believes that metallothionein (MT) dysfunction is one of the primary bases for ASD. 85% of children he studies exhibit elevated copper/zinc ratios in blood compared to healthy controls. He tests for plasma zinc, serum copper, plasma ammonia, urinary pyrrole, and ceruloplasmin to help him balance the body chemistry of his patients with minerals, especially zinc, and other nutrients.

MT protects cells from the harmful effects of oxidative stress, DNA damage, and toxicity of excess heavy metals. As it is an intracellular protein, only the cellular activity is important for the assessment of metal-induced toxicity; plasma analyses of MT levels are not relevant. I use the functional MT assay which analyzes the cellular level of MT expression before and after stimulation with metals as performed by Immunosciences Lab in Beverly Hills, CA to assess effectiveness of MT protection. This test along with hair analyses and RBC minerals guides me in determining the need for chelation work for my patients.

Like all of us working with ASD children, Dr. Walsh has found the greatest treatment challenge is the high incidence of severe gut problems. He reported ASD outcomes in his chemical rebalancing nutrient therapy protocols dramatically improved with regular use of special diets, digestive aids, probiotics, and sugar elimination.[3]

Laboratory Testing in Chelation Therapy

The primary tests to prepare for chelation therapy (see Chapter Seven for a discussion of the chelation protocol) are:

- Standard preliminary tests as outlined above to check general health

- Urine and/or stool tests to make sure gut is healthy, e.g. OAT and CDSA.

- Hair analysis (see above)

- Porphyrin test, urine (read details in Chapter 7)

- Red Blood Cell mineral analysis to help in mineral/ nutrient plan

- Pre and post-challenge urine test for toxic elements

The challenge tests are often unnecessary and are ordered when desired by parents or the referring doctor who may not be convinced that the child would benefit from chelation therapy. A regular morning urine sample is taken (pre-challenge), and then one or two doses of the chelating agent are given, usually DMSA (Chemet, or 2,3-dimercaptosuccinic acid), as calculated per weight of the child and administered the night before and the next morning or if once just before the urine collection starts. The post-challenge is obtained by catching a urine sample usually for six hours or 1st morning urine after the morning dose. The chelating agent binds to the metals that are in the urine and the pre and post-challenge tests are compared to help see what the response to chelation may be. Further details of this test are given in Chapter Seven.

Immunology Testing

Because of its highly technical nature, the discussion of immunology testing is included in Chapter Eight where the immune system is discussed in greater detail.

Which Laboratories to Use

The question of which laboratory to use is an important one. The preliminary tests are pretty standardized and can be done anywhere. If the practitioner has his or her own venipuncturist in the office that is ideal. If not, it is important to help the patient locate a lab nearby that is willing to draw blood for specialty labs and work with special needs children. These laboratories often specialize in autism, and perform tests not usually available locally. In this case, kits are either given to the patient by the practitioner or sent to them upon the doctor's request by the lab. The primary laboratories I personally use for specialty work are:

GEORGIA
Meta-Metrix Lab (MML)   **800-221-4640**

ILLINOIS
Doctors' Data Lab (DDL)   **800-323-2784**

OTHERS
WISCONSIN
Neuroscience/Immunology Lab   **888-342-7272**

KANSAS
Great Plains Lab (GPL)   **888-347-2781**

NORTH CAROLINA
Genova Diagnostics (GSL)   **800-522-4762**

All of these labs are willing to send kits to the clients upon the doctor's request. Most send duplicates of results to the ordering practitioner so the patient can have one for their files.

I'm sure there are other good laboratories out there; each practitioner has to experiment and find the ones with which they like to work. Using the same lab for a certain test with all my patients helps me relate test results to the symptoms I'm seeing clinically. This approach also helps me become familiar with the lab personnel so I can get my questions answered. Ease of reading the reports, timeliness of getting results back, and the accessibility of the lab directors to talk to me about results are often important to me in choosing between equally good labs.

References

[1] Comi A.M. et al. "Familial clustering of autoimmune edisorders and evaluation of medical risk factors in autism," J. Child. Neurol. 1999 Jun;14(6): 388-94, Johns Hopkins Hospital Div of Ped Neurology, Baltimore MD

[2] Cutler, Andrew "Amalgam Illness Diagnosis and Treatment," Minerva Labs, Jun 1999

[3] Walsh, William J. et al., Booklet "Metallothionein and Autism." Oct 2001, Pfeiffer Trtment Cntr, Naperville, IL

FIVE

GASTROINTESTINAL HEALING

Gastrointestinal Health is a Key Issue

The "take home" message of this chapter is that the majority of autistic children suffer from impaired gastrointestinal health. Many of our children are unable to verbally express the pain or discomfort they may feel, yet intestinal problems may be obvious from patterns of persistent diarrhea, constipation, abdominal pain with bloating or abnormally appearing stools. In some children, intestinal pathology may be less obvious and detectable only via appropriate lab-tests, (e.g. mild inflammation due to undiagnosed food hypersensitivity). Parents and physicians often focus on the more obvious cognitive impairments and may not realize that correcting their child's underlying intestinal imbalances can lead to significant overall improvement.

Among autism-spectrum children, self-restriction of their diet to a few usually non-nourishing foods is common. Yet even the rare child who is willing to eat vegetables and other nutritious foods may not be able to get these nutrients to benefit his/her brain adequately because of the inability to properly digest, absorb, and/or utilize the nutrients taken in. In some cases, nutrients may be prevented from nourishing the brain cells because of viral infestations or other toxins in the brain. PCR (polymerase chain reaction)-based studies have shown that certain viruses can migrate into small areas of the brain, remain dormant for long periods of time, and do so without generating an obvious encephalitis. Prolonged diarrhea could enable viruses to enter tissues of the gut in some children, from where they would be capable of migrating into the central nervous system.[1]

The impressive shift in cognition in many children during heavy metal chelation treatment definitely implicates toxic metals as interfering with the brain's ability to take in adequate nutrients for proper function. In nutritionally preparing children for chelation when laboratory tests indicate mercury poisoning, there is very often an obvious improvement in cognition and language with the nutrient program alone. A state of impaired nutrient status in blood, intestines, liver, and kidneys could allow for metals accumulation injurious to those tissues and, if the metals level is sufficient, then some metal may enter the central nervous system and disrupt neuronal function.

To repeat, unavailability of breast feeding, persistent colic in infancy, frequent use of antibiotics, certain immunizations, and inability to detoxify heavy metal or other environmental toxins are all known to contribute to impaired gut function. Food allergies, intolerance to wheat and milk products, evidence of immune impairment such as frequent ear infections in infancy, and chronic yeast or viral infections all point to a need to have the gastrointestinal system evaluated in our ASD children. Family history may implicate genetic or environmentally shared factors, since digestive disturbances are common in the parents and siblings of children with autism. Dysfunctions such as "leaky gut" syndrome (excessive permeability), fungal, bacterial and parasite overgrowth, malabsorption (incomplete uptake of nutrients), maldigestion, inflammation (enterocolitis), and liver detoxification impairment are frequently noted by the clinicians working with these children. Histological studies done on a study of 36 children with autism showed evidence of reflux esophagitis in 69.4%, chronic gastritis in 41.7%, chronic duodenitis in 66.7%, and low intestinal carbohydrate digestive enzyme activity in 58.3%.[2]

Some parents have related to me that when they asked their pediatrician for remedies for their child's bowel problems, they were told that "it is normal; it is a stage that will pass." Untreated, some of these children may gradually get better, but many of them continue severe bowel dysfunction into adulthood. On the other hand, when their GI ailments are treated successfully, most autistic/ASD children respond favorably, not only with improved digestive health and function, but also by exhibiting improved behavioral and developmental responses. Chronic diarrhea, constipation, gaseousness, and abdominal discomfort are obvious to the caretakers of these children. However, we are finding that many children even in the absence of these overt intestinal symptoms have significant gut problems that often must be addressed as the first step in their healing journey. Part of the challenge in dealing with the gut disorder is the inability of many children to tell us how they are feeling along with their commonly observed high pain threshold.

Research has shown that 60-70% of the immune system in humans is located within the intestinal tract and its digestive organs, easily making the gut the largest immune system organ in the body. Because the immune system is so involved with the gastrointestinal tract, intestinal pathology can contribute to immune dysregulation, and vice versa. Regardless of whether the immune impairment is acquired or genetic, many of these children are susceptible to multiple infections, especially ear infections, and are often repeatedly treated with antibiotics—without considering the possibility of viral otitis, for which antibiotics are ineffective. Antibiotics not only irritate the intestinal wall and cause gut inflammation, but also destroy the beneficial bacteria, creating an opportunity for Candida, (a yeast), Clostridia (an anaerobic bacteria) and other pathogens normally kept in balance by the "good bugs" to overgrow and cause further damage. Pioneering researchers including Dr. William Shaw have shown that many autistic patients tend to have elevated yeast levels in their intestines.[3]

As we have mentioned in earlier chapters, yeast overgrowth interferes with the absorption of nutrients (the yeasts take them for their own growth and multiplication, particularly the sugars); this is often the cause of the diarrhea and/or constipation. Yeast species can excrete chemical byproducts that are absorbed through the intestinal wall and enter the blood stream to circulate throughout the body. Furthermore, yeast cells can convert to an invasive colony form, imbedding themselves into the lining of the intestinal tract and, via secreted enzymes, destroy intestinal tissue. This type of injury creates "holes" in the intestine through which undigested food molecules can pass. This hyperpermeable state is called "leaky gut syndrome." In many children with leaky gut, the undigested food is apparently detected by the immune system, causing antibodies of both IgE (immediate reaction) and IgG (delayed reaction) to be produced. This process leads to greater allergic susceptibilities. Effective treatment of yeast or bacterial overgrowth often decreases or eliminates these allergic reactions.

Treatments That Can Be Implemented by Parents

THE GF/CF/SF (GLUTEN, CASEIN, SOY FREE) DIET

As we indicated in Chapter Two, well-respected researchers have shown in their studies that casein, which is found in milk, breaks down in the stomach to produce a peptide known as casomorphine. Morphine is a powerful painkilling drug. The peptide casomorphine has "morphine"-like or opioid properties. Similar opioids called gluteomorphins are formed in the stomach when these children try to digest gluten from wheat and other grains like rye and oats. Though other researchers have not found the same results with their studies, and therefore dispute the "opioid theory" there is no doubt that parents often say of their children with autism that they appear "spacey" and that they don't seem to feel pain in ways similar to someone under the influence of opioids.

Scientific studies are pointing to inflammation in the gut being caused by gluten, casein, soy and other foods. This is not an "allergy" from the perspective of a traditional allergist, but what is called T-cell inflammatory response to these foods. In a study conducted by Dr. H. Jyonouchi from the University of Minnesota, it was shown that 75% of the children with autism spectrum disorder have T-cell reactivity to foods.[4]

Regardless of the theories, clinical experience of many DAN! physicians has identified the GF/CF/SF diet as the single most effective action you can take on your own to begin to help your child. In my practice, I have found that almost every child with autism placed on this diet benefits from it. Many parents of my young patients have reported that their children's chronic diarrhea stopped and the appearance of formed stools began after successful implementation of the GF/CF diet, particularly when any current yeast infection was treated at the same time. Many other parents report that potty training was finally achieved within a few weeks after the child began a GF/CF/SF diet.

Many parents also report that their children are better able to mentally focus and show improvement in their capacity to learn as a result of the diet. For instance, Janie, the mother of an autistic child named Kelly, told me, "We are having great results on this diet. Kelly is much more aware, alert, and curious about her environment. She also has better eye contact and is more affectionate since starting it." Improvements such as these may be due to the fact that intestinal pathology has an effect on brain function; gut-brain interactions have been well described by numerous researchers.[5]

When I first recommend the GF/CF (and recently, SF or soy-free) diet to parents, most mothers (and some fathers) protest, "My child will starve, he (or she) won't eat anything else." The majority of ASD children have very limited diets. They refuse most foods and fixate on only a few favorites, generally foods such as pizza, chicken nuggets, cakes, cookies, and ice cream, foods rich in gluten or casein. They seem to be addicted to exactly the foods they need to stay away from. I understand that it seems like an almost impossible task to change your child's entire diet, and I cannot deny it affects the whole family. However, many families find that the child is not the only person with hypersensitivity to gluten, casein or soy. Some families have ultimately found that they all feel better after eliminating wheat, milk and soy products from their diet. This is not easy especially when there are older siblings who have established eating habits and resist changes. It took me nine months to finally convince myself and my daughter Elizabeth, Chelsey's mother, to initiate the GF/CF diet in 1998. However, she now swears by it. I encourage parents by assuring them that the benefits to the child will outweigh the difficulties, and hopefully as the children heal, they will be able to tolerate some gluten and casein. To repeat, the majority of the parents of my young patients report significant improvements in sleep patterns, behavior, language, eye contact, attention span and ability to focus and a decrease in "stimming" in their children after starting this regimen.

Many parents report seeing physical, emotional, or even cognitive improvements a few days after dairy is removed from their child's diet. Some parents make the same point about gluten. However, gluten takes longer to disappear from the digestive tract than casein. Urine tests reveal that casein can disappear from the body within three days, whereas it can take months before the gluten leaves. In fact, urine tests have revealed gluten in the urine of some children for as long as eight months after it was removed from the diet. However, if it shows up in the urine after that time, it may be that not all hidden sources have been identified. Some parents find their child didn't improve until hidden sources of gluten (or casein) were discovered and removed. When I used to ask parents to eliminate just casein and gluten, many children improved to a certain point and then plateaued. When a subsequent IgG food test showed other hypersensitivities, the removal of these substances would lead to a further spurt in progress. As more and more of the hypersensitivity food tests showed that soy was a frequent allergen, I suggest at the outset of the diet that soy also be eliminated, which has led to even better results.

A word of warning: Illogically, the U.S. Food and Drug Administration maintains that casein is not a dairy product. Therefore, many foods marked as "non-dairy" contain casein. It may be listed on food labels as sodium caseinate. Any food with that ingredient should be eliminated from your child's diet. Adhere to the diet strictly for at least six months. Almost all of the parents of my patients have reported improvement from the diet. As I have said, I have come to the realization that for most autism-spectrum children, until the inflamed gut is healed, pathogen overgrowth corrected, and nutritional status improved, other treatments will be far less effective.

How to Start the Diet

I recommend that parents start the process of a casein/gluten free diet slowly. Sometimes taking away the offending foods one meal at a time while gradually introducing new ones works the best for some families. Often, parents find that removing milk products is easier than the removal of wheat. Take straight milk away first, then over the course of several weeks, remove other milk and dairy products. Use substitutes such as rice, potato, almond, or coconut milks if food sensitivity testing has shown that your child is not allergic to any of these substances. Then start removing the wheat-based products. Have the rice or potato bread substitutes handy, and slowly let the children acquire a taste for them during the period of casein removal. Many mothers (and a few dads too!) learn to make breads from non-offending flours. I have recently begun recommending that parents avoid soy-based products completely unless a food sensitivity test demonstrates that the child is not allergic to soy. It used to be one of my standby substitutes until I learned from experience (lack of success on the diet with using soy as the main milk substitute) that soy comes high on the list of foods likely to cause adverse reactions, right after wheat and milk.

Be strict about the diet. Tell your friends and other family members not to weaken and give the child a regular cookie or cracker. Even tiny amounts of gluten or casein can cause a child to regress and have diarrhea for days. I learned that "Just a little can't hurt anything" can lead to a real setback until the gluten finally gets out of the system again. Not a few children learn that these foods will make them sick, and so will refuse them if offered by a friend or relative who just can't believe pizza or cookies are bad for anyone.

Unfortunately, we have learned that gluten is hidden in many products and ingredients. Therefore, when you go grocery shopping you have to be vigilant. Become a detective and ferret out hidden sources of gluten and casein. Be warned: Hidden sources of gluten will not be immediately recognizable by just reading the label of foods. For instance, many labels may state "natural and artificial flavors, food starch, malt, and vinegar." Those are only a few of the ingredients that can be derived from wheat.

Where to Get Help

So what are you going to do? Do not get discouraged. Manufacturers are very consumer conscious and the demand for foods free of casein and gluten is increasing steadily as more and more parents realize that curtailing these offending foods makes their children healthier. If you have any doubts, phone the manufacturer (most have toll-free lines) and ask the customer service representative to check if the suspect food or any of its ingredients contains gluten or casein. If they blithely and automatically claim that their product is GF/CF, explain that gluten or casein can be used in preparation of the labeled ingredients and specifically ask if they know for sure whether any of those ingredients have had contact with wheat or milk. If the customer service representative is uncertain, ask to speak to a supervisor and ask that he or she check with the food manufacturer's chemists. The more calls like that they get, the more conscious they will become about the issue. Although acquiring this knowledge and checking ingredients may at first seem overwhelming, once you invest the initial effort you will quickly learn which foods are safe and which are not.

You will also learn where to buy GF/CF/SF foods. For instance, GF/CF foods like Heinz Ketchup, Bush's Baked Beans, Ore-Ida Golden Fries, and Starkist Chunk Light Tuna (although we are now recommending ASD children not eat tuna because of the mercury levels) are available at most local supermarkets. Other GF/CF foods such as Erewhon cereals and GF/CF-free yogurts can be found at local health food stores. Kosher markets that sell products marked "Pareve" are GF/CF/SF. Many Internet and mail order sources sell GF/CF/SF products There are two books that I recommend to all parents planning to put their child on the GF/CF/SF diet. One, written by Karyn Seroussi, mother of a son formerly diagnosed as autistic who has now lost that diagnosis, is entitled, *Unraveling the Mystery of Autism and Pervasive Developmental Disorder: A Mother's Story of Research and Recovery*, published by Simon & Schuster, 2000. Another mother of an autistic child is Lisa Lewis, who authored *Special Diets for Special Kids*, 1998, same title #2, 2001, published by Future Horizons. Lisa Lewis and Karyn Seroussi also founded ANDI, the Autism Network for Dietary Intervention, an organization devoted to helping families get started and maintain the GF/CF/sf diet. They produce *The ANDI News*, a quarterly newsletter with articles written by parents and health professionals regarding the diet. Contact ANDI at P.O. Box 1771, Rochester, NY 14617-0711, or email: AutismNDI@aol.com. Also check http://www.AutismNDI.com for similar information.

Another resource for help in implementing a GF/CF diet is *The Gluten-Free Baker Newsletter* which is published quarterly and provides recipes for flavorful baked goods. Write the newsletter for subscription information at 361 Cherrywood Drive, Fairborn, Ohio, 45324-4012. Still another resource is Autism Educational Services (AES) in New Jersey. Phone and ask for Nadine Gilder at 732-473-9482 or email her at ngilder@worldnet.att.net.[6] AES has developed a recipe book of GF/CF/SF foods ranging from pancakes and waffles to mock Graham Crackers and has also developed a cassette tape, "How to Survive a Gluten-and Casein-Free Diet" that further explains why you should put your autistic child on such a diet. The tape contains many timesaving tips on how to maintain such a diet.

An excellent cookbook with delicious GF/CF recipes is *The Cheerful No Casein, No Gluten, Sugar Optional Cookbook* by Sally Ramsey, a professional chemist who is a gourmet cook. It is available from the Autism Research Institute, San Diego, CA.

Many parents ask me if their child should have certain testing done before going on the GF/CF/SF diet to see if their child really needs this kind of special treatment. Tests for urinary peptides may sometimes be useful, though there have been many false negatives reported. A morning urine sample can be tested and will often identify peptides in the urine of these children if done before they start the restricted diet. These tests are not perfect, and as yet are considered "investigational." Studies show that at least 50% of people with autism who are tested appear to have elevated levels of these opioid-like peptides, thought by prominent researchers such as Paul Shattock in England and Karl Reichelt in Norway to result in abnormal stimulation of opiate receptors in the brain. The effects of this stimulation can be a reduction in pain threshold along with other opiate-like reactions such as impaired perception, learning and motivation. I believe a food-hypersensitivity panel is extremely useful for most of these children, though it does not check for peptides.

In my clinical experience, some children have produced negative results on these lab tests, but my assessment of the child was more correct as there was remarkable improvement when the child was placed on the GF/CF diet. I believe that even if the gut pathology has not progressed to the point of a leaking gut, there is still a lot of evidence that these foods irritate the gut and cause other digestive and immunity problems. The large peptides contained in wheat and milk are very similar. Many children do best when both gluten and casein are avoided. Yet for some children, gluten is the primary culprit; for others, casein must be removed, and for others, soy too offends. Each autism-spectrum child is uniquely individual, even at the level of food hypersensitivity.

The GF/CF/SF diet is an important treatment that can be instituted by parents without any prior laboratory tests. At first in my practice, I accepted all of the families who sought my help. It took me a while to learn that the children who were on the diet generally responded to treatment more successfully than those who had not had the casein and gluten removed. Then I and other clinicians began realizing children with yeast overgrowth were not responding as well as we hoped for to the chelation therapy; in fact, the yeasts, clostridia, and other pathogens seemed to be thriving on the oral chelation agents and rendering our administration of them ineffective for detoxification purposes. These lessons clarified a general principle: *gut healing has to come first*, and gut healing cannot take place if foods that are not being properly absorbed and digested are keeping the gut inflamed. I have for many years had a waiting list of parents who want their children to be evaluated for treatment. One of the ways I screen my acceptance of new clients is by their parents' willingness to implement the GF/CF/SF diet; that's how strongly I feel about healing the gut first. I have no way to prove that all the children have inflamed guts and need the diet, but research evidence is coming in steadily that the majority of these children studied do have inflamed guts. Clearly, removing irritants and toxins from the diet and environment as much as possible is the first step in allowing the gut to heal.

One way parents may do their own evaluation without any laboratory testing is to implement what we call the rotation diet. Foods or food classes are systematically removed for at least 4 days and then restarted with close observation of changes in behavior, toileting, or other parameters such as sleep patterns, learning capabilities, and eye contact. Through hard-earned clinical experience, Defeat Autism Now! doctors have found that each child presents a unique treatment challenge based on his or her biochemical status, immune needs and sensitivities to foods and chemicals. I ask parents to impose the diet for at least four and preferably six months strictly before abandoning it.

ENZYMES

Parents ask me: How long should I keep my child on the GF/CF/SF diet? Several years ago, many of us working with these children would have said "Probably forever!" However, that hopefully may be changing as we are learning more. One of the factors affecting this change is the increased understanding of the importance of digestive enzymes as part of the healing regimen in ASD. Another encouraging factor is the observation that some of the children who have been undergoing chelation long enough to lower their toxic metal load have become able to tolerate previously offending foods. This treatment-related progression back to a more ordinary diet is being helped by the addition of enzymes to help reduce the inflammation in the intestinal lining that can be associated with the leaky gut syndrome. Digestive enzymes diminish both the number and size of inappropriate molecules which in turn tends to reduce inflammation. Reducing inflammation helps heal the leaky gut that was initiated by yeast-excreted enzymes that allow the organisms to burrow deeply into intestinal tissue. Impairments in digestion and absorption (often accompanied by gut inflammation) contribute to the child's impaired nutritional status, which can in turn contribute to and further impair immunity, detoxification and brain function. Furthermore, the proper breaking down of foods minimizes the residue of undigested food that encourages the growth of pathogenic organisms.

Many researchers have done studies showing the incomplete breakdown of protein peptides from casein and gluten (Shattock[7], Reichelt[8]); other researchers have shown the inflammation of the gut lining (Wakefield[9], Horvath[10]) found in the majority of ASD children studied. These as well as further studies have documented and described enzyme deficiencies.[11] The studies reveal a complex range of enzyme deficiencies: pancreatic enzymes, stomach lining enzymes, and brush border membrane enzymes secreted by the small intestine.[12] These and many other studies suggest that these enzyme deficiencies and especially carbohydrate malabsorption may explain many of the significant intestinal problems that the ASD children have.

Regardless of whether the deficiency of pancreatic enzymes starts with a toxic injury such as a mercury-laden vaccination at birth, arises from antibiotics or adverse colonization, or derives from a difficult to define genetic predisposition, the bottom line is that the gut impairment clearly needs to be treated for these kids to improve. There are many different enzyme formulations to handle the special needs of ASD children. Trial and error with safe plant-based enzyme preparations is the best way to find out what most benefits your child. I advise parents in the beginning of the gut-healing program to use enzymes only for dietary infractions that are likely to occur during large family gatherings and birthday parties at friends' houses where restriction is difficult. When the new improved enzymes started coming out, parents were enthusiastic and began replacing the diet with enzymes, with some children becoming very ill. My current approach is to use enzymes in combination with dietary restrictions until children are well on the road to intestinal health. I do not agree with enzyme makers who advertise that enzymes can replace dietary control. My clinical experience early on indicated that in the beginning of treatment for the children where I tried enzymes alone I found only 50% improvement over what a restricted diet based upon food hypersensitivity testing achieved. Before the gut has at least partially healed, some enzymes may be irritating. I advise parents to start with very small doses given just before meals, working up to an optimal level and sometimes with every meal or snack. Many children benefit by removal of items such as soy and corn along with casein and gluten products; enzymes may help them handle these foods if total removal is difficult. For at least some children, appropriate use of digestive enzymes may eventually supplant or even replace dietary restrictions, but not without considerable gut healing first according to my experience.

I find that most children benefit by a broad-spectrum enzyme formulation. My current recommendations (2004) are Klaire Labs, recently improved Vital-Zymes Complete high-potency broad-spectrum digestive enzyme formulation[13], and Kirkman Labs, Enzym-Complete/DPP-IV, also a broad-spectrum formula.[14] Both formulations are SCD compliant. As all children are unique, I advise parents always to try different formulations to see what works best for their child.

PROBIOTICS

Probiotics are beneficial microorganisms ("good gut bugs") that normally inhabit the healthy intestine. Probiotic supplements are often used to prevent or counteract the overgrowth of pathogenic organisms in the gut such as yeast, bacteria, and parasites. We try to "crowd out" the pathogenic bugs ("bad gut bugs") by giving large numbers of beneficial ones. For most autism-spectrum children with intestinal challenges, probiotic supplements are important in bringing the diseased gut back to health. Clinicians becoming more aware of the increasing incidence of yeast infections regularly recommend that patients taking antibiotics also take probiotics, which can minimize the likelihood of overgrowth by pathogens. Fortunately there are numerous preparations available of these essential gut denizens that have proven effective in diminishing diarrhea and constipation, particularly in conjunction with a GF/CF diet. Clinically, probiotics are effective in reducing allergic symptoms, regulating bowel function, and enhancing the immune system. They are remarkably safe and can be purchased by parents without a prescription.

However, a few parents have reported adverse effects of probiotic supplementation, particularly when the gut is severely inflamed. Apparently probiotics can increase gut inflammation in some children. Your child may respond well to one kind or brand of probiotic and negatively to another. It is a case of trial and error, based on astute observation of the child's responses, always starting with small doses and gradually building up. I routinely recommend a broad-spectrum formulation; my favorite is Klaire Labs' new high-potency Ther-Biotics Complete, which contains 12 synergistic colonizing and transient probiotic strains that provide a high degree of intestinal support. Another favorite is Ther-Biotics Detox. These products need to be mixed with cool (not warm or hot) beverages or food such as pear sauce before meals to retain the new InTactic technology for delivering far higher functional potency than other probiotic formulations.

Nutritionist Mark Brudnak, formerly a consultant to Kirkman Labs' Technical Staff, believes probiotics play a pivotal role in detoxification. He provides scientific support regarding the ability of probiotics to detoxify methyl mercury by sequestering it and propelling it along the gastrointestinal tract toward elimination.[15]

Generally, commercially available formulations contain the most well recognized strains of probiotics that address those various populations of pathogens that might be causing or contributing to the gut problems. Though some manufacturers state their probiotics need not be refrigerated, I recommend they always be kept cold to maintain maximum potency. It is also important to keep track of expiration dates and use only fresh products.

Yogurt is a good natural source of the Lactobacillus acidophilus strain of bacteria that research studies have shown counteracts yeast overgrowth and reduces the toxic by-products that overgrowth produces. Many health-conscious adults ingest yogurt regularly, but since almost all of the children in my practice are on a milk-free and usually soy-free diet, parents need to make sure that the probiotic formulations they use are dairy and soy free as well.

Numerous studies have been published showing the role of probiotics in promoting the immune function of the gut, both by strengthening immunological barriers and stimulating immune function.[16] This is not surprising when we understand the huge part the gut plays in regulating the entire immune system.

Both animal and human studies have shown that infants are much more susceptible to persistent yeast infections than adults. In very persistent infections, large doses of probiotics are essential to help crowd out the offending pathogens and help the child's immune system combat the infectious process. When yeasts colonize the gut, they produce toxins that can get into the blood stream and travel to other organs such as the brain. These circulating toxins create even more damage to the gut, producing substances such as ammonia and phenols that need to be counteracted in the child's overall nutrient program.

BASIC NUTRIENT SUPPLEMENTATION

Though choosing supplements that directly address deficiencies targeted by laboratory testing is ideal, parents should not wait for these tests to start supplying their ASD children with the basic nutrients they are likely to need. Before any testing is even necessary, I believe parents should give their child a good Basic Multiple Vitamin and Mineral—without copper—at least daily; Vitamin B6 in the P5P+Magnesium form, 50mg once/day; Vitamin C 100-1000mg, as much as you can get your child to take in divided doses (Vit C does not stay in the body very long) without causing loose stools; and Calcium 500—1000mg per day. Dimethylglycine (DMG) is an important non-toxic supplement and comes in a small sublingual form (125mg) that tastes good, as glycine is naturally sweet. In some children, DMG will start activating greater language ability. Every child should be given a trial of DMG, starting with one a day always given in the morning, building up to three or four all taken at once in the morning if hyperactivity isn't a problem. Giving folinic acid 800mcg along with DMG will often prevent hyperactivity. DMG does double duty in providing the brain with a valuable and important amino acid, and also helps raise immune system efficiency. In about 15% of children, DMG causes agitation as well as hyperactivity, even with folinic acid. Some parents have found that TMG (trimethylglycine) is more tolerable, even though the compounds are very similar, and a few children can tolerate neither DMG nor TMG. (Folinic acid is the biologically active form of folic acid.)

In the next chapter called "Feeding the Starving Brain" I will describe in more detail tests that help target your child's specific nutrient needs, and will also describe those nutrients I have found to be helpful for most autism spectrum children.

In summary, parents need to educate themselves about these treatment modalities that help most autism-spectrum children along the road of recovery—even before finding a physician qualified in autism. Besides *diet restriction* (eliminating casein, gluten, soy and all refined sugars) and *appropriate supplementation* with plant-based digestive enzymes, almost all ASD children need probiotics and a good basic nutrient program. Often, parents who have read about and studied the biomedical-treatment options may know more than their family doctor or pediatrician, whose views about autism are likely to have been formed in medical schools that taught the "must necessarily be genetic" model of autism. So I advise parents to do the homework. As outlined above, you can pursue initial aspects of your child's healing yourself; this saves you money and time, and allows the doctor to focus on testing and prescription medications that may facilitate further treatments. If these preliminary steps are already well along, then lab-tests and treatments that require medical supervision such as anti-fungal, anti-viral, and detoxification protocols can be instituted much sooner.

When you do start the dietary, probiotic, nutrient and enzyme treatments, don't try everything at once. I advise you start one thing at a time and give each a good week to stabilize before you add anything else to the regimen. Keep a journal of what you are doing and how the child is responding. Record the dates and doses of nutrients, so if there is any reaction it will be easier to find the culprit. Record the dates of diet changes, infractions and their consequences. Learn to keep good records of your child's progress and insist on getting a copy of every test taken to keep for your medical files.

Gastrointestinal Treatments That Require Physician Participation

As described in the last chapter, when treatment moves beyond the GF/CF diet, digestive enzymes, probiotics and basic nutrients, laboratory tests that must be ordered by a doctor are needed to guide your child's further treatment. It would be ideal if every family could find a sympathetic and knowledgeable doctor to guide the healing program. However, the fact of the matter is that the complex needs of these children, the newness of the biomedical approach and the epidemic proportions of autism have created a drastic shortage of such physicians. Thus, as I have emphasized, parents must become not only their children's educational advocates but their medical advocates as well. It is imperative that parents read, study, join support groups, peruse the incredible resources now available on the internet, and start the child's healing work even while searching for the doctor oriented towards the biomedical aspects of ASD children.

If parents have already implemented a restricted diet supported by a program of probiotics and enzymes, started a good basic nutrient program, and have been willing to cut out excess sugars and junk food, the child will be well along in the healing game by the time a physician needs to participate in further stages of evaluation and treatment. Yet in moving beyond the child's initial phases of healing, not only must the tests be ordered and interpreted by the doctors, but the prescriptions for advanced drug therapeutics such as anti-fungals, anti-virals, antibiotics, chelation, and specialized medicines for behavior, seizures, and sleeping difficulties if indicated require a doctor's participation.

Learning from the internet and from books is helpful. However, in my opinion some treatments should NOT be tried as home remedies. Chelation is one such treatment. Some parents have felt they can't afford chelation or have been unable to find a physician who will supervise the process and have tried going it alone. This course of action is unwise as behavioral deterioration (i.e., regression) is possible if the child gets a severe gut pathogen infestation. Chelation must be supervised by a physician and augmented by appropriate lab tests.

ANTI-FUNGAL TREATMENT

Along with foods that act as toxins, the accumulation of mercury and other heavy metals also stresses the gut and opens the door to yeast overgrowth. As I have emphasized, for many autism-spectrum children, injury by vaccinal ethylmercury may have been the trigger that set off the whole cascade of problems—including the child's chronic susceptibility for gut dysfunction. The oral chelation agents which I will describe in Chapter Seven have unfortunately shown themselves to be an encouragement for yeasts and anaerobic bacteria such as Clostridium difficile. I have found my biggest delays in the chelation process are caused by the necessity of stopping chelation to treat these pathogenic overgrowths.

Just as the gut needs to be as healthy as possible to start the chelation process, similarly dietary approaches that minimize the yeast burden need to be enacted before starting anti-fungal medication. For example, eliminating foods with sugar should be done for at least two weeks before starting an antifungal medication. Why take medicine to kill the yeasts and feed them their favorite food (sugar) at the same time? Sucrose, glucose, fructose, galactose, honey, brown sugar, maple syrup, rice syrup, etc. are all sugars that feed yeast, and therefore are not beneficial for kids with yeast infestations (or perhaps any kids, certainly in excess or at the expense of healthier foods!). In my opinion, aspartame is not good for anyone, and especially not for ASD children. Nothing is without its drawbacks, but at the moment the sugar substitutes I recommend are stevia and xylitol. Unfortunately, fruits contain high levels of various sugars and must be strictly limited or preferably cut out altogether when yeast is an issue. This includes fruit juices, except for pear juice which yeasts don't seem to crave as they do apple and grape products. Dr. Bruce Semon in his book *Feast Without Yeast*, says "In clinical experience, apples, apple juice, grapes and grape juice wreak havoc in children sensitive to yeast. Pears substitute well for apples; fresh berries substitute well for grapes."[17] Semon only recommends cranberry and pear for fruit sauces. Other clinicians and I have wasted precious time trying to treat yeast with anti-fungal remedies while the child continues to feed the yeast colonization by eating sugary foods, fruit, and fruit juices. Anything that negatively affects immunity is likely to help yeast overgrowth, and sugar (by any other name!) is well known to be injurious to the immune system, especially to one that is already impaired.

In addition to being willing to restrict sugar, parents have taught me that rotating natural anti-fungals such as Lauricidin, grapefruit seed extract, oregano, garlic extract, sacro-B and undecyn can often help in keeping children free of yeast overgrowth. Homeopathic treatments along with continuous probiotics are often a part of this alternative or "natural" yeast control.

When we start anti-fungal treatments, natural or prescription, parents need to know that their child may experience what are called "die-off" side-effects. In medical lingo this is called "the Hexheimer reaction." As the yeasts are starved by lack of sugar and/or are killed by anti-fungal agents there's abnormal release of toxic by-products, creating side-effects that often seem like those of "flu." Symptoms may include fever, irritability and body aches and pains as well as an increase in hyperactivity, "stimming," and other autistic behaviors.

Even though these natural remedies can be quite effective, severe cases of fungal colonization often require a prescription medication; both need to be accompanied by probiotics and sometimes enzymes.

Nystatin is the most well-known prescription anti-fungal medication. It is very safe as it does not enter the blood stream but stays within the gastrointestinal system. Besides safety, readiness of most doctors to prescribe it and insurance companies' willingness to pay for it (relatively inexpensive) are a few of Nystatin's best features. Some of its worst are that it works best if given four times a day and is much less effective for more serious infestations than some of the systemic anti-fungals. For the child who cannot swallow capsules, Nystatin powder tastes quite bitter but can be mixed with stevia and dye-free flavorings by a compounding pharmacist.

The prescription anti-fungal that I have found the most useful is Diflucan (Fluconazole), reported to have the best central nervous system penetration. Though all systemic anti-fungals present a small possibility of liver toxicity, I never have seen that in my practice. I order a CBC and Comprehensive Metabolic Panel before starting any prescription anti-fungal other than Nystatin, which is not absorbed by the gut except in rare cases of extreme gut inflammation. If tests are within normal limits, I prescribe 4-5mg/Kg a day of the Diflucan divided into two doses, and administer for 21-30 days. There is a 40mg/ml variety which is most convenient, as it creates a smaller amount that has to be given per dose. I obtain an OAT (organic acid test) to check for yeast in the week following this course of treatment unless the child still has obvious clinical symptoms of yeast infestation. If the latter is true, I give one week off and ask the parents to obtain another serum chemistry with liver enzymes to assure that the liver is not showing stress from the treatment. If this test is normal I do not have to check again for two months unless there is some clinical indication of liver stress.

The other prescription anti-fungals I use are Nizoral (Ketoconazole) and Sporanox (Itraconazole), but only if treatment with Diflucan does not seem effective and if lab-tests indicate the child's colonization would be more responsive to other agents. Sporanox is one of the few antifungals that eradicate Candida parapsilosis, a dangerous pathogen. If rarely the child has elevated liver enzymes on the "safety" blood tests, I resort to the safer Nystatin while giving nutrients to strengthen and regenerate the liver. Note that liver health is extremely important regardless of other treatments.

OTHER GUT PATHOGENS AND TREATMENTS

Sometimes extremely large amounts of probiotics are required to crowd out the yeasts and bacteria, especially Clostridia. Clostridia are anaerobic bacteria commonly present in small amounts in the gut, but capable of creating a dominant colonization. Unfortunately, Clostridia overgrowth can be very resistant to treatment and very destructive to the gut wall. Some children have been noted to have an amazing improvement in their cognition and behavior during a treatment course of the antibiotic Vancomycin, which kills Clostridia. However, because it is spore-forming, the child's impairment almost always returns after the course of antibiotics is completed. When a child has severe Clostridia, even more strict adherence to diet and probiotics is in order. I have learned that clostridia must be treated before or concomitantly with anti-fungal treatment when both are present, as it has been noted that when one is treated, the other can sometimes flourish with less competition for the food available. I have recently started the use of anti-bacterials and anti-fungals concomitantly for several months at a time along with high potency probiotics such as Klaire's Ther-Biotics Complete, a frequent combination being Diflucan with Vancomycin or Flagyl.

Flagyl (Metronidazole) is a powerful antibiotic that is effective against bacteria such as Clostridia and protozoa or other common parasites. This medicine is very bitter, although a compounded form tastes somewhat better. Heavy use of probiotics upon cessation of the drug is recommended as Flagyl will destroy "good bugs" too. In extremely resistant cases of Clostridia, the antibiotic Vancomycin HCl just mentioned is very effective, but also must be followed by adequate probiotics to replace the good flora that this medicine destroys.

Anything that enhances the immune system helps the child combat yeast overgrowth. Anytime a child starts erratic and unusual behaviors (and there is no obvious cause such as starting a new nutrient or a dietary infraction), yeast or other pathogenic overgrowth should always be suspected, tested for, and adequately treated.

Anytime a child acts "drunk" you can bet they have the "auto-brewery syndrome"—alcoholic intoxication due to the overgrowth of Candida albicans in the G.I. tract.

The Secretin Story

Parents are the experts for their own children in most ways. I have noted that if a mother has an eating disorder herself she may find it doubly hard to deny her child the foods that are part of her addiction, especially sugar. Yet I continually see the nobility in parents who supersede their own limitations and do what helps the child, no matter how hard it is. Here's a real-life story.

The desire of one mother to get a certain test for her child with autism led to the development of a useful treatment for a substantial subset of autistic children and provided even more convincing evidence that autism is a gut-related illness. This mother (not a patient of mine) was an early guiding light, someone who was not willing to accept her child's severe gastrointestinal problems as something to be disregarded just because he was autistic. The "secretin story" provided important evidence that helped many professionals to recognize that in autism the gut and the brain are connected.

Secretin is a natural hormone that has been used as a diagnostic tool to check pancreatic function. Victoria Beck, the mother of an autistic child troubled by severe diarrhea and gut pain, had read about this test. She convinced a medical doctor to give an infusion of secretin to her son, Parker, to see if it would yield a clue as to why he had constant bowel problems. It only takes 10 or 15 seconds for the infusion to go in. After just that small amount of time, Parker startled both the medical doctor and his mother by speaking directly and coherently to his mother. Victoria's son had not spoken for months.[18]

Victoria was totally elated. The medical practitioner, K. Horvath, MD, of the department of Pediatrics at the University of Maryland, was totally mystified, but intrigued and decided to study the hormone further. After years of exploration he now postulates that secretin helps the leaky guts of some autistic children at least temporarily.

In one double-blind, placebo-controlled study, Dr. Horvath and colleagues measured the intestinal permeability of 20 autistic children after a single dose of secretin. "Double-blind, placebo-controlled" simply means that a similar number of patients were infused with a fake hormone and neither the researchers nor the patients knew who was getting the secretin until after the study was over. Thirteen out of 20 autistic children who had exhibited high levels of intestinal permeability showed significant decreases in gut leakage after the infusion of the real hormone.[19]

Research continued. In November of 2001, at the annual meeting of the Society for Neuroscience and the International Meeting for Autism Research, scientists reported animal studies demonstrating that secretin specifically activates neurons in the amygdala, a part of the brain known to be important in social interactions. Several studies in other laboratories had previously established that people with autism do not show normal activation of the amygdala when engaged in such social interactions as recognizing emotions from facial expressions. A long-held theory about secretin is that the hormone stimulates proper digestion and assimilation of foods, which may help to increase a child's detoxification potential while enhancing the availability of nutrients necessary for proper brain function.

Though studies have repeatedly shown that secretin therapy is safe, it is recognized that only a subset of autistic children may be significantly responsive. Younger children aged three or four seem to be more responsive than older children with a few notable exceptions. Among the findings presented at a recent international medical meeting:

A. Dr. R. Sockolow and colleagues from the department of pediatrics at Winthrope University Hospital, Mineola, NY, conducted a six-week study on 34 autistic subjects to assess the safety of secretin treatment. Each child had two secretin injections and no serious side effects were seen immediately after the treatments nor during the six-week follow-up. Four of the patients showed "dramatic improvements" in sociability. All four had had low baseline secretin levels before the therapy.[20]

B. In another 12-week double-blind, placebo-controlled study, Dr. Cynthia Schneider and her colleagues at the Southwest Autism Research Center, Phoenix, AZ, evaluated the effects of a single dose of secretin on 30 children with PDD. The children, ages two to 10, were randomly assigned to receive either a high or a low dose of the hormone. Again, neither the researchers, the patients nor their parents knew the size of the dose each child received. The children were given psychological, language and GI assessments at the beginning of the study and at three, six, and 12 weeks after the infusion. The researchers reported that the children who had the most severe PDD symptoms exhibited greater improvements at the six and 12-week points with the high-dose, rather than the low-dose of secretin. Single doses of secretin were generally ineffective in children with mild or moderate levels of autism.[21]

C. When a study is not "blinded", it is called an "open-label" trial. J. R. Lightdale and his colleagues evaluated the effects of single-dose secretin on the gastrointestinal functioning of 20 young autistic children who had a history of GI problems. Prior to treatment, 80% of the children had loose stools. Parents of 15 of the 20 children reported fewer and more normal stools during the five weeks following secretin treatment. Although not confirmed by clinical testing, 83 percent of the parents reported moderate to significant language improvement in their children following the treatment. Lightdale and his colleagues concluded that a subset of autistic children may indeed suffer from pancreatic dysfunction.[22]

Unfortunately, a roughly equal number of studies have failed to find positive effects from secretin infusions. Still, an increasing number of parents claim that secretin helps their children. Why do so many researchers continue to do studies that show negative results? Dr. Bernard Rimland suggests a "negative placebo effect" may be occurring. A "negative placebo effect", he explains, "is the tendency for researchers who believe that a certain treatment doesn't work to conduct research that "proves" just that. As an example, Dr. Rimland cites a study published a few years ago in the *New England Journal of Medicine* in which the researchers reported they found no benefit to autistic children after administration of secretin. Yet, the same authors reported that 69% of the parents wanted their children to be continued on the hormone. Could the parents be better at seeing improvements in their children than the researchers?

I'm a firm believer in parent wisdom. If parents say that their child is improving on the therapy, I'll bet they are usually right. I hope research on secretin will continue, and I believe that it will prove to be an effective therapy for about 25% of autistic children below 4 years of age.

While secretin is a promising treatment to some children with autism, it obviously isn't a "magic bullet" for all. We keep finding out that there is no one treatment that works for all ASD children. However, secretin was the first treatment to appear in a long time that had such a dramatic effect. Hopes in the ASD community ran high about secretin until we reluctantly realized that most children didn't have the amazing response exhibited by a few. However, the secretin story gave us more clues to the importance of healing the "leaky gut" and helped inspire a lot of investigation into the gut-brain connection that is continuing to this day. Of course, for the small population that benefits by secretin therapy, it is used regularly and in a cyclical manner. When parents who have their child on this treatment see their child revert to earlier or regressive behaviors, these symptoms are signaling that another secretin treatment is needed. Some parents have continued having IV injections given to their children every 5-6 weeks for many years now, and many others continue to use the transdermal form nightly or a few nights a week.

Although meta-reviews have concluded that secretin is not an effective treatment for autism (1-2), a small number of parents report that secretin treatment is beneficial for their autistic child. Since a CpG island in the secretin gene is contributes to gene-expression regulation (3), the fact that many autistic children have hypomethylation (4) suggests another pathway whereby secretin function may be dysregulated in some autistic children. Furthermore, secretin is a member of the G protein family (5), which has been hypothosized as relevant to autism and treatable with vitamin A (6). The Megson theory (6) is enhanced by the fact that vitamin A is a precursor for retinoic acid (7), which participates in secretin gene-expression, including within neurons(8-9). Intestinal pathology is frequent in autism (10). Secretin deficiency and/or secretin receptor nuances may incline toward pathologies involving intestinal lymphocytes (11-12) and thereby might contribute to a child's suboptimal nutritional status, impaired detoxification, and weakened immunity.

Importantly, pancreatic function was found to be normal in a subgroup of autistic children despite "low intestinal carbohydrate digestive enzyme activity" (n= 36; 13), and no weak alleles were found in the secretin gene of autistic children (n = 29; 14). Therefore, we speculate that secretin helps some autistic children (eg, 15) by non-intestinal pathways and/or while improving digestion and absorption by alleviating intestinal pathology. Noteworthy are recently published studies about secretin's role in various parts of the body, including cerebellum, hypothalamus, hippocampus, and amygdala (16-19). Intriguingly, "After administration of [intravenous] secretin, the Autism Diagnostic Interview-Revised (ADI-R) score improved" in 7 of 12 autistic children (20).

Circa 2006, secretin therapy does not seem prudent as an initial tool for most autistic children, but recent findings are encouraging. More research is needed, and researchers may be well served to use experimental designs wherein analysis identifies very small subgroups of autistic children who are secretin responders.

The secretin story is important because it illustrates the value of parental observations and because secretin's efficacy calls attention to the importance of healing intestinal pathologies and leaky guts.

References for Secretin

[1]   Esch BE, Carr JE. Secretin as a treatment for autism: a review of the evidence. J Autism Dev Disord. 2004 34(5):543-56.

[2]   Williams KW et al. Intravenous secretin for autism spectrum disorder. Cochrane Database Syst Rev. 2005 20;(3):CD003495.

[3]   Lee LT et al. Regulation of the human secretin gene is controlled by the combined effects of CpG methylation, Sp1/Sp3 ratio, and the E-box element. Mol Endocrinol. 2004 18(7):1740-55.

[4] James SJ et al. Metabolic biomarkers of increased oxidative stress and impaired methylation capacity in children with autism. Am J Clin Nutr. 2004 Dec;80(6):1611-7.

[5] Dong M et al. Possible endogenous agonist mechanism for the activation of secretin family G protein-coupled receptors. Mol Pharmacol. 2006 70(1):206-13.

[6] Megson MN. Is autism a G-alpha protein defect reversible with natural vitamin A? Med Hypotheses. 2000 54(6):979-83.

[7] Duester G. Families of retinoid dehydrogenases regulating vitamin A function: production of visual pigment and retinoic acid. Eur J Biochem. 2000 267(14):4315-24. http://www.blackwell-synergy.com/doi/abs/10.1046/j.1432-1327.2000.01497.x

[8] Lee LT et al. Retinoic acid activates human secretin gene expression by Sp proteins and nuclear factor I in neuronal SH-SY5Y cells. JNeurochem.200593(2):339-50.

[9] Lee LT et al. Retinoic Acid-induced human secretin gene expression in neuronal cells is mediated by cyclin-dependent kinase 1. Ann N Y Acad Sci. 2006 1070:393-8.

[10] Reviewed elsewhere in this volume.

[11] Mihas AA et al. Effects of gastrointestinal hormonal peptides on the transformation of human peripheral lymphocytes. Res Commun Chem Pathol Pharmacol. 1991 73(1):123-6.

[12] Rindi G et al. Sudden onset of colitis after ablation of secretin-expressing lymphocytes in transgenic mice. Exp Biol Med (Maywood). 2004 229(8):826-34.

[13] Horvath K et al. Gastrointestinal abnormalities in children with autistic disorder. J Pediatr. 1999 135(5):559-63.

[14] Ng SS et al. The human secretin gene in children with autistic spectrum disorder: screening for polymorphisms and mutations. J Child Neurol. 2005 20(8):701-4.

[15] Pallanti S et al. Short report: Autistic gastrointestinal and eating symptoms treated with secretin: a subtype of autism. Clin Pract Epidemol Ment Health. 2005 15;1:24.

[16] Koves K et al. Secretin and autism: a basic morphological study about distribution of secretin in the nervous system. Regul Pept. 2004 15;123(1-3):209-16.

[17] Lee SM et al. Expression and spatial distribution of secretin and secretin receptor in human cerebellum. Neuroreport. 2005 16(3):219-22.

[18] Yung WH et al. The role of secretin in the cerebellum. Cerebellum. 2006;5(1):43-8.

[19] Chu JY et al. Endogenous release of secretin from the hypothalamus. Ann N Y Acad Sci. 2006 1070:196-200.

[20] Toda Y et al. Administration of secretin for autism alters dopamine metabolism in the central nervous system. Brain Dev. 2006 28(2):99-103.

Summary—Gut Health and Healing

In my opinion, when all biomedical factors are considered, restoring intestinal health is a primary key to healing the autistic child's immune system and brain function. A leaky or permeable gut allows peptides, those incomplete proteins that are short chains of amino acids, to leak through the intestines and invade the bloodstream.

The bloodstream carries them throughout the body to locations where they are not supposed to be including the brain. Some of the peptides seem to act as opioids that apparently "drug" our children. However, even non-opioid peptides can be dangerous. The body may perceive those peptides as neurotransmitters. These peptides can bind to normal neurotransmitter receptor sites and block, or at least impair, normal transmission of nerve signals. Naturally, this adversely affects brain cognition and development.

Leaky gut syndrome is a subset of intestinal pathology, and not all autism spectrum children have demonstrated increased permeability in their evaluation. Many children do not show the elevated peptides on the tests we now have available, but when they are elevated it is always an extra incentive to the parents to place their child on the restricted diet. Eventually so many children improved on the diet even with negative peptide tests that I no longer do this test and place every child with autism and many with ADHD on a restricted diet with improved recovery rates. However, other types of gastrointestinal pathology can induce the gut inflammation and nutrient deficiencies described previously in this chapter and further in Chapter Six. We know that the leaky gut syndrome causes a long list of vitamin and mineral deficiencies because the inflammation process damages the various carrier proteins normally present in a healthy GI system. My own clinical experience and study after study has shown that these children are deficient in various vitamins, minerals, amino acids, essential fatty acids, enzymes and co-enzymes. That's why I recommend a comprehensive program of nutrient supplementation in conjunction with the GF/CF and now Soy/Free diet. Besides replacing depleted nutrients, a more recent addition to my supplementation program consists of enzyme therapy to improve the gut's ability to break down proteins. Even on a strict diet there are peptides in foods other than milk, soy and wheat that do not get broken down properly in many children's diets. Many parents are starting to supplement the diet with the use of enzymes and several nutrient companies are working to make better enzyme compounds that are helpful for differing needs. Many parents use them only for dietary infractions, some use only enzymes in conjunction with a regular diet, and others use both. The use of both diet and enzymes at this point appears to be the most beneficial, though some children who are losing their autism diagnosis through detoxification and other biomedical interventions are gradually converting back to a regular diet with the transitional help of enzymes.

For some children who do not respond to the GF/CF/SF diet and continue to have gut problems, parents have gone on to implement even more restricted diets. One of these, the Specific Carbohydrate Diet (SCD) is based on Elaine Gottschall's book, "Breaking the Vicious Cycle," originally intended for those suffering from Crohn's Disease, Ulcerative Colitis, Celiac Disease, IBD, and IBS.[23] This diet is a strict grain-free, lactose-free, sucrose-free dietary regimen that works by severely limiting the availability of carbohydrates to intestinal microbes leading to the formation of acids and toxins which can injure the small intestine. SCD is based on the principle that specifically selected carbohydrates requiring minimal digestion are well absorbed, leaving virtually nothing for intestinal microbes to feed on. At the present time, some ASD parents are transitioning their children from GF/CF/SF to SCD with generally good and some exceptional results. Adjustments have had to be made for the autism population, as many parents found they could not rapidly give their children dairy and honey until after a period of several months or more on the SCD. A website with much information on this diet as well as recipes and lists of "legal" foods is available[24].

References for Chapter Five Other Than Secretin

1   Binstock, Teresa, Common Variable Immune Deficiencies, http://www.jorsm.com/~binstock/cvid.htm

2   Horvath, K. et al., "Gastrointestinal abnormalities in children with autistic disorder." Journal of Pediatrics 1999 Nov., 135(5): 533-5

3   Shaw, William PhD Biological Treatments for Autism and PDD, New revised 2002 edition

4   Jyonouchi H. et al., "Proinflammatory and regulatory cytokine production associated with innate and adaptive immune responses in children with autism spectrum disorders and developmental regression." J. Neuroimmunol 2001 Nov1;120(1-2): 170-9

5   Binstock, Teresa, Medical Hypotheses, Volume:57, Issue:6, Dec. 2001 pp. 714-717 "Anterior insular cortex: linking intestinal pathology and brain function in autism-spectrum subgroups"

6   Nadine Gilder, pamphlet, "The Importance of a Gluten-and Casein-Free Diet," Autism Education Services, published by Autism Educational Services, 1218 Steeplechase, NJ.

7 Shattock, P., Lowdon, G., "Proteins, peptides and autism, Part 2: Implications for the education and care of people with autism." Brain Dys 1991;4(6): 323-34

8 Reichelt, K.L. et al. "Gluten, milk proteins and autism: dietary intervention effects on behavior and peptide secretion." Jour Applied Nutrition 1990;42(1); 1-11

9 Wakefield, A.J. et al. "Enterocolitis in children with developmental disorders." American Jour Gastroenterology 2000 Sep; 95(9): 2285-95

10 Horvath K. et al. "Gastrointestinal abnormalities in children with autistic disorder." Jour Pediatrics 1999 Nov;135(5): 533-5

11 Brudnak, M. "Application of Genomeceuticals to the Molecular and Immunological Aspects of Autism", Medical Hypotheses, 2001

12 Beck, Gary and Victoria, Rimland, Bernard "Unlocking the Potential of Secretin", Autism Research Institute, 1998, San Diego CA

13 Klaire Laboratories, www.Klaire.com, 866-216-6127

14 Kirkman Laboratories, www.kirkmanlabs.com, 800-245-8282

15 Brudnak, MA, "Probiotics as an Adjuvant to Detoxification Protocols." Medical Hypotheses, July 2001

16 Cross ML. Microbes versus microbes: immune signals generated by probiotic lactobacilli and their role in protection against microbial pathogens. FEMS Immunol Med Microbiol. 2002 Dec 13;34(4):245-53.

17 Semon, Bruce MD & Kornblum, Lori, Feast Without Yeast, Wisconsin Institute of Nutrition, LLP, 1999

18 Victoria A. Beck, Confronting Autism: The Aurora on the Dark Side of Venus —A Practical Guide to Hope, Knowledge, and Empowerment, 1999, New Destiny Educational Products, Bedford, NH

19 K. Horvath, R. H. Zieke, R. M. Collins et al., "Secretin Improves Intestinal Permeability in Autistic Children." Presented at the World Congress of Pediatric Gastroenterology, August, 2000.

20 R. Sockolow, D. Meckes, K. Hewitson, and V. Atluru, "Safe Use of Intravenous Secretin in Autistic Children." World Congress of Pediatric Gastroenterology, August, 2000.

21 C. K. Schneider et al., "Synthetic Human Secretin in the Treatment of Pervasive Developmental Disorders." World Congress of Pediatric Gastroenterology, August, 2000.

22 J. R. Lightdale et al., "Evaluation of Gastrointestinal Symptoms in Autistic Children." World Congress of Pediatric Gastroenterology, August, 2000.

23 Gottschall, Elaine, "Breaking the Vicious Cycle: Intestinal Health Through Diet," Kirkton Pr, Dec. 1994 **www.pecanbread.com**

SIX

FEEDING THE STARVING BRAIN

Vital Nutrients

It is now generally accepted that vitamins, minerals and other supplements have important roles to play in promoting optimal health, reducing the risk of chronic disease, and extending the life spans of adults. It thus escapes me why anyone would question the vital role nutrients have in healing the ailing gastrointestinal systems of children with autism spectrum disorder, especially when laboratory tests have revealed vitamin and mineral deficiencies in almost all of the children tested. I will continue to emphasize that children with autism almost always have underlying physical medical problems, especially gastrointestinal problems that must be treated. A child's state of health reflects his or her state of nutrition. When minerals, vitamins, amino acids, or enzymes are deficient in a child's system, the result can be a "disturbed biochemical homeostasis" or imbalance that causes impairment of nutrition to all parts of the system, including the brain. This, in turn, can cause an inability to focus, concentrate, and stay on task. Unfortunately, many mainstream physicians still tell parents that diet changes or supplements are of little use. Many doctors remain locked in a paradigm that says treatment means prescription drugs; once out of formal medical training physicians depend primarily on the pharmaceutical industry to provide their continued medical education.

Woody McGinnis, MD, an autism researcher from the Tucson, AZ area conducted a study of ASD children and found that 69% of the children suffer from esophagitis, 42% suffer from gastritis, 67% suffer from duodenitis, and 88% suffer from colitis. The frequent nighttime awakening of ASD children is thought by some clinicians to be due to irritating reflux problems; persistent bowel problems are obvious in years-long intractable diarrhea, constipation, or both at various times in the child's history.

A common denominator in all these conditions is gut inflammation. For example, duodenitis is inflammation of the duodenum. Colitis is inflammation of the colon. Esophagitis is inflammation of the esophagus, and yes, gastritis simply means inflammation of the stomach.

If mainstream medicine will not provide relief for our ASD children suffering from those chronic conditions, we must turn to alternative medicine. By the way, just because "alternative medicine" includes the modifier "alternative," one shouldn't necessarily think of it as "lesser medicine." Although the popular press has made a big deal about the dichotomy between so-called "mainstream medicine" and "alternative medicine," this artificial division blurs considerably if one takes the long view. Many treatments once considered "alternative" have become "mainstream" once their effectiveness became proven. The use of antibiotics to cure ulcers is one example. Furthermore, some therapies once considered "mainstream" are now considered "alternative." The use of herbal therapies is one such example. For hundreds of years, mainstream doctors used herbs as the mainstay of their treatments. It was only with the rise of modern pharmaceutical companies that herbal preparations fell out of favor. Ironically, some herbal therapies may be on the way back to the mainstream. Two examples are the use of the milk thistle herb to strengthen the liver, and the use of St. Johns' Wort, sometimes referred to as "herbal Prozac" for the treatment of depression.

University researchers tell us that the "gold standard" for evaluating medical therapies is the double blind, placebo-controlled study —the type of study where neither the patients nor their treating physicians know which is the treatment being evaluated and which is the placebo. However, as anyone who is familiar with the history of medicine can attest, most medical treatments in current use were originally validated over a period of time by the "silver standard" of clinical trials without the rigorous double blind, placebo-control study to back it up. Once a treatment is known to work it often becomes unethical (especially in lifesaving situations) to do a double blind, placebo-controlled study because one segment of the population being tested will get the placebo, not the needed treatment.

In the absence of large scale, double-blind studies, how does one separate the wheat from the chaff in treating this complicated disorder we call ASD? There are reasons Defeat Autism Now! practitioners take a pragmatic view in prescribing the treatments they do. A large number of biochemical and biological abnormalities have been identified in autistic children and adults, and many Defeat Autism Now! doctors have found that treatments directed at these abnormalities are likely to be helpful. One of my inspirational and favorite mottos is Dr. Bernard Rimland's emphatic "Do what works!" Many of the successful Defeat Autism Now! treatments were learned through trial and error, since few researchers have been interested in looking for funding for studies on nutritional deficiencies, nutrient supplementation, special diets, or detoxification protocols. Informed parents and concerned physicians are not willing to wait until extensive formal studies are done to use methods that are safe, make a lot of sense and are already showing benefit for many children.

NUTRITIONAL DEFICIENCIES IDENTIFIED IN OUR CHILDREN

What are the biochemical imbalances generally present in ASD children? According to a Defeat Autism Now! study on the "Nutritional Status of Autistic Children,"[1] most autistic children demonstrate the following abnormalities:

- Low vitamin B6 levels and poor B6-binding combined with low or low-normal amounts of intracellular magnesium

- Low intracellular zinc

- Low blood levels of vitamin A and D

- Low biotin, B1, B3, and B5 function, according to microbiological assays

- Low urinary vitamin C
- Low Red Blood Cell (RBC) membrane levels of eicsapen-taenoic acid (EPA is a derivative of omega-3 fatty acids)
- Elevated RBC membrane levels of archidonic acid (one cause of inflammation)
- Low levels of taurine (vital to nerve cells)
- Elevated casomorphine and gliadomorphine levels (opioid peptides)
- Elevated urinary yeast metabolites
- Elevated IgG antibodies to milk
- Imbalance of the bacterial flora of the gut

In addition, many autistic children demonstrate:
- Low serum selenium (50% of subjects)
- Low folate and B12 on microbiological assay
- Elevated Red Blood Cell membrane trans fatty acid levels
- IgG antibodies to grains
- Elevated urinary bacterial metabolites (50% of subjects)
- Overly acidic stools

Furthermore, studies by Dr. William Walsh, Dr. William Shaw and others reveal that large numbers of autistic children are deficient in Zinc, B6, and GLA (Gamma Linolenic Acid), as well as low methionine levels usually due to poor-quality protein intake.

THE USE OF VITAL NUTRIENTS

The above listed imbalances are what I and many other Defeat Autism Now! practitioners are attempting to treat with biomedical protocols that use specific vitamins, minerals, and other nutrients. Although these treatments are only now starting to be formally evaluated by large double-blind, placebo-controlled trials, the vital nutrients employed have been used safely for years to treat these and similar abnormalities in patients with other ailments. In other words, we know from long-term clinical practice that these supplements are safe and effective. Still, it is important to point out here that often a great deal of trial and error is involved in determining optimal nutrients and appropriate dosage levels for each child. Even though we know certain substances may be deficient in most of the children in the spectrum, individual tolerances and sensitivities require that we start with low doses, build slowly toward what we feel are adequate levels to correct deficiencies, and observe closely for reactions. In very sensitive children, occasional testing must be done to evaluate specific deficiencies and help guide us in our nutrient program. There are even brand sensitivities in some children, and certain additives or tablet coverings can sometimes make the difference as far as tolerability for a particular child.

The vast majority of my patients, particularly the younger ones, show enormous benefits from their nutrient/vitamin/mineral program. Typically ASD children's food choices have been so limited that almost all of them have long-standing vitamin and mineral deficiencies. If they were not using vitamin supplements before, the reaction is sometimes quite dramatic, taking the form of greater speech, more eye contact, and better behavior and sleeping patterns within days to a few weeks after starting their nutrient program. My advice to parents is to start with low doses, using one new nutrient at a time until the child adjusts to the recommended dose before starting the next nutrient, all the while carefully observing and recording reactions.

Parents are often dismayed at the number of nutrients they are asked to give to their children, and some creative ways have been devised by vitamin dispensers and parents to hide bad flavors. Giving the child a feeling that they are doing a very important job in getting them down (and resisting making a face when you smell them yourself!) often helps. Sometimes nothing but a compassionate but firm, "There's no choice; we have to do this, so let's get it over with" approach is necessary. Following the nutrient brew with a favorite drink or a favorite chewable clearly in sight is sometimes helpful. There is a lot of incentive for the parents to teach the children how to swallow capsules, which makes life easier for everyone. To facilitate this, parents may purchase very small empty capsules at their pharmacy and practice with these to get the child used to swallowing small objects before moving on to the regular or large sized capsules.

When parents fully understand the seriousness of their child's nutritional deficiencies, it makes this daunting task of taking supplements more tolerable, just as in the case of the GF/CF/SF diet when parents recognize the damage certain foods are doing to their child's gastrointestinal tracts and brains. Some parents who felt that their children did have a fairly good diet were quite surprised at the beneficial reaction to the nutrient program. These cases demonstrate that due to maldigestion or malabsorption problems even a child that is not so picky still may not be providing the proper nutrition to the brain because of his or her gut inflammation.

PRIMARY RECOMMENDED SUPPLEMENTS

Primary

- Vitamin B6, preferably the activated form P5P` + Mag, 50mg under 5yrs/day, 50-100mg/day over 5yrs. Pyridoxine up to 20mg/kg.

- Magnesium, glycinate form is most absorbable, 200-400mg/day.

- Zinc, picolinate form is most absorbable, but I also give zinc monomethionine (vrp) and zinc citrate at certain times and for certain children: 20-50mg/day (up to 1mg/lb + 20 for chelating).

- Calcium, at least one gram daily divided into several doses

- Selenium, doses up to 150-200 mcg daily for the larger children; 75-150 mcg under 5 (unless testing shows levels very low—high doses can be toxic, but rarely and unlikely)

- Vitamin A, 1000-2000iu/day; beta-carotene does not convert to A in most children. Recent recommendations by the Vitamin D Council caution that Vitamin A may be opposing Vit D and causing Vit D deficiencies in many children in Developed Countries as the US. Because of the variable rates of Vit A in the different products, Cod Liver Oil is not currently being recommended - if this changes I will post it on my lists and my website www.starvingbrains.com.   Recommended ratio now is 5:1 D3 to A for most children on the spectrum.

- Vitamin D–Test child for serum 25-hydroxyvitamin D; ideal level 60-70 ng/mL; current recommendations 5000iu daily for breast-feeders, dark-skinned children, children who do not get much sunlight, or in wintertime. Otherwise, 2000-5000iu daily.

- **Important note about Vitamin A and Vitamin D:** Recent newsletters and reports by the Vitamin D Council caution that Vitamin A may be opposing Vitamin D and causing Vitamin D deficiencies in many children in Developed Countries such as the US. Apparently this situation is not true in Developing Countries where Vitamin A deficiencies may be rampant, particularly in regard to measles for which Vitamin A is the only known therapy; current Vitamin A treatment is showing great benefit in those countries that were beset by high rates of measles death prior to the administering of adequate Vitamin A to young children. The Vitamin D Council group headed by Dr. John Cannell is against any Cod Liver Oil being taken by adequately nourished children, as the Vitamin A levels oppose proper absorption of Vitamin D. He posits a near universal Vitamin D deficiency considered to be secondary to the avoidance of sunshine and the use of sunblocking agents, and many recent scientific articles are attesting to the importance of Vitamin D in much higher levels than current RDAs suggest for almost all of us. Dr. Cannell particularly feels that Vitamin D deficiency may be playing an important role in the current autism epidemic. Though many questions still remain and further elucidation may be coming, at the present time there are too many agreements from highly respected scientists that Vitamin D levels need to be higher than we thought in the past, and I am giving Dr. Cannell's current recommendations for Vitamin D for children (and adults) with autism:

(Below excerpted from October 2008 Vitamin D Newsletter)

Says John Cannell MD, www.vitamindcouncil.org: "I have come up with a protocol for diagnosing and treating vitamin D deficiency in autistic children but it can be used in any child. Remember, the worst thing that can happen is that children will have stronger bones:

1. Advise parents to stop giving children all preformed retinol, such as cod liver oil, and all vitamins or supplements containing retinyl palmitate and retinyl acetate. Preformed retinol antagonizes the action of vitamin D, probably at the vitamin D receptor site. Beta carotene does not have this same effect but children only need extra beta carotene if their diet is poor in colorful fruits and vegetables, dairy products, or fortified breakfast cereals.

2. Order a 25-hydroxy-vitamin D [25(OH)D] blood test. Do not order a 1,25-dihydroxy-vitamin D as it is often elevated in vitamin D deficiency and will mislead you. Note: A new home test kit for Vitamin D3 with a heel or finger stick can be ordered by parents (cost $65) directly from ZRT Labs to keep track of their Vit D3 levels, www.zrtlab.com

3. If the 25(OH)D level is less than 70 ng/ml, the mid range of American references labs (30 - 100 ng/ml), give your child vitamin D3 supplements. Generally children require 1,000 IU per 25 pounds of body weight per day. However, great individual variation exists and autistic children need to be retested and the dose adjusted about every month until levels are at least 50 ng/ml in healthy neurotypical children and at least 70 ng/ml in any child with autism, diabetes, frequent infections, or any chronic illness.

4. Test for 25(OH)D every several months and treat with enough vitamin D until 25(OH)D levels are stable. Vitamin D toxicity has never been reported, in adults or children, with 25(OH)D levels below 200 ng/ml."

Per Dr. JM: In testing many children for serum Vitamin D over the last two years in my practice, most are low, and I have yet to test one who is close to 70ng/ml, so for now I am going along with Dr.

Cannell's suggestions as to Vitamin D dosing. As to Vitamin A, he states: "I don't think these kids with autism need more than 1000 to 2,000 IU daily of preformed retinol as supplements. For your High Dose Vitamin A Protocol for children thought to have measles in their GI tracts, instead of giving them 200,000 IU of vitamin A as a push dose, give 200,000 IU of vitamin D, you'll be happy with results and there is 0% chance of toxicity with this dose."

If this changes, I will post it on the CSB e-list/files and put the information on my website.

- Vitamin B12 as methylcobalamin 750-2500mcg injectables (64.5mcg/Kg) 2X/wk; daily injections help 40% of kids. Nasal spray with or without folinic acid created by parent Stan Kurtz now can also be compounded, 1-2 sprays 2X weekly or daily per response, 1250mcg + 300mcg of folinic per spray.

- Vitamin C, up to 1000mg/day to tolerance, better given 3 or 4 x/day (doesn't stay in the body very long), buffered forms better tolerated.

- Vitamin E, 200iu/day for under 5yrs, 400iu/day for over 5yrs, high gamma tocopherol best.

- Essential Fatty Acids, Omega-3's 750-2000mg, minimum essential for all–500mg EPA, 750-1500 DHA/ and GLA 50-100mg/day. DHA especially important for brain development.

- DMG (125mg caps or sublinguals 1-6/day) or TMG (500-2000mg/day + Folinic Acid (800-mcg/day)

- Vitamin K–children are very sensitive to Vit K, and it can be toxic. Decent diet will provide all children who do not have coagulation disorders plenty of Vit K, especially dark leafy vegetables are rich in K.

Miscellaneous

- Additional Minerals e.g. Manganese, Chromium, Molybdenum, Boron, Vanadium

- B-vitamins e.g.Thiamine, Riboflavin, Niacin, Biotin, Pantothenic Acid. Ecological Formulas Co-Enzyme B-Complex is good

- Amino Acids, essential and non-essential, Klaire's Essential Aminos good.

- Minerals, B-Vitamins, and Amino Acids are usually included in a comprehensive multiple vitamin/mineral compound. With amino acid testing, some children receive an individualized formula, which is optimum, but usually balanced formulas are available that serve many children adequately. Recommend Klaire's VitaSpectrum.

- Specific nutrients may sometimes be given based on test results showing deficiencies or in special circumstances such as chelation which may require extra nutrients to compensate losses. Special nutrients may include those with strong anti-oxidation benefit, such as idebenone (the biological form of CoQ10.)

- Most children are low in L-glutathione; reduced L-glutathione in capsules, liquids and transdermal creams are available and advised for many children. For children who do not have elevated cysteine (about 15%), reduced L-glutathione precursors are good preparation for chelation and actually begin the process slowly and safely. New lipoceutical forms of oral GSH are now available and are more effective than the powder in capsules.

- Milk thistle compounds for liver health and immune enhancers also raise glutathione levels. Nutrient immune modulators such as IP6 or arabinogalactans are also utilized for children whose immune impairment results in frequent illnesses.

Metallothionein Dysfunction

Dr. William Walsh at the Pfeiffer Treatment Center in Naperville IL has been working on metallothionein dysfunction in ASD children and reports significant improvements in nutrient programs designed to correct this dysfunction. (see Causation Models in Chapter One and Testing in Chapter Four). His medical system includes extensive laboratory testing, diagnosis of chemical imbalances, identification of nutrients that are in deficiency or overload, and biochemical therapy aimed at balancing body chemistry. Though some of his nutrient protocols are patented and presently not generally available except to those working with his staff, he has shared some of his findings. He states that "45% of our autistic population exhibit undermethylation which can be effectively treated with supplements of methionine, magnesium, DMG, SAM(e), and calcium, along with strict avoidance of DMAE and folic acid. In contrast, 15% of autistics exhibit overmethylation and benefit from liberal doses of DMAE, folic acid, and B-12, along with strict avoidance of methionine and SAM(e)."[2] Undermethylation is thought to be the predominant state in most ASD children. What seems like "over methylation" may indicate a trap in the complex folate cycle where important enzymes and co-factors are not available to keep the cycle functioning properly.

The Rationale Behind the Use of Specific Nutrients

B6 AND MAGNESIUM

Bernard Rimland has for many years championed Vitamin B6 (pyridoxine) and magnesium as helpful treatments for ASD children deficient in those substances. According to Dr. Rimland, 18 studies evaluating vitamin B6 as a treatment for autistic children have provided positive results. Dr. Rimland collaborated on two such studies; in one double-blind, placebo-controlled study with Drs. Enoch Callaway of the University of California, San Francisco, and Pierre Dreyfus of the University of California, Davis, 16 autistic children were treated with B6 and magnesium. The magnesium was added because it enhances the effects of B6 and protects against possible B6-induced magnesium deficiency.

There were statistically significant positive benefits to children who were on daily doses of between 300 and 500 mg of B6 (8 mg of

B6 per pound of body weight) combined with several hundred mg of magnesium (3 or 4 mg of magnesium per pound of body weight). The benefits included increased eye contact, less self-stimulatory behavior, more interest in the world around them, fewer tantrums, and expanded speech. While no patient has been "cured" with the vitamin B6 and magnesium treatments, many parents report the treatments produced calming effects and resulted in improved, more normal behavior.

In a survey of over 3,500 parents of autistic children, the parents were asked to provide rating on a variety of treatments and interventions. Among the biomedical treatments, the use of vitamin B6 and magnesium received the highest rating from 318 parents with 8.5 of them reporting behavioral improvement to every one reporting behavioral worsening. Those results were better than what parents reported for drug treatments.

ZINC

Zinc is present in over 200 body enzymes, and its deficiency results in a weakened immune system. It is well known that most ASD children are deficient in zinc and excessive diarrhea is known to be one of the leading causes of zinc depletion. In fact, at the 2001 Defeat Autism Now! conference biochemist William Walsh, PhD reported that a study of 503 children with autism revealed that 85% had high copper-zinc ratios. In other words, they had abnormally high levels of copper and low levels of zinc in their bodies. Zinc is an essential micronutrient that the human immune system needs to function at peak performance. Zinc deficiency affects a range of functions including growth, immunity, and brain development. Controlled trials have shown that zinc supplementation is associated with improved growth, particularly among stunted children. Zinc also reduces the severity and duration of both acute and chronic diarrhea. In fact, the World Health Organization recommends giving zinc supplements to children as part of managing severe protein energy malnutrition and persistent diarrhea.[3] Though a dosage of 25-50mg of zinc is usual, in those with high copper levels, higher doses may be needed to oppose and get the copper level down. Zinc is so important that when I have children in chelation and their copper levels are high, I usually suggest 1mg per pound of body weight or more depending on test levels. Levels may need to be monitored for certain children to keep their levels within a normal range.

CALCIUM

Calcium is a major constituent of bones and teeth, and is crucial for nerve conduction, muscle contraction, heartbeat, blood coagulation, the production of energy, and maintenance of immune system function. A calcium deficiency can contribute to ADD/ADHD behavior. Children deficient in calcium are more likely to exhibit irritability, sleep disturbances, anger, and inattentiveness. According to the American Academy of Pediatrics, the current dietary intake of calcium by children and adolescents is well below the recommended optimal levels.[4] The first signs of a calcium deficiency include nervous stomach, cramps, tingling in the arms and legs, and painful joints. Children need from 800-1200mg of calcium daily, particularly those on the GF/CF diet.

SELENIUM

Selenium is a mineral with antioxidant properties that works with vitamin E in preventing free radical damage to cell membranes. Selenium deficiency causes depressed immune function and a resulting increase in susceptibility to infections due to decreased levels of white blood cells and natural killer cells. Selenium is antagonistic to heavy metals in the body, and is an important mineral to supplement especially during chelation therapy. Care must be taken not to overdose since it can be toxic in excess and the multiple mineral supplements usually already contain selenium. I recommend 100 to 200mcg/day total intake.

VITAMIN A AND HIGH-DOSE VITAMIN A PROTOCOL

Vitamin A is an antioxidant and general immune enhancer, specific against measles. Infants and many children are not able to convert non-toxic beta-carotene to A, so though important for itself carotenes cannot be relied upon as a source of A. Current RDA's for A are probably too low generally and more so for our population, though rare cases of A can be toxic, usually in long-sustained high doses or mega-doses in the millions. Some parents have been using (upon my recommendation) a 2-day mega-dose to combat gut measles in their ASD children no more often than every 6 months. Recent new findings show that Vitamin D is now considered deficient in most of our children, but because Vit A can oppose Vit D it is questionable how beneficial Vitamin A is now generally. For those who do want to still do the mega-dosing with Vitamin A it is better done with the palmitate (I recommend Klaire's Mycelized Vit A 5000iu/drop). My criteria for mega-dosing (and some doctors and parents still find it very beneficial using 200,000iu (up to 35#) or 400,000iu (over 35#) for 2 days in a row every six months) are: Elevated IgG serum rubeola titers, evidence of auto-immunity per high myelin basic protein (MBP) and other neural elements antibodies, history of regression after MMR, and persistent gut problems.

Dr. Mary Megson, a pediatrican in Richmond VA, showed that certain children susceptible to autism are genetically at risk from a G-alpha protein defect. She posits a progression of injury in these susceptible children starting with exposure to wheat, followed by exposure to measles antigen, and then addition of the pertussis toxin, which takes them into a disconnection of the G-alpha protein pathways. The retinoid receptor pathways are critical for vision, sensory perception, language processing and attentiveness. Sideways glancing may indicate poor rod function and may be a tip-off to the G-alpha protein defect, especially if family history shows others with night-blindness and hypothyroidism. A trial of Cod Liver Oil followed by a trial of Urecholine for stimulating acetylcholine receptor blockage (shown by decreased bile and pancreatic secretions) might be therapeutic in this subset of ASD children.

VITAMINS C AND E

Vitamins C and E are important antioxidants which work together to fight free radicals, those unstable oxygen molecule outlaws that can literally pierce cell walls and oxidize or destroy brain cells. Since brain cells are very vulnerable to oxidative stress, adequate supplies of both vitamins C and E are essential. The body cannot manufacture Vitamin C so it has to be taken in through food or supplements, Vitamin C also protects against the harmful effects of pollutants and enhances immunity. Mothers of autistic children with constipation will be happy to learn that Vitamin C also helps regularize bowel movements because of its cathartic properties. In fact, Vitamin C is so important that we ask parents to increase it to gut tolerance, determined by increasing the dose until it causes diarrhea, than backing off just a little. We suggest parents give C in divided doses, as it does not stay around very long in the body. Vitamin C works synergistically with Vitamin E, so these two should be given together. C is recommended up to 1000mg or more/day and Vitamin E from 200-600IU/day according to the size of the child. Vitamin E is an especially important antioxidant, protecting cell membranes from oxidative damage. This important vitamin promotes proper metabolism and reception of vitamin D and calcium, improves circulation, and repairs tissue. E also prevents cell damage by inhibiting lipid peroxidation and formation of free radicals.

ESSENTIAL FATTY ACIDS

Factors contributing to an almost universal shortage of essential fatty acids in most Americans are: Soil depletion, excessive food processing, (e.g. chemical processing and refinement of foods with removal of certain oils to extend shelf life), and the widening use of antibiotics with the consequent alteration of intestinal flora. Children with attention problems and autism have been shown to be more deficient in essential fatty acids as a group than neurotypical children. Fish oil is rich in a special type of fatty acid called Omega-3. These fatty acids are labeled "essential" because our bodies don't make them. They must enter the body through our diets or from supplements. Furthermore, many autistic children have defects in fatty acid metabolism. Fish oil supplements work to correct that deficiency and are recommended for all children, not just those in the ASD spectrum. New deodorized forms of fish oils are becoming available, so it is important for parents to experiment until they find one their child will tolerate. I recommend 500-750mg EPA/day and 500-1000mg of DHA/day. Some children also need GLA 50-100mg/day; some forms of fish oil supplements contain all three of these together. DHA is particularly important for brain growth.

Omega-3 fatty acids are vital for normal neural development and the maintenance of neurotransmitter, cellular, and membrane

integrity. Neurotransmitters affect behavior and learning. Any neurotransmitter deficiency or blockage will have a dramatic effect on
a child's (or an adult's for that matter) ability to learn and function
optimally. These essential Omega-3 fatty acids also help improve the
immune response, work against inflammation in the GI tract, and
help keep the blood flowing by preventing blood clots.

Please see information on testing for fatty acids deficiencies in
Chapter Four.

DMG AND TMG

DMG (Dimethylglycine) benefits about half of the ASD children who take it, with notable language improvement in some after
only a few days or weeks. Since it is non-toxic and also known to be
an immunity enhancer, I suggest all parents give their child an experimental DMG trial. I prefer the small sublingual 125mg tablets
because the children usually love glycine's natural sweetness, (I am
always looking for nutrients the children like.) Morning dosages are
preferable as some children show some hyperactivity until they get
used to it; I suggest starting with one tablet and working up to 6 or
more (all taken in the am) if benefit is shown. The hyperactivity that
occurs with DMG in some children can be moderated by giving
folinic acid along with it up to 2400 mcg/day. If the hyperactivity
persists even with the folinic acid, the DMG should be discontinued, as approximately 15% of children are reported to be intolerant
of methylating agents such as DMG and TMG (the "overmethyla-
tors.") Some mothers state that TMG does not cause the hyperactivity that DMG does; TMG is DMG with one more methyl group,
increasing serotonin through a precursor called SAM(e) (S-Adenosylmethionine), an enzyme important in acetylcholine synthesis.
However, other mothers report that when they changed from DMG
to TMG they noticed hyperactivity and returned to the DMG without problem. Children's chemistries are so unique that trial and
error with these non-toxic substances is the only way to find out
whether they are beneficial. Both DMG and TMG have a tremendous safety record.

B-VITAMINS

The B vitamins are coenzymes involved in energy production and help to maintain healthy nerves, skin, eyes, hair, liver and mouth as well as muscle tone in the gastrointestinal tract. B vitamins should be taken together as they work as a team, but a larger amount of any one may be given additionally when necessary, such as B6 or folic acid.

A. **B1 or thiamine** is important for blood formation, the production of hydrochloric acid, and carbohydrate metabolism.

B. **Vitamin B2 or riboflavin** is necessary for red blood cell formation, antibody production, and is essential for the metabolism of tryptophan.

C. **Vitamin B3 or niacin, niacinamide, or nicotinic acid** is necessary for proper circulation. It plays an important role in the formation of tryptophan in the liver. Niacin aids in the metabolism of carbohydrates, fats, and proteins and in the proper functioning of the nervous system.

D. **Vitamin B5 or pantothenic acid** is known as the "anti-stress" vitamin. It is important in the production of the adrenal hormones, the formation of antibodies, and helps convert fats, carbohydrates, and proteins into energy. B5 is essential for production of vital steroids and cortisone in the adrenal glands.

E. **Vitamin B6 or pyridoxine (in its biologically activated form, pyridoxal 5' phosphate, or P5P)** is involved in more bodily functions than any other single nutrient. This vitamin maintains sodium and potassium balance, promotes red blood cell formation, and is necessary for normal brain function and the synthesis of RNA and DNA. These are the nucleic acids containing genetic instructions for the reproduction of all cells and for normal cellular growth. Multiple studies have shown the importance of Vitamin B6 for ASD children. Magnesium enhances the absorption and reduces hyperactivity which some children show with B6; I prefer the P5P compounded with magnesium for optimum benefit (P5P+Mag) available at Klaire Labs.

F. **Vitamin B12** (preferred form methylcobalamin) is necessary for cell formation, proper digestion, absorption of foods, protein synthesis, and metabolism of carbohydrates and fats. A B12 deficiency is most often due to a defect in absorption and not a dietary lack except in strict vegetarians, since it is only available from animal sources. Deficiency is common in those with digestive disorders, and is present in almost all ASD children. Symptoms of deficiency include abnormal gait, memory problems, eye disorders, and anemia. Many ASD children show a mild anemia which can be caused by other nutrient deficiencies, especially zinc, as well as heavy metal intoxication. If the anemia is mild, I try to rebalance with nutrient support and gut healing before giving iron, which can increase oxidative stress. If more severe, insufficient B12 levels as a cause may be shown (but not always) by a urine or blood measurement of methylmalonic acid (MMA), but there is no completely reliable test for Vitamin B12 adequacy. A trial with a methylcobalamin injection showing a good response qualifies as a positive test. If doses are adequate, we will usually see a positive response within the first few days. If the initial B12 shot does benefit the child, parents can be taught to administer the injection in varying schedules depending upon how long the benefit lasts. After a while parents can experiment to see if high sublingual or oral doses will accomplish the same results. Please see Chapter 10 for more on MB-12

G. **Folic acid (folate):** Folic acid functions as a coenzyme in DNA synthesis and is essential for the formation of red blood cells. It works best when combined with Vitamin B12. The anemia caused by folic acid deficiency is similar to that of B12 deficiency, "large cell" or macrocytic anemia. Folic acid deficiency is common in those with chronic diarrhea, and does not store in the body for many years as does Vitamin B12. Folinic acid is the biologically active form and thought in recent years to be the preferable folate to give for most of our children and in general. It is important to receive folinic acid along with methylcobalamin for almost all children; this is the form Dr. Neubrander says helps the most children. A small percent of children cannot handle very much folinic acid and must use Folopro or rarely none at all of any form.

AMINO ACIDS

Amino acids are fundamental building blocks for muscle and brain tissue and for hormones, neurotransmitters, hormones, and digestive enzymes. They are molecules connected together to form peptides or proteins, which can contain hundreds to thousands of amino acids. When vegetable or animal proteins are ingested, our digestive tract breaks them down to single, free-form amino acids or to very short-chained peptides (two or three aminos) which can be absorbed through the mucosal cells of the small intestine. Further digestion takes place by peptidase enzymes in the blood, liver, kidney and other organs. The resulting pool of free-form amino acids can then be reassembled in specific sequences to make human proteins and peptides used for tissue growth and repair and for a multitude of physiologic functions. The essential amino acids are: leucine, iso-leucine, valine, methionine, phenylalanine, tryptophan, lysine, and threonine. Important nonessential (the body can make them) amino acids especially in autism are taurine, cysteine, and glutamine. It is estimated that at least two-thirds of ASD children show abnormal amino acid patterns as shown by urine or fasting plasma amino acid analyses. Some of these abnormalities are of genetic origin, such as Phenylketonuria, but most of them seem to be related to maldiges-tion and subnormal uptake. Some labs which perform the amino acid analysis offer a customized amino acid powder to address the deficiencies, and adequate B-Vitamins and essential minerals must be provided with these supplements.

ADDITIONAL MINERALS

Vitamins and minerals are cofactors that activate amino acids and fatty acids in metabolic processes; they catalyze reactions in the mitochondria of the cells and are synergistic, meaning there is a co-operative action among them. Calcium, magnesium, sodium, po-tassium and phosphorus, are the "major" minerals and are needed in larger amounts than what are called "trace minerals": zinc, iron, copper, manganese, chromium, selenium, molybdenum, boron, germanium, sulfur, vanadium and iodine. Except for specially tested deficiencies or extra needs due to absorption problems or chelation, minerals are usually given in a multiple compound designed for the typical balance needed.

Nutrient Interactions

Although I have listed each of the above nutrients individually and explained the principal roles of each, it must be emphasized that there is a synergistic interaction or "dance" between the various vitamins, minerals, and other nutrients. In this dance, vitamins, minerals, and other nutrients partner with each other, changing partners often as they work together to enhance the health of the body and mind. That's why deficiencies in one vitamin or mineral often affect the role other vitamins and minerals play. For instance, deficiencies in Vitamins A, C, E, or of the B vitamins niacin, panothenic acid, B6, and folic acid and/or deficiencies in minerals like zinc, magnesium, calcium and selenium impact on numerous gastrointestinal and neurological processes. In particular, deficiencies in any of the vital nutrients just discussed can interfere with the body's ability to metabolize essential fatty acids. That can affect the immune and gastrointestinal systems and interfere with neurons, the message signaling transmitters to the brain. Study after study has revealed that not only autistic children, but also children with ADD and ADHD are lacking in key nutrients. When these nutrients are not present in the body or diet, cognitive function and behavior is adversely affected. If parents want their child to get better, it is absolutely vital to identify and correct nutritional deficiencies that interfere with the metabolism and functions for which certain nutrients are known to be necessary for optimal functioning.

Testing for Nutritional Deficiencies

Testing, as described in Chapter Four, usually starts with a routine complete blood count, urinalysis, a metabolic profile, and thyroid panel. This helps me see an iron deficiency as well as overall kidney, liver, thyroid and general health status. I list here again the particular tests that help to determine the optimum nutrient program for the ASD child (together with the medical and dietary history and clinical assessment):

- Fasting amino acid analysis (plasma), 40 better than 20.
- Organic acid analysis (OAT—urine), also called Organix.
- Fatty acid analysis (plasma)
- IgG (delayed) 90-food sensitivity test (serum)
- Red blood cell essential minerals (whole blood)
- Vitamin Panel, homocysteine, serum Vit D 25(OH) level

Red cell membranes can also be tested for fatty acid levels, but since we know almost all of our children are deficient, it is sometimes more prudent to provide the fatty acids and clinically observe the child's reactions. An RBC essential minerals analysis is performed as a monitoring test every few months when the child is undergoing chelation to make sure the mineral levels remain properly balanced. Occasionally, specific elements must be checked in a certain child such as cysteine, sulfates, and stool pH to help us fine-tune their supplement intake. Hair analysis is useful as a screen and can show overall imbalance patterns; this test serially can then be corroborated with more specific urine and blood testing if the child is not responding to the nutrient program in the way we had hoped.

Parents Say Nutrients Help Their Children

Some of the parents who come for evaluation seeking detoxification for their children from mercury reluctantly agree to the nutrient program when they find out it is a prerequisite to get to the magic "chelation therapy" they have heard about (see Chapter Seven). Many children improve so much on the nutrient program that some parents have questioned whether their child needs chelation. Actually, we know that the body will begin a detoxification process as the metabolism starts getting balanced, but this may be a very long process for most children. Since the parents want to maximize brain-healing without being required to indefinitely create special diets and give large doses of nutrients, almost all go on to a full supplement program to prepare their children for chelation. As they are also required to maintain the optimum diet for reducing gut inflammation and yeast overgrowth as well as administer probiotics regularly, they find the combination of this regime plus the supplements provides noticeable improvement in bowel function, cognition, and overall behavior. These parents did not realize the extent to which their children's brains were starving!

Here are some comments from just a few of those parents:

Sarah, the mother of 5 year-old Aaron reports, "In the past five or so days Aaron has taken a large leap forward. We see this mainly in language and abstract thinking. We are amazed at some of the things he is coming up with. We find ourselves just looking at each other with each new comment that he makes. We feel it is due to the supplements."

Janice, mother of 3-1/2 year old Terry, "We are faithfully following your recommendations since Terry has done nothing but improve dramatically since starting the supplements. He has been responding very well, with increased verbal skills which are surprising all of his therapists. He is listening better, repeating what I say as if he's absorbing new learning. It's very gratifying. Pronunciation is still rough, and he still has attention and processing issues. It will be exciting to see if we get even better results with the chelation process."

Darlene, mother of 4 year old Danny: "I think with all these supplements, Danny's overall performance has improved a lot already. Just this week, he started to use his gestures when he talks. This is something we have trained him to do for so long, and he just couldn't do before."

Joan, mother of 3 yr old Julia: "Within a week to ten days of starting the supplements, Julia has added 50 new words to her vocabulary. Her teachers are amazed and every day she seems to be coming up with new words we didn't even know she knew."

Marilyn, mother of 5 yr old Jimmy: "I never thought I'd be able to get all these pills down Jimmy, but once he knew he had to do it, he's being surprisingly willing. I think it's because he feels better and cares more about pleasing me and relating to all of us more than he ever has. He's definitely trying to talk more since we started the program. We are so pleased."

In summary, nutritional supplements can help alleviate the deficiencies so common in autism spectrum children. Nutritional imbalances are known to contribute to immune system abnormalities, pathogenic intestinal overgrowth, and impairment in detoxification. For those parents who do not choose to test their children, there are excellent neutraceutical companies that provide vitamin and mineral supplements specifically for ASD children. Supplement mixes are already made up that cover the most frequent types of deficiencies in the doses appropriate for the child's age, and I encourage all parents to get their child started on basic nutrients. Klaire Labs' recently developed Vita-Spectrum Complete which is my current favorite multiple and works well for many children; their probiotic line (Therbiotics) is excellent. To order directly from Klaire, call 888-488-2488 to get 20% off of all purchases by telling them I sent you - part of all profits go to basic autism research. Kirkman's Labs has dedicated itself to working with the autistic community to provide nutrients especially for this population. Kirkman's also provides a website with a compendium of autism information that may be downloaded for free. The nutrient companies I personally use the most are: Klaire Labs, Ecological Formulas, VRP (Vitamin Research Products), and Thorne Research. I am sure there are many good products and neutraceutical companies that I have not tested, but over the years I have worked out nutrient programs that experience has shown me will help most of the children I evaluate using the sources mentioned. Supplementation is emerging as an increasingly important means of treating autism, as we are learning more about the role of the affected gastrointestinal tract in this disorder.

References

[1] Reported by Woody McGinnis, MD, during presentation at October, 2001 Defeat Autism Now! conference, San Diego. For a review of published medical studies on the nutritional status of autistic and ADHD children see www.autism.com/mcginnis

[2] Walsh, William J. et al., Booklet, "Metallothionein and Autism," Pfeiffer Trtmt Ctr, Naperville IL, Oct. 2001

[3] Statement at the WHO Conference on Zinc and Human Health, Stockholm, 14th June 2000.

[4] Policy Statement, American Academy of Pediatrics, in the journal *Pediatrics*, 104, Number 5, November 1999, pp. 1152-1157.

SEVEN

REMOVING THE HEAVY METALS

Heavy Metal Toxicity

Imagine you are standing on a pier. Your child is drowning (he or she has developed autism or one of the other autism spectrum disorders) and you can't swim. You desperately look for help or a life preserver (a physician or treatments that might work). You find a rope tied to the pier (special diets, nutritional supplements, anti-fungal/anti-viral treatments, secretin, methylation, detoxification (formerly called chelation) for heavy metal toxicity—all of which you have learned are safe and help many of these children). However, authorities warn you not to use them because it has not been proven that the rope is strong enough (the treatment options have not received final approval by "authorities" who are waiting for reports of completed scientific studies appearing in peer-reviewed journals). Meanwhile your child is still drowning (exhibiting autistic/ASD symptoms).

If you were that parent on the pier you wouldn't wait for the completion of double-blind clinical trials to assure you that that rope is strong enough. You would pick it up and throw it to your child. The worst that could happen is that the rope would break with your child closer to the pier! In real life, numerous parents, some of whom are physicians, have been finding that removing toxic metals is an effective treatment for their children. Parents of ASD children cannot afford to wait for approval of the guiding agencies appointed to protect our children's health to try treatment options these agencies consider "alternative medicine," particularly when the "traditional experts" have nothing better to offer. This is especially true as the parents learn that the very actions they dutifully followed on the recommendation of these authoritative agencies may have been the cause of their child's autism, such as accepting the mandate that their newborn be vaccinated with unsafe levels of ethylmercury via the HepB vaccine. The case for mercury-triggered ASD has been made in Chapter Three; further details are provided in Appendix B and C provided by researcher Teresa Binstock.

There is tremendous variability among individuals in the capacity to naturally eliminate toxic metals. Hence a similar level of exposure can result in very different levels of net retention among different people; in some the exposure might be benign whereas in others it may have catastrophic effects. There must be some threshold level of retention of metals before toxicity is expressed. Importantly, toxicity is exhibited for an individual when the level of retention exceeds the individual's physiological tolerance. As we discussed in Chapter Three, many and probably most ASD children have impaired detoxification capability. This means that the child has reduced ability to sequester and/or eliminate toxic substances. Heavy metals merit special concern because they are present in increasing amounts in the environment of our technological society. The child's impaired detoxification appears to derive from several possible sources, including genetic susceptibility to toxic influences, especially early immune injury, and "mild" or not so mild intestinal pathologies with subsequent effects on nutritional status and immune function. Chelation-efficacy studies already presented to the Institute of Medicine and at an international conference support a new model: many autism-spectrum children have impairments causally related to the child's excessive accumulation of toxic metals. Also important is the fact that, along with removing excess accumulation of heavy metals, many children's biomedical profiles often reveal other underlying pathologies (e.g. methylation defects) that, when treated, improve the child's gastrointestinal health, immunity, and capability for further detoxification. As stated before and probably many times in this book, the most likely cause of autism is a combination of genetic vulnerability and environmental triggers, e.g. toxic adjuvants in vaccinations.

A Practical Approach to the Removal of Mercury

Although occasionally described as an "alternative" therapy, oral detoxification with the use of oral chelating agents has been well studied and found to be both safe and effective for children. However, many physicians are not even aware that detoxification mechanisms are impaired in almost every autistic child evaluated, and very few physicians are trained to conduct or oversee a chelation protocol. It is important to stress that the use of chelating agents to detoxify ASD children should always be preceded by gut-healing, nutritional correction, and as much general improvement in the child's immune system as is possible. In fact, the preparation for chelation often enables the detoxification mechanisms to start improving on their own. I have seen this happen many times in my practice; the desire for this kind of treatment will finally motivate the parents to do a strict diet and place their children on the nutritional supplements they need to start getting better. Almost all children improve on the preparation process even before actually starting the detoxification protocol.

Currently, DMSA[1] is the primary substance that I and other Defeat Autism Now! practitioners use to remove mercury and other heavy metals from our children if testing shows they are heavy-metal poisoned. DMSA binds toxic metals, especially lead and mercury, and enables them to be eliminated from the body, primarily through the urine. Also known as Chemet, the prescription form made by Sanofi Pharmaceuticals, DMSA was approved in 1998 by the FDA for the removal of lead from the bodies of children; its safety in children is well studied and documented. Fortunately, DMSA also binds other heavy metals, particularly mercury, although the process must be carried out with caution, since chelation also may remove other essential minerals needed by the body. If a child's medical history supported by laboratory testing indicates the presence of heavy metals, I use a protocol of oral chelation with DMSA in the first phase of the detoxification process. The child needs to be well mineralized prior to starting; during chelation, nutritional status and metal-profiles are monitored with regular lab tests.

I was moved to start using chelation therapy in my practice after hearing reports about the success that Dr. Amy Holmes and Dr. Stephanie Cave were having in improving the health and behavior of autistic children through the removal of mercury and other metals by chelation. The mother of an autistic son, Dr. Holmes left retirement not long after her son was diagnosed with autism to join Dr. Stephanie Cave's medical practice in Baton Rouge, LA.

In October 2000, Dr. Cave spoke at an autism conference prompted by Bernard et al's autism/thimerosal paper (see Appendix B) and hosted by the National Institute of Environmental Health Sciences. The meeting's primary focus was the possible role of mercury in the causation of autism. She told the group that in her experience over a number of years of treating over 400 autistic children with various modalities, she had found no treatment more effective in a great many of those children than removing toxic metals via chelation.[2]

I had been corresponding by e-mail with Dr. Holmes about other treatments we were both using or considering around the time she was starting to chelate her own son and was impressed with her candor and courage as well as her careful and scientific approach to this new and exciting protocol. I knew she would not do anything that would harm her son who was her first chelation patient. Dr. Holmes inspired me to start chelation therapy with my granddaughter Chelsey, who was my first chelation patient and already six years old by that time. Evidence indicates that the older the children are, the slower they excrete the metals, but I believe it is better late than never to get their toxic load down as much as possible. Chelsey's progress was slow compared with the very young children I began chelating subsequently. We still use chelation with Chelsey and have off and on through the years, with several long breaks along the way for other treatments. Chelsey was not one of the dramatic responders to this intervention as she was to dietary restriction; autism is extremely complex and responses to various therapeutic interventions is very different with different children.

Detoxification is not simple, and though there are various chelation protocols available for adults, there were no well-known chelation protocols in place for treatment of children prior to 1999 except for lead removal. Despite Stephen Edelson's 1998 study, only a few people were beginning to realize that mercury probably played a role in our current epidemic of "regressive" autism.[3] In response to that situation, Dr. Bernard Rimland, director of the Autism Research Institute (ARI), convened a Consensus Conference on the Detoxification of Autistic Children in Dallas, Texas, February 9-11, 2001. The attendees included 25 carefully selected physicians and scientists knowledgeable about mercury and mercury detoxification, including Dr. Holmes and Dr. Cave. The fifteen physicians present included seven who were parents of autistic children who had detoxified their own kids with excellent results. The physicians present had treated well over 3,000 patients for heavy metal poisoning, about 1,500 of them being autistic children. The chemists, toxicologists, and other scientists present had a combined total of almost 90 years of experience in studying the toxicology of mercury. The purpose of the meeting was to arrive at a consensus document that would delineate the safest and most effective methods for detoxifying autistic children; this document was revised in 2005 and will soon be undergoing another revision.[4]

The oral chelation protocol I have been using is based on the consensus information gathered 1st at the 2001 conference and enlarged upon for the 2005 revision. It is called simply the Defeat Autism Now! consensus for chelation. Of course, since each autism-spectrum child is unique, we all use the protocol simply as a guide. Each physician needs to integrate the protocol's guidelines with considerations specific to the child being chelated. In other words, this consensus-protocol was written as guidance and not as law. I make allowances for differences in response, age, desire of the parents, and other individual circumstances in the child's history and current medical status to alter the protocol as my clinical judgment dictates. The chelation-protocol's authors emphasize that the treatment of autism is in a state of continual flux and recommendations concerning the protocol will continue to evolve as more is learned about autism's various biomedical subgroups. As mentioned before, I ask the reader to take the recommendations in this book in the same spirit. The protocol document also states that the evidence that chelation is beneficial is largely based on clinical experience although the theories and medical models on which the therapy is based are being vigorously studied by a number of researchers. An oral DMSA chelation study is currently underway being conducted by Dr. James Adams at the University of Arizona; the results of that study will have to appear in a future edition.

Even if the child's initial evaluation indicates the presence of mercury, I do not initiate chelation therapy right away. Often parents hearing of this treatment want to bring their child in to just "get the metals out." Sometimes they are impatient when they find that much work has to be done to ready the child for this kind of treatment. The child's intestinal health, nutritional status, and immunity must be optimized. These goals need to be achieved before the child can be considered for chelation. Many of us have learned the hard way that unless the child is at least relatively free of gastrointestinal pathogen overgrowth when we start, chelation with DMSA is likely to make the situation worse (as sulfur agents support yeast growth), to the point of making our chelating efforts less successful. This effect of the overgrowth of yeast and other intestinal pathogens is one of the factors leading to a search for other means of handling the toxicity issue and will be discussed further at the end of the chapter. For the children with more mature gastrointestinal systems who do not succumb to gut pathogen overgrowth problems in the process, I still believe at this time that the process I am about to describe is the safest and best way for most Defeat Autism Now! practitioners to get the metal load down in a way that leads to improvement in most children given this treatment. However, recently much work has been done with rectal suppository and intravenous chelation protocols in addition to the oral use of Ca-EDTA and DMPS, and with DMSA for the suppository route (DMSA cannot be given IV). The IV treatments are often followed by glutathione infusions and sometimes nutrients, especially Vitamin C, as well. More will be said about these protocols later. For a period, many parents were trying the transdermal use of DMSA and DMPS to chelate their children, but repeated urine output studies showed very little excretion with this route compared to the oral, rectal, and IV methods. Though these agents are still available at compounding pharmacies in transdermal forms, relatively few doctors or parents want to continue this route even though it is easy and non-invasive when they find out the success the community is having with the other approaches. The consensus of most of the Defeat Autism Now! group now is that the transdermal approach is not the best and most efficient method of chelating our children.

Pre-Chelation Testing

I often include the hair analysis with the routine tests I order for the evaluation. The CBC and Chemistry Panel must be repeated just prior to starting chelation unless they have been done within the previous two months and results are within normal limits. If there is any evidence of abnormal values, these must be corrected prior to starting the detoxification process, e.g. the use of milk thistle to regenerate liver, iron supplementation for severe anemia, and mineral replacement for any other deficiencies. In addition to the routine evaluation tests (if not already done), I recommend the following:

- **Hair Analysis**: This is an informative, non-invasive and inexpensive screening test (around $50 if paid when sample submitted). Hair elemental analysis provides a qualitative assessment of exposure, and if collected from about one inch of the scalp, can indicate exposure that occurred over approximately the preceding 3 months. I order this from Doctor's Data Lab (DD) for several reasons: They have the biggest data base of hair analyses in the world, and Dr. Andrew Cutler taught me how to interpret their particular way of reporting. Dr. Cutler's reading is based on what is known about heavy metals' effects on essential minerals in the body. As a screen, if the lab results do not concur with what I am seeing clinically and historically, I can use further testing to corroborate the finding. *Anecdotal data from Dr. Holmes' large data base indicate that many ASD kids have lower levels of toxic metals in hair as compared to siblings and parents, which may turn out to be an indication of impaired detoxification.* This corroborates mineral evidence of toxicity with no or little mercury showing in the hair excretion.

Technique: Parents are given a kit with a small scale they use with very clear instructions about what hair to cut. The hair sample is mailed directly to the lab for analysis. Doctor's Data will send reports to the ordering physician, who receives two copies, one to give to the parents for their child's medical file.

- **Porphyrin testing:** The urinary porphyrin test is newly being explored by the Defeat Autism Now! group now as a biomarker of environmental toxicity. This test measures the presence of porphyrins, a chemical ring structure that the body uses to make hemoglobin. It is the "heme" of hemoglobin. Hemoglobin is a porphyrin ring with iron in the middle. Mercury and other toxins interfere with the production of porphyrin at specific places on the ring. The result is malformed or incompletely formed porphyrin that the body excretes because it cannot use it to build hemoglobin. Mercury is thought to interfere with porphyrin production at the fifth and sixth step, resulting in excretion of the unfinished porphyrin. The urine test detects specific incomplete, unusable porphyrins discarded before the disrupted step which denote the presence of mercury. Other toxins disrupt production at other junctures, resulting in the elevation of different porphyrins. An article in March 2006 by Dr. Robert Nataf et al at the Philippe Auguste Laboratory in Paris, France written in Toxicology and Applied Pharmacology described studies comparing porphyrin levels on autistic and control groups. The coproporphyrin levels were elevated in children with autism relative to controls. Following treatment of the autistic group with oral DMSA a significant drop in urinary porphyrin excretion was shown. U.S. labs (Lab Corp, Quest Labs, Metametrix, and Great Plains) now offer tests that measure porphyrins in both blood and urine, but at this point they have limited experience with the test. Philippe Auguste Laboratory in Paris has broader experience with the testing and provides clearer results, and most of us are sending our children's urine samples to this lab for analysis so far. Some Defeat Autism Now! clinicians believe that when chelation is thought to be completed because no mercury is still being excreted in the urine, that a porphyrin test will give even better evidence that chelation is ready to be terminated than our usual post-provocative test. Parents or doctors may send a urine sample by regular air mail and it takes a week to 10 days to process. Contact them for kits at: contact@labbio.net. At this time, the test costs about $125 plus shipping.

- **Pre- and Post-Challenge Urine Toxic Elements Test**: This testing is not actually necessary for many children, but it can be convincing for parents who doubt that their child could possibly have mercury poisoning. It is the most definitive test for estimating the net retention/body burden of toxic metals. Urinary testing is more reliable than hair which can pick up environmental contaminants in shampoos, for example, or copper in swimming pools. The "provocation tests" work because the agents are able to bind metals that are sequestered in deep tissue stores, those that are not in circulation. The most productive agents for mobilizing mercury are DMPS and DMSA, and both work well when given orally. For DMPS, IV is thought by many clinicians to be even better than oral for the provocation testing. Since the mid 1950s, the CDC has advocated the use of post-Ca-EDTA urinary lead for the diagnosis of lead toxicity; this agent is starting to be used for treatment for lead toxicity in autistic children more and more now as well, with excellent results being reported. A tragedy in the community occurred last year when a human error in judgment was made and the incorrect solution of EDTA was given a child, Sodium-EDTA rather than Ca-EDTA, and the child went into heart failure and died. For awhile many in the community were intimidated from using IV methods, but as we all learned more, the success and the huge dumps of mercury and lead with the IV methods are bringing more and more parents and doctors to this method of lowering the heavy metal loads in their children. All of these agents are very safe when used correctly.

Pre-Challenge Technique: A urine sample is collected in the morning in the kit provided by the lab and placed in the refrigerator.

Post-challenge: A one-time dose of oral DMSA (10mg/kg) or 5-10 mg/kg rectally, or DMPS 5-10mg orally or l.5mg/kg rectally or, or IV DMPS or IV Ca-EDTA is administered and urine collected for six hours in a large orange plastic bottle, carefully measured and recorded. A portion of the urine is placed in the small bottle in the second kit and both bottles clearly labeled are put back into the kits along with the physician's requisition specifying which tests are wanted. All samples are kept refrigerated until Airborne Express comes to pick them up in the plastic bags provided in the kits by the lab.

- **RBC Essential Elements:** Many ASD children are depleted in essential minerals. This test helps assess whether the child is low in magnesium, selenium, zinc etc. and helps guide the nutrient program. The child needs to be well mineralized prior to starting chelation and monitored periodically (every 3-6 months) during chelation. Meta-Metrix and Doctors Data Labs do this test.

- **Cysteine:** This can be done as part of a Great Smokies Lab (name has now been changed to Genova Diagnostic Labs, same phone number) Detoxification profile and helps determine whether the child would benefit from glutathione, N-acetyl cysteine (NAC), or high sulfur foods in the diet. Those with high cysteine levels may have negative reactions to sulfur compounds and sulfury foods and sometimes to oral or transdermal glutathione. For those low in cysteine (the majority of ASD children) there is much benefit from NAC because it can rapidly elevate intracellular glutathione levels which are essential in detoxification processes. However, some children become very hyperactive on NAC or on glutathione; for some kids it may be better to use these later in the chelation cycle after the load of mercury is down.

Gut Readiness Before Starting Chelation

In Chapter Five we discussed the high occurrence of intestinal yeast colonizations and other intestinal pathologies in ASD children. In fact, medical histories suggest that early immune impairment is almost ubiquitous among these children, as indicated by repeated ear infections and/or gut dysfunction. In the Defeat Autism Now! chelation consensus document it states that attempting heavy metal detoxification before the patient's underlying gastrointestinal and nutritional problems are corrected will likely be disappointing. Please refer to Chapter Five for details about treating gut dysfunction.

- **Organic Acid Test (OAT):** If the child has had overgrowth of yeast or other pathogens, he/she will already have been placed on a strong dietary and probiotic program to get this controlled. A repeat OAT is highly recommended just prior to starting chelation to make sure the gut is in good shape for the process. I personally use Metametrix Organix and feel it gives me the most information for treatment guidance than almost any other test in my armamentarium (though Doctor's Data is preferable for toxicity testing).

- **Comprehensive Microbial Digestive Stool Analysis:** If difficulties in overgrowth of pathogens occurs, stool studies may reveal sensitivities and help determine which anti-fungals, anti-bacterials, and anti-parasitic medications are appropriate for the child's treatment. Earlier in my work with ASD children, if the OAT (Organic Acid Test) was normal (which is unusual), I would not usually order fecal studies unless the child had bowel dysfunction in the form of diarrhea, constipation, excessive gas or bloating, reflux, or stomach pain. However, I have recently had some cases where this testing showed parasites that do not put out known metabolites in the urine as yeast and many bacteria do, and more often now I may routinely order this in my evaluation. ASD children tend to put things in their mouths excessively and are apt to pick up parasites that can set up residence in the already compromised gut; these infestations need treatment. I like Doctor's Data for this analysis, though different doctors have their own preferences, sometimes based on insurability.

Nutrient/Mineralization Readiness

Children with mercury or other heavy metal accumulation need early biomedical intervention to help their gastrointestinal, immune, and neurological systems to heal and begin functioning properly. As I have explained in previous chapters, this often means special vitamins and minerals are needed to offset the chemical aberrations associated with the mercury-induced injuries and the subsequent neurological dysfunction. Because of poor nutrition and absorption, many ASD children have numerous mineral deficiencies, zinc and selenium being two of the most important ones.

- **Zinc** needs to be given prior to, during and after detoxification therapy along with all the other vitamins and minerals. (Please see Chapter Four for specific recommendations and specific testing to guide supplementation.) Supplementation with 1-2mg/kg/day of zinc is recommended; more may be needed if testing shows a marked deficiency. Many children are worked up to one mg per pound plus 15-20mg of zinc a day in preparation for chelation. The RBC essential minerals test allows such judgments to be made more precisely. It is preferable for zinc to be given alone (not with calcium or other minerals) for most efficient absorption.

- **Selenium** is one of the few nutrients that can cause toxicity if given in excess and should be limited to 1-4mcg/lb/day unless there is laboratory evidence of a profound deficiency. Again, occasional RBC minerals lab-tests allow monitoring of selenium levels and staying at or under 200mcg a day is safe.

- **Other minerals** may be deficient in ASD children. Molybdenum, manganese, vanadium and chromium, along with zinc, can be obtained in a multi-mineral supplement. For a comprehensive trace mineral product I use Thorne's Pic-Mins. Excessive copper is neurotoxic and often elevated in ASD children. Any multiple vitamin should be free of copper. Extra molybdenum along with adequate zinc may help children with high copper levels. There are many good multi-vitamin/mineral supplements; my favorite is Ecological Formulas Hypomultiple (without copper or iron). Iron levels are often somewhat low in many of these children, but unless excessively so, I do not usually supplement it, as too much iron can stress the oxidative mechanisms and the deficiency is seen by some as the body's way to conserve energy.

To repeat: All supplements important to a good and balanced nutritional program should be well in place prior to chelation. If nutritional deficiencies have not been corrected, important physiological mechanisms that support detoxification may not function properly. Because the ASD child's diet is often limited, mineralization with supplements becomes even more important as some necessary minerals may be taken out of the body through the chelation process.

- **Vitamins:** Many ASD children are deficient in vitamins for the same reasons they are low in minerals: poor diet, and poor absorption. Tests show that many children are deficient in Vitamin B6, B12, folic acid, and niacin. These should be given routinely, beginning with the child's preliminary work-up (after testing) recommendations. Please see Chapter Four for guidelines. Vitamins C, E, and B6 and other B vitamins are particularly important to keep well supplied during chelation. Vitamin C is known to be an aid to detoxification and is non-toxic other than causing loose stools; I usually recommend C be given at least 3X/day in as high a dose as tolerated short of diarrhea.

Heavy Metal Detoxification per 2005 Defeat Autism Now! Consensus, Summary

Though DMPS (2,3 dimercaptopropane sulfonate) is known to be a good mercury chelator, it has never been formally tested on children. Therefore until safety testing has been done on DMPS, DMSA remains the primary chelator recommended by the Defeat Autism Now! Protocol for the beginning phase of the chelation process and the agent I routinely use, either orally or rectally. DMSA is safe, effective, and has been tested rigorously for use in children. However, I have occasionally used oral DMPS with good results in some of my older children whose progress has slowed down on DMSA, sometimes with a notable spurt in mercury elimination per urine testing. In 2004 many parents began using transdermal DMPS and DMSA; as I mentioned transdermal forms eventually were shown to be less effective with much less excretion of mercury in most children given this protocol. Oral and rectal routes have been shown to be more effective and IV infusions have become much more popular and more effective than transdermal methods of chelation at the present time. IV CA-EDTA and DMPS are particularly useful for challenge testing to reveal the degree of mercury and other heavy metal toxicity, and are being used more and more for treatment as well as provocation. All practitioners do not feel comfortable using IV medications, with varying enthusiasm for the suppository protocols, but for those who do use either of these, the evidence of metal excretion and reports of improvement are impressive.

After DMSA has cleared the body of "loose" mercury or other toxic metals as shown by lab testing (usually urinary), some clinicians begin a second phase of chelation therapy by adding another chelator, Alpha-lipoic acid (ALA) in an amount usually 1/6 to 1/2 of the dosage of DMSA. Unlike DMSA, ALA is believed to cross the blood brain barrier (BBB) and bind with mercury to remove it from the brain, though there remains controversy on this point. ALA is a nutrient in many foods and can be purchased from any good health food store, although it can also be compounded in exactly the strength needed for the weight of the child. Currently, most Defeat Autism Now! practitioners feel that ALA should not be used prior to DMSA chelation, because ALA can bind to a toxic metal in the body's periphery, some of the ALA-bound metal may cross the blood-brain-barrier, thereby possibly reentering the child's brain. In other words, ALA therapy should follow thorough DMSA chelation. Some practitioners do not agree with this and prefer to give ALA throughout chelation; some parents (usually those who do not have access to a supervisory doctor) have chosen to use ALA only, without clearing out the body mercury with DMSA. ALA has been noted to cause increased "stimming" in some children, probably due to it's yeast encouraging potential; transdermal ALA may help with this problem.

Phase I, DMSA Dosages and Timing: I basically use the 3 days on, 11 days off schedule for chelation except for special situations. This allows the parents to give the first dose on Friday around noon for children who are not in school, and in the afternoon for those who are, continuing either every 4 or 8 hours as directed for the particular child. There is some difference of opinion as to which of these timing schedules are the best, with some very substantial arguments by knowledgeable persons advocating each timing. I find myself often using the more frequent timing with smaller doses for smaller children and the lower frequency with larger doses for larger children, unless side effects or lack of progress indicate it may be better to give more frequent doses. I usually explain the different points of view to the parents and let them decide since there is evidence that both schedules work. I make it clear that we can always change the timing if experience indicates more frequent dosing might work better or longer periods between doses (much easier for all concerned) will work just as well. Again, there are differences of opinion about dosing; I tend to start very low and gradually work upward to the suggested amounts in the protocol per clinical results and lab testing, based on weight of the child. The point of the first phase is to remove as much body mercury and other toxic metals as possible, as DMSA cannot cross the blood brain barrier to remove it from the brain.

- **Dosages, DMSA:** Doses based on weight for 8 hour schedules are as follows for three days on and eleven days off: (Divide in half for 4 hour dosing frequency)

  20-40 lbs. : 100mg.
  (especially for the smaller children, I start with half)
  40-50 lbs. : 200mg.
  50-60 lbs. : 250mg.
  60-70 lbs. : 300mg.
  70-80 lbs. : 350mg.
  80-100 lbs. : 500mg.
  >100 lbs. : 500mg.

- **Lab Monitoring:** I recommend urine testing (Urine Toxic Elements done by Doctor's Data Lab) after the 1st or 2nd two-week cycle, then every 3rd or 4th two-week cycle done on the 2nd day of the 3-day cycle several hours after the morning dose. I have found the random urines are as useful as the 6-hour collections I used to get, and much easier on the parents and child. Urine collection bags must be requested from the lab for children that are not potty-trained. This testing continues until the body mercury or other toxic metals are gone or extremely low and it is safe to give ALA without the danger of carrying ALA-bound toxic metal or "loose mercury" back into the brain. Usually after 10-12 two-week cycles the child's body is free of mercury, some are free after 7-8 cycles, and some take longer than 12 cycles. If pathogen overgrowth occurs, chelation must stop until that is addressed.

  Every 2-3 months while chelating I order "safety" testing: a CBC and Chemistry Panel performed to make sure blood, liver, kidneys etc are not being harmed. An RBC Essential Elements Test is helpful every 2-6 months throughout the process to help monitor mineral status; this can be done along with the routine tests every 2nd or 3rd time. (When aluminum is high, the nutrient Malic Acid is reported to be very effective in reducing aluminum levels; food from metal cans is to be avoided.) ALA is the best chelator for arsenic.

- **Readiness for Second Phase: Adding A-lipoic Acid (ALA):** It is time to go on to the second phase when little or no more mercury is coming out as assessed by the Urine Toxic Elements test. DMSA pulls out most heavy metals in no particular order. If there are large amounts of lead or tin coming out, DMSA should be used until these are not being excreted in large amounts, as they may be "hiding" mercury and have been shown to slow down Phase II if not reduced to low level before starting the ALA. (If very large amounts of lead are starting to come out, sometimes showing up only after quite a few cycles, I sometimes give a long course of DMSA (17 days straight) to get the lead down before proceeding to Phase II. It is important that the parents become detectives to make sure their child is not being exposed to lead anywhere in his or her environment.) In addition to the metals mercury, tin, and lead being low, the child must have good metabolic test results and the gut must be in good shape, because ALA is notorious for "feeding intestinal pathogens," and severe yeast and Clostridia overgrowth can take place if not carefully monitored. Signs of pathogen overgrowth include bowel dysfunction or plateau or even regression in chelation effects. In my experience diligent probiotics, GF/CF diet, and sugar removal from the diet really pay off in terms of shortening the time for the chelation process. Many children have to endure long delays to take care of the "bad gut bugs." Many practitioners have abandoned the use of ALA for this reason.

- **Second Phase, Laboratory Monitoring:** DMSA dumps metals into urine, making lab testing fairly simple with the Urine Toxic Metals test. Once we add ALA, most metals are sequestered into the bile and then excreted through the stool. During the ALA phase, urine tests tend not to show mercury any more; thus the best way to test for excretion is through the Fecal Metal test also done by Doctor's Data Lab. Stool transit times vary and catching the metal output by stools is difficult. The test is done on Day 4, the 1st day after completing the three day cycle. Once children are out of diapers and particularly with bigger children, collecting stool samples can be fairly daunting for the parents. However, we only ask parents to do this test every 4-6 months. Recently I have been using serial hair analyses for the Phase II testing and, though it is less accurate than the stools test (if you happen to catch a sample at the right time!), I get useful information that combined with assessment from the parents and teachers help us to see what is happening. "Safety testing" is done every few months routinely. As time goes on I mainly do testing when there is a plateau in improvement or a regression (often caused by gut bugs). In addition to the lab test data, other useful information often comes from parents and teachers, whose assessments of the child's behavior and learning abilities provide an additional monitor about the effectiveness of the child's chelation therapy. Occasionally, a child experiences a regression while undergoing chelation. Many clinicians report that the regression is most likely due to a resurgence of intestinal pathogenic colonization. Albeit rare, other regressions have been noted for which we have no ready explanation. Parents and physicians need to be alert throughout the chelation process.

For ALA doses, use 1/6 to 1/2 the amount of DMSA for the child's weight; ALA and DMSA are given together either every 4 hours or every eight hours as the parents and I have agreed, 3 days on,11 days off. Be watchful of gut issues.

- **Completion of the Chelation Process:** Chelation is usually terminated when the child has "plateaued" and is no longer showing obvious changes in behavior and language. For some autism-spectrum children, this improvement is sufficient so that the child can be "mainstreamed" in school. Many children have outgrown their diagnoses as autistic. We usually say the detoxification work takes six months to two years and maybe longer for older children. Parental and clinical assessment is more important here than mercury excretion dropping below detectable limits as measured by lab testing.

On rare occasions, an autism-spectrum child undergoing chelation experiences an unexplainable but sustained regression. Though this may be confused with regressive episodes or traits (mainly hyperactivity, increase in self-stimulatory activity) at the beginning of DMSA treatment and also at the beginning of the ALA treatment, there are often improvements in language and sociability simultaneously that make parents want to keep going. Several children in my practice (as in those of other clinicians) have had difficulty when starting ALA; our first thought was that metals were being moved around. We came to discover that the most common reason was pathogen overgrowth, though we were not certain of this being the cause in every case. Sometimes we just cannot find out why the children stop improving and start regressing to previous levels, reminding us that there is still a lot unknown about this complex process. Treatments to eradicate pathogens in difficult cases can take months, and parents who had been seeing remarkable gains with their children prior to the pathogen invasion find themselves impatient to get on with the chelation. New therapeutic approaches are being explored and created as fast as possible to deal with these pathogen episodes. Many different patterns have emerged, such as keeping children on anti-fungals for months at a time, and many explorations of new anti-bacterials and anti-fungals.

Obviously the younger the children the easier it is to treat them and the faster they are able to excrete the metals. Sometimes the gains are uneven; some children become more sociable as their first improvement, others show expansion of language capabilities with receptivity (understanding what is being said to them) being one of the first improvements that many parents report. Expressive language and improvements in pronunciation seem to be the most difficult to achieve as noted in many other ASD treatments. It is very helpful to compare reports by the child's teacher as a check on the parents' and doctor's assessment as to progress.

In the name of safety, chelation, as we are learning to do it right now, usually needs to be a long, sometimes drawn-out process. Though I tell parents it may take from 6 months to two years for the younger kids and even longer for the older children, every child is so different that this period varies considerably. Many of the children the Defeat Autism Now! clinicians have been working with currently are markedly improved or have recovered or improved so much that the parents and I feel they are well on their way toward recovery. Some children respond very quickly, others move much more slowly. I cannot predict how any particular child may respond.

Alternative Detoxification Treatment

ALLITHIAMINE: TRANSDERMAL THIAMINE TETRAHYDROFURFURYL DISULFIDE (TTFD)

Recent research has shown that a chemical closely related to allithiamine is useful in treating autistic children.[5,6] Derrick Lonsdale, M.D. has described beneficial effects in ASD children with thiamine tetrahydrofurfuryl disulfide (TTFD), the synthetic counterpart of a naturally occurring disulfide derivative of thiamine (vitamin B1) found in the allium species of plants. The best known of these plants is garlic. Other disulfides of the vitamin (S-S) have been synthesized and TTFD is the most modern of these. The naturally occurring molecule is known as allithiamine, named thus because of its presence in these plants.

Thiamine is composed of two rings, one of them being 5-sided, called a thiazolium, because it contains a sulfur atom. This ring can open and a number of different prosthetic groups can be attached to the sulfur atom. Hence there are several other synthetic compounds that are not disulfides, known as S-acyl derivatives (SAT). The best known of these is S-benzoylthiamine monophosphate (Benfotiamine).

Lonsdale et al suggest three possible sulfur-related mechanisms to account for TTFD's beneficial effects in autism. First, TTFD may improve energy metabolism in the CNS. Second, TTFD functions as a chelating (more properly, extracting) agent; several metals—with arsenic the most common—were documented at increased levels in urinary excretions. Third, 3 of the 10 children had indications of "intracellular thiamine deficiency," which the TTFD may have alleviated.[6]

Lonsdale's view is that it is TTFD's disulfide bond that is broken at the cell membrane. The thiamine molecule, consisting of a pyridinium ring and a thiazolium ring joined by a methylene bridge, passes through the membrane and the thiazolium ring closes. TTFD does not require the transport system needed for water-soluble thiamine that is rate limiting for the usual method of getting thiamine into the cell. Thus, a large concentration of thiamine is built up inside the cell where it is capable of stimulating thiamine-dependent activity. This includes the formation of thiamine triphosphate which is essential as a phosphate donor in synthesizing ATP and is important for mitochondrial energy synthesis. The tetrahydrofurfuryl moiety stays outside the cell and becomes a mercaptan. It is probably this that binds the SH-reactive metals and is the "business end" of the molecule. Though it is clear that TTFD is "chelating" SH-reactive metals, we still do not know about redistribution of the mercury:mercaptan complex into brain tissue with this agent any more than is the case with the other commonly used "chelators." Notable excretion of metals appear on urine testing, especially arsenic, cadmium, nickel, lead, and mercury.

Why is there an important difference between S-S and SAT compounds? To answer this requires a little history, for the great interest in thiamine was generated in Japan because of the disease known as Beriberi. Lack of thiamine is the major cause of this disease and for centuries it had been occurring mainly because of the ingestion of white rice as a staple in the diet. Thiamine and other B group vitamins are contained in the rice husks that surround the grain. Milling removes the husks to create white rice and this was done because it looked better when served.

In the middle of the 20th century, after the discovery of thiamine, an organization known as the Vitamin B Research Committee was formed and this resulted in a book that provides details of research performed in both human subjects and animals. A chapter in this book describes the detailed research applicable to the differences between the S-S and SAT derivatives[7].

First, it must be stressed that absorption from the intestine, by diffusion, of both the S-S and SAT compounds gives rise to greater blood concentrations of thiamine than the original thiamine from which they are constructed. The major difference between them is the disulfide bond since this is an important factor in normal cell membrane physiology. When TTFD comes into contact with cell membranes the S-S bond is fractured. One fragment passes through the membrane and the thiazolium ring closes to form an intact molecule of thiamine inside the cell where its action is needed. The prosthetic group, the tetrahydrofurfuryl moiety is left outside the cell and becomes a thiol known as a mercaptan. Enzymatic cleavage in liver is required for the similar breakdown of SATs and there is no resulting mercaptan produced. The released thiamine molecule then has to be absorbed into the cells that require its action, using the same less efficient transport system that enables the absorption of ordinary thiamine as it occurs naturally in foods. To our knowledge, no work has been published as to the fate of the prosthetic group resulting from the cleavage of the SATs.

Japanese investigators found that this made a major difference in the clinical behavior of these two groups of thiamine derived vitamers. The term vitamer is used to indicate a formula that gives rise to a vitamin in its normal course of action. They researched these biological effects in detail. Animal studies revealed that the S-S vitamers provided partial protection from the toxic effects of trichloroethylene, carbon tetrachloride and cyanide. The SAT vitamers did not have this effect and they concluded that it was the S-S bond that created the difference[7].

We can think of TTFD as an easy delivery system for incorporating vitamin B1 into cells. Thiamine normally requires a transport system for its absorption across cell membranes. The disulfide enables the vitamin to pass into cells without the requirement of this transport system which has a rate limiting ability. Administering TTFD therefore makes it possible to concentrate thiamine inside the cell, giving it a therapeutic range that cannot be achieved as easily with ordinary thiamine.

What happens to the mercaptan moiety that is left outside the cell when TTFD comes into contact with cell membranes? The Japanese investigators did a great deal of research on this. They found that it was non toxic and was broken down by a series of enzymes to sulfates and sulfones and excreted in urine[8-11].

How does this relate to the treatment of Autistic Spectrum Disorder (ASD)? Since there is evidence that mercury and other SH-reactive heavy metals play an important part in the underlying cause, we have to look at the ways and means of chelating these metals and excreting them. Their SH-reactivity is the key to understanding their toxicity. Animal studies have shown that EDTA, a well known chelating agent for lead, given in conjunction with thiamine, removes experimentally induced lead from sheep through excretion via bile and urine[12]. The combination of the two agents was better than one of them alone so it can be said that thiamine does indeed remove this SH-reactive metal although the exact mechanism is unknown. A pilot study, using TTFD in the form of rectal suppositories, showed that there was a measurable clinical improvement in 8 of 10 children so treated[6]. Studies of urine samples showed concomitantly increased excretion of one or more of the SH- reactive metals, lead, mercury, arsenic and cadmium.

Although the therapeutic effect of TTFD certainly depends on the intracellular action of thiamine[8], the prosthetic group may play a part in its role as a mercaptan. One of the side effects of transdermally administered TTFD, but not when it is taken by mouth, is a skunk-like odor emitted from the patient. The secretion of skunks that gives rise to its characteristic odor is because it consists of several organic mercaptans. Their olfactory stimulation is caused by vanishingly low concentrations, as we all know. Several observations have been made by clinicians using transdermal TTFD. The skunk-like odor is considered to be due to the action of a mercaptan, a logical deduction in view of what has just been said. The odor seems to occur in specific patients and is not completely predictable. Furthermore, it gradually decreases as the patient improves clinically, thus suggesting that the reaction is tied to the abnormal biochemistry of the patient. The administration of 10 mg of biotin by mouth, a member of the B group vitamins, often will remove the odor rapidly. Another observation made by the parent of a child with ASD is that lemon juice applied to the skin also will reduce the odor. The mechanism is unknown.

It is possible to suggest that TTFD has a special role because of the formation of a thiol mercaptan in the prosthetic group. There is much evidence that ASD is causatively associated with what is known as oxidative stress, a phenomenon that is known to be related to a number of diseases, particularly of the central nervous system and brain. Put into ordinary language, it means that the utilization of oxygen in body cells is inefficient. The primary biological counterpart to oxidation by reactive nitrogen species (RNS) and reactive oxygen species (ROS) is reduction (i.e. antioxidation) by thiols, also known as mercaptans (9). This author goes on to note that these sulfur-containing molecules can donate an electron in order to quench a free radical, themselves becoming oxidized in the process. They are therefore potent antioxidants, a term that we associate with the actions of vitamins C and E, for example. In addition, although experimental evidence is unfortunately lacking, it is probable that at least part of the increased urinary excretion of SH-reactive metals is due to the chelating action of the prosthetic mercaptan derived from the cleavage of the S-S bond in TTFD.

Finally, as already indicated above, it must be understood that the major effect of TTFD comes from the increased intracellular content of thiamine. The place of this vitamin in energy metabolism is of vast importance and there is still much to be learned about its manifold actions, particularly in the brain and nervous system (8). On clinical grounds it appears to be a very important addition to the many different nutrients that have been found to be beneficial in this alarming epidemic of ASD affected children. Observations by a number of physicians have suggested that TTFD is more potent and more effective when administered by transdermal application. The skunk-like odor never occurs when it is given by mouth and it is thought that this is because the molecule breaks down prematurely in the acid secretions of the stomach, thus losing its disulfide reaction in the absorption of thiamine into body cells. The small yellow tablets made by the manufacturers in Japan are protectively coated to ensure that TTFD will be absorbed in the small intestine where a more alkaline medium exists. They are sold in Japan as a prescription item known as Alinamin F (odorless) to indicate that it does not give rise to the penetrating odor that was produced by earlier disulfide derivatives of the vitamin. These are not available in the U.S.

As the autism community embraced this new weapon in our armamentarium to help our children, there were some reports of a few children having pale stools and/or constipation when starting to use TTFD. A few using the oral allithiamine also have noted this. (This actually is not an uncommon finding in ASD children aside from the use of TTFD). Dr. Lonsdale told me he had not experienced this in his studies (nor did I in my patients) and suggested I check with Dr. Jon Pangborn. Dr. Pangborn informed me that TTFD has cysteine oxidase activity, and can cause cysteine to be broken down into the sulfite rather than the taurine branch of metabolism. Since biliary function needs taurocholic acid for bile formation, he informed me that in his opinion giving taurine along with the TTFD would probably take care of this problem.[14]

Over 60% of our ASD children are found to be low in taurine on testing. If cysteine is insufficient, also often found through testing, there would be even more taurine insufficiency and adequate supplementation would be even more important. Taurine functions as a neuromodulator and is known to be a very important amino acid for thinning bile and preventing gallstones. It has also been shown to help decrease epileptic seizures in some children at doses between 400 and 1200 mg per day, and can be given up to 2000 mg or more per day (in divided doses) without toxicity, starting low and building up. Vitamin B6 along with magnesium is known to be necessary for taurine to be metabolized from methionine to cysteine to taurine.

Since all of my patients were using optimal levels of vitamins and minerals as needed per testing, this may have been why I did not see the problem of pale stools and constipation in my group. Diligent use of Vitamin C seems to help constipation, and needs to be administered preferably three or four times a day but at least twice daily, since it stays in the blood stream for a very short time after administration. (Most of our children need at least 750-1000mg a day and some of them need and benefit from much more, especially during any chelating process). I am now advising parents to make sure B6, magnesium, Vit C, and taurine are well in place before starting TTFD. As Dr. Lonsdale has said, "We have to remember that no nutrient works alone—if you push the metabolism through the use of TTFD at the mitochondrial level, you may well uncover vitamin deficiencies that have remained latent previously. In over some 30 years of almost continuous use of TTFD, I have never seen any major toxicity. It has a very powerful vector force in stimulating aerobic metabolism and these kids are notoriously bad eaters so their vitamin deficiencies can easily become overt if metabolic processes accelerate."[8] Dr. Lonsdale has emphasized that his study was a PILOT study and still needed more research in a clinical setting.

SUMMARY

The use of transdermal TTFD is new, and more controlled studies will be needed before we understand all the dynamics of this process. I believe the agent is benign and beneficial and a welcome addition to our treatment armamentarium, particularly for those children susceptible to the "gut-bug" overgrowth we struggle with so often with the use of DMSA and ALA (less so with DMPS in my experience). I do not consider any chelation process a "first-line" treatment, but believe it needs to be preceded and then accompanied by work on healing the gut and the administration of necessary nutrients based on proper testing. I advise good gut health measures such as probiotics, judicious use of enzymes, and dietary restrictions to be in place before and while doing chelation.

According to parental reports, it appears that those children who can tolerate the glutathione especially benefit from the combination of GSH with TTFD. Almost all my patients have shown rare evidence of negative side effects so far except for the unpleasant odor of the cream and the occasional pale stools and constipation that some children experienced before we learned that co-administration of taurine along with the TTFD was important. (Note: TTFD now available as Authia from Ecological Formulas.)

General Comments on Detoxification Treatment

Although it would be great to have a number of conclusive research studies to direct each of the protocols we use, neither I nor parents of ASD children are willing to wait for such research if a treatment makes sense and is safe. In the case of chelation, preliminary data are too compelling to wait for long-term verification studies. Many of my patients are drawing on every tool I have in my armamentarium that we think will help them. I'm constantly on the lookout for even more information and new treatments to help Chelsey and the other ASD children to have a better life.

In the beginning of my learning curve about chelation I discovered, through a process of trial and error, that if certain children developed an overgrowth of yeast or other gut pathogens, positive effects would plateau or even in some cases they would start to regress. Dr. Amy Holmes was the first to help me realize that the chelating agents we were using not only seemed to be feeding the yeast, but even encouraged bacterial overgrowth, especially Clostridium difficile, an anerobic bacteria very difficult to eradicate. (The OAT test identifies Clostridia through elevations in urinary metabolites such as HPHPA [dihydroxyphenylpropionate])[14]. We knew all along that chelation might remove some needed nutrients, so we have been very diligent in making sure each child is properly mineralized and nutritional deficiencies corrected as much as possible. We also follow a conservative process of chelating for only a few days and giving the child's system (and the parents!) a rest of at least as many days off as on. Generally now with a few exceptions I follow the 3-days on, 11-days off cycle, which seems to provide a safe steady course to which most children respond positively without any evidence of harm. If there is evidence of "bad gut bugs" as shown by diarrhea, constipation, or severe regression in behavior—or if the child's metabolic signs deteriorate—chelation is stopped until the problem is taken care of by appropriate testing and treatment. I have come to immediately regard a plateau in improvement as a tip-off that gut pathogens may be affecting the child's ability to respond, and take appropriate measures to correct the situation.

In my chelating experience, the children suffering the most with gut pathogens during chelation have been those not on the GF/CF/SF diet. Recent studies support evidence that 75-80% of children with ASD have immune reactivity to dietary proteins including soy, milk, and wheat. Dr. Harumi Jyonouchi, pediatric immunologist and allergist at the University of Minnesota, has tested the immune responses of autistic children and compared them to healthy controls. Her scientific research supports parents' claims that autistic children have abnormal immune responses to gluten, casein, and soy.[15] I have begun requiring the GF/CF and now SF (soy-free) diet as a prerequisite to chelation for children with delayed onset or "regressive" ASD, particularly those who received the HepB vaccine as newborns, very likely triggering the early gut and immune injury, frequent infections, antibiotics, and "leaky gut."

Confusion has arisen in the autism community at times over the dosing and frequency of administration of chelating agents. Studies have shown DMSA or DMPS (some controversy here) do not cross the blood-brain-barrier, nor do they release the mercury once they bind to it, so mercury removal as shown by urinary testing during chelation is presumed to come from body stores other than the brain. Yet thousands of ASD children have unarguably improved with chelation. Suggestion that "redistribution of metals" causes damage with longer dosing intervals is scientifically unproven, yet clinical experiences show us that about 50% of children do better with 4 hr dosing and lesser amounts of chelating agents vs 8 hr intervals with larger doses. Many of us doing this work now believe that there are other as yet unproven mechanisms at work relating to the sulfation/methylation chemistry and provision of sulfur by the chelating agents for its various uses in the body, including formation of cysteine and its role in helping the body detoxify itself. I tend to give smaller more frequent doses to younger or more damaged children and every 8 hr larger doses to the older kids, with readiness to move to the 4 hr dosing if side effects or lack of improvement dictate; either schedule works for some children.

In a recent query to some of the practitioners who contributed to the Mercury Detoxification Consensus Group Position Paper in 2001[4], I learned that a few clinicians prefer now to only use DMPS (oral, TD, IV), feeling it is a better chelator with less incidence of gut pathogen overgrowth than DMSA. Several prefer only the 4 hour schedules, a few more only use the 8 hr schedule, and most vary schedules according to the individual situation. Many doctors (including myself) are using transdermal TTFD (allithiamine) as an accelerator or adjunct to our usual chelating agents. I want to emphasize once again that safety is of the utmost concern. Appropriate testing to monitor the status of the blood and urine should be done periodically. In addition, periodic urine and/or fecal tests to determine which metals are being removed are helpful in guiding treatment. Chelation therapy for ASD children as delineated by the Defeat Autism Now! group is relatively new and much is still to be learned by all of us in this field. Most but not all children undergoing chelation have benefited, and to the best of my knowledge, there have been no reports of irreversible medical damage from this treatment when based upon Defeat Autism Now! guidelines[4].

Additional notes re: chelation: Those of us who have been using the Defeat Autism Now! protocol have noticed that many children improve when we begin with a strong nutrient program even before introducing the chelation agents. It is possible that we have been helping the child's own detoxification mechanisms to function better through improved nutrition even without understanding all the underlying cellular mechanisms. I usually start my nutrient program with anti-oxidant vitamins such as A, C, D, Co-Enzyme Q & E, calcium, and mineralization (usually including extra zinc, an avoidance of copper, and P5P' plus magnesium). Once those are in place, I add other B vitamins, omega-3 oils, and oral and transdermal reduced glutathione with a glutathione precursor formula including NAC (N-acetyl cysteine), ALA, glycine, inosine and selenomethionine as a preliminary "natural" chelation. I start this very cautiously as some children cannot tolerate too much NAC, at least until appreciable chelation has been done. Some practitioners have started administering IV's, both DMPS and CA-EDTA, often following with IV Glutathione with many ASD children showing great benefit. The glutathione-zinc relationship is known to be an essential aspect of effective metallothionein function, along with adequate selenium to support the delivery of zinc to cells and the sequestering of mercury and other heavy metals. The addition to my detoxification regiment of gentle steady detoxification with transdermal allithiamine (TTFD) or thiamine tetrahydrofurfuryl disulfide has been of great help to many children.

As in all our detoxification protocols, our biomedical therapies aim to eliminate toxic metals, protect against both present and future toxic exposures, normalize the gut, improve immune function and behavior, and enhance development of brain neurons and synaptic connections. As has been emphasized, much of the Defeat Autism Now! chelation protocol and my personal approach to treatment includes healing the gut and obtaining optimal nutritional status. Clearly, further research and documentation is needed and is occurring. At this time, the bottom line is that many children are being helped by the protocols delineated in this book. As the data already presented to the NIH and IOM indicate, the earlier detoxification therapies as well as behavioral therapies are begun—simultaneously with gut healing and nutritional support—the likelier the child will significantly improve.

Questions and challenges relating to detoxification continue. Opinions on optimum frequency and dosage amounts of chelating agents continue to differ among well-respected practitioners. More doctors are using DMPS and CA-EDTA than before even though they have not been formally tested in children. Many of us agree that small oral or rectal doses are safe and effective. Discovering new ways to turn on the detoxification mechanism inherent in all of us is definitely exciting research which we will learn more about in future study and research. Clearly, the jury is still out on some of these issues, and different subsets of children according to age, gut status, toxicity level and other factors may respond more favorably to one or another protocol as we are finding for most biomedical treatments for ASD children.

References

1 DMSA, trade name Chemet made by Sanofi Pharmaceuti-cals, is 2,3-dimercaptosuc-cinic acid

2 Autism Research Institute: Defeat Autism Now! Mercury Detoxification Consensus Group Position Paper, May 2001, Background and In-troduction by Bernard Rim-land, PhD Director of ARI http://www.autism.com/ari/mercurydetox.html

3 Edelson, S.B., Cantor, D.S., "Autism: xenobiotic influences." Toxicol Ind Health 1998;14: 553-563

4 ARI Defeat Autism Now! Mercury Detoxification Consensus Group Position Paper, May 2001, Background and Introduction by Bernard Rim-land, PhD Dir. of ARI http://www.autism.com/ari/mercurydetox.html. 2005 revised version now available.

5 Lonsdale D. Summary of TTFD clinical results. Research Conference sponsored by Autism Research Institute, San Diego CA, October 24, 2002.

6 Lonsdale D, Shamberger RJ, Audhya T. Treatment of autism spectrum children with thiamine tetrahydrofurfuryl disulfide: A pilot study. Neuroendocrinology Lett 2002;23(4):303-8.

7 Fujiwra M. Absorption and fate of thiamine and its derivatives in [the] human body. Inouye K, Katsura E, eds. In: Beriberi and thiamine. Tokyo, Igaku Shoin Ltd; 1965:179-213.

8 Fujita T, Suzuoki Z. Enzymatic studies on the metablolism of the tetrahydrofurfuryl mercaptan moiety of thiamine tetrahydrofurfuryl disulfide . I Microsomal S-transm-ethylase. J Biochem 1973;74:717-22.

9 Fujita T, Suzuoki Z Kozuka S. Enzymatic studies on the metabolism of the tetrahy-drofurfuryl mercaptan moiety of thiamine tetrahydrofurfuryl disulfide. II sulfide and sulfoxide oxygen bases in microsomes. J Biochem 1973;74:723-32.

10 Fujita T Suzuoki Z. Enzymatic studies on the metabolism of the tetrahydrofurfuryl mercaptan moiety of thiamine tetrahydrofurfuryl disulfide. III Oxidative cleavage of the tetrahydrofurfuran moiety. J Biochem 1973;74:733-8.

11 Fujita T, Teraoka A, Suzuoki Z. Enzymatic studies on the metabolism of the tetrahy-drofurfuryl mercaptan moiety of thiamine tetrahydrofurfuryl disulfide.IV Induction

of microsomal S-transmethylase, and sulfide and sulfoxide oxygenases in the drug-treated rat. J Biochem 1973;74:739-45.

[12] Olkowski A A, Gooneratne S R, Christensen D A. The effects of thiamine and EDTA on biliary and urinary lead excretion in sheep. Toxicol Lett 1991;59:153-9.

[13] Pangborn J. Personal correspondence, 11-16-02.

[14] Shaw, William, 2002, New revised edition of Biological Treatments for Autism and PDD

[15] Jyonouchi H, Sun S, Itokazu N. Innate immunity associated with inflammatory responses and cytokine production against common dietary proteins in partients with autism spectrum disorder. Neuropsychobiology 2002;46(2):76-84

EIGHT

IMMUNITY, AUTOIMMUNITY, AND VIRUSES

An Overview of Immune Dysregulation in ASD Children

GENETICS

In 1997 when I first began searching for information about the biomedical aspects of autism, most of the medical literature referred to this disorder as genetic and stated that autism begins in the womb. My explorations revealed an enormous diversity for the etiologies of autism and acknowledgment that the underlying pathologic mechanisms were unknown in most cases. I found there was no clear proven identification for any one exclusive chromosome carrying a gene for autism, though several studies showed that 5% of autistic children possessed an identifiable array of chromosomal aberrations. Still, there is general consensus among researchers and clinicians working with the autistic spectrum disorders that family and twin studies give enough evidence to indicate that hereditary factors play a role. In Bernard Rimland's 1964 study of monozygotic (identical) twins with autism, he concluded that genetic components seemed strong, yet were significantly affected by the existence of modifying factors.

IMMUNE ABNORMALITIES

The infectious and toxic etiologies would seem to be exceptions to the genetic influence. However, an individual's susceptibility to such injuries can be heightened by genetic predisposition, as well as by environmental factors, so that the timing of an insult can be crucially important. In an informal survey of one of the internet autism groups in which I was a participant in 1999, 30% of the mothers of children with autism who participated reported having autoimmune diseases, which is consistent with Comi, et al. Such studies have shown an increased incidence of hypothyroid disease and diabetes as well as rheumatoid arthritis in the parents of children with autism compared to parents of matched controls.[1] Many immunological studies of individuals with autism have found atypical immune function of one type or another, the results often depending on the age of the individuals in the particular study. Such studies included:

- Abnormalities in T cells and T cell subsets (Stubbs, et al. 1977, Warren, et al. 1990, Yonk, et al. 1990. Warren, et al. 1995, Gupta, et al. 1998)

- Depressed responses to T cell mitogens (Stubbs, et al. 1977, Warren, et al. 1986) decreased natural killer cell function (Warren, et al. 1987)

- A lower percentage of helper-inducer cells (Denney, et al. 1996)

- Elevation of interleukin-12 (Singh 1996)

- Elevation of interferon-gamma (Singh 1996)

- Elevation of alpha-interferon levels (Stubbs 1995).

Immunological signs of food allergy have been found to be higher in patients with autism compared to healthy controls.

The major histocompatibility complex (MHC) has a group of genes that control the function and regulation of the immune system. One of these genes, the C4B gene, encodes a product that is involved in eliminating pathogens such as viruses and bacteria from the body. A deficient form of the C4B gene, termed the C4B null allele (meaning no C4B protein produced) has an increased frequency in autism, ADHD, and dyslexia.

AUTOIMMUNITY AND AUTISM

In a review of the literature in the emerging field of "psychoneuroimmunology" van Gent et al hypothesizes that autoimmune and/ or viral processes in some way affect the nervous system and alter central nervous system activity.[2]

Antibodies to myelin basic protein (MBP) and neuron-axon filament protein (NAFP) have been found to be positive in children with autism compared to healthy controls.[3] Singh et al have reported that positive measles virus or HHV6 titers were related to autoantibodies, especially those of anti-myelin basic protein in children with autism but not in controls.[4]

PATHOGENS AND AUTOIMMUNITY

An infection with a pathogen that triggers an abnormal immune response to self-tissue can be an important component of the development of autoimmune disorders. Some infectious diseases identified in autistic children are rubella, herpes simplex encephalitis, varicella, cytomegalovirus, and roseola (caused by the HHV6 virus). In very young children, an inherited but mild deficiency of the immune system may prevent the patient from clearing a pathogen in a timely and normal fashion without the child necessarily seeming to be very ill. This situation places him or her at higher risk for the pathogen to interfere with brain development or function and/or to trigger autoimmune responses, both of which are strongly identified as major ASD symptoms.

Uta Frith says in her book, *Autism: Explaining the Enigma,* "If the central nervous system becomes infected at a critical time, either before or after birth, autism may result. Of special interest are certain types of virus called retrovirus, which totally integrate themselves in genetic material in the body cells. Other viruses that have been suggested as possible causes of autism are herpes and cytomegalovirus.

These can remain dormant for years but from time to time can be reactivated."[5]

GASTROINTESTINAL DISEASE AND AUTISM SPECTRUM DISORDER

MMR and Development Regression

As mentioned in previous chapters, Dr. Andrew Wakefield, formerly a research gastroenterologist at Royal Free Hospital and School of Medicine in London and the Inflammatory Bowel Disease Study Group there, identified measles virus (MV) particles in the ileal lesions of some children with autism. The complicated politics with the vaccine industry and the official rejections of Wakefield's excellent research that led to his departure from Royal Free Hospital would make a dramatic movie. Recently, important parts of Wakefield's work have been duplicated by Dr. Timothy Buie of Harvard, who identified a group of autistic children with ileal hyperplasia. Subsequently, a respected virology group in Japan used a DNA/RNA sequencing technique to demonstrate that the MV present in the children with ileal inflammation was indeed the vaccine strain.[6] This finding leaves little doubt in the minds of many parents and professionals that a certain subset of children are susceptible to developmental regression from the MV component of the MMR. Dr. Wakefield has said all along that there was no need for all the furor. All the vaccine makers had to do was to separate the three components (Measles, Mumps, and Rubella) and allow them to be given as separate single vaccines spaced in time, with the parents taking care to make sure their children were not suffering from some infection or illness at the time of the shot.

Fungal Infections and the Immune System

Cell-mediated immunity has been shown to be an important host defense mechanism against Candida albicans infections. A switch from Th1 to Th2 type responses has been noted to increase susceptibility to mucosal candidiasis.[7] Several studies have documented Th2-like shifts in certain groups of autistic children.

ATYPICAL ELEVATIONS OF COMMON VIRAL TITERS

Examples of these include Epstein-Barr Virus, Cytomegalovirus, Herpes Simplex Viruses 1 & 2, HHV6, and MV. Although interpreting viral-titer lab data is complex, the various titer elevations suggest to Teresa Binstock and others that an ASD subgroup has chronic, low level viral infections that are etiologically related to the child's autism.[8] These children have enough overall immunity to keep from appearing sick, yet they have an underlying immune-impairment that permits an atypical chronic infection to exist. During the 1990s, polymerase chain reaction (PCR) studies demonstrated that certain viruses can invade and migrate into small areas of the central nervous system without necessarily generating an obvious encephalitis, where they can remain dormant for long periods of time even as cell function is altered.

It has been shown in rats that the ubiquitous Herpes Simplex Virus (HSV) is capable of entering gastrointestinal nerves and of migrating into the spine from various peripheral locations. Furthermore, Gesser et al showed that this migration could occur all the way into the amygdala and that HSV's migration in humans can follow the same pathway as identified in rats.[9] We hypothesize that, in at least some autism-spectrum children who respond favorably to acyclovir or Valtrex, HSV may have migrated into crucial brain regions and done so intraneuronally, without creating an obvious encephalitis. This model is consistent with the amygdala's role in anxiety, emotions, appetite, the processing of sensory information, and reaction to faces. In fact, the amygdala have neurons specific for eye contact and are linked with seizure disorders and certain emotional nuances of language.[10] Other autism-spectrum children who respond favorably to acyclovir or Valtrex may have HSV persisting within other tissues such as the pancreas, liver, and spleen.[11]

ALLERGY AND IMMUNITY

In babies that are bottle fed, a milk-based formula would cause children allergic to milk to have very early gut inflammation and indigestion problems. Breast fed babies generally have better immunity because they receive antibodies from their mother's milk and are rarely allergic to it. Some mothers have reported their child's descent into autism began shortly after cessation of breast-feeding and the introduction of cow's milk into the diet. Of course, other events may take place around that time also, like the injection of toxin-laden vaccines, but there is a lot of evidence that breast-fed babies generally fare better in ASD than bottle-fed babies. These findings would seem to corroborate the growing realization that casein is toxic to many and perhaps most ASD children when taken together with all the studies that have shown a higher incidence of allergies in ASD children than in controls.

CHRONIC LOW-GRADE INFECTIONS

A long-standing model of autoimmunity posited that autoimmune syndromes could be induced in some individuals by a "hit and run" pathogen (since ordinary laboratory studies at the time could find no evidence of the pathogen). However, more recent PCR-based evidence increasingly demonstrates that several subgroups of multiple sclerosis patients may have reactivated or chronic, low level infections.[12] Similarly, clinical lab data suggest that there are subgroups of ASD children in whom a low-level or a reactivated infection may be etiologically significant.[13]

When considering an individual child (not in the context of a general epidemic), it is always difficult to know whether he or she is part of the ASD infection-subgroup because of a predisposition due to mild immune impairment, because the infection was prenatal or congenital, or whether lingering infection continues to inhibit immune capacity.

Diagnostics–Immune Testing

"What tests to order" in immunologically diagnosing ASD children is not easy for several reasons. This is a relatively new field for clinicians, and it is difficult for parents to find a doctor willing to order and even be qualified to evaluate the lab data. Understandably, parents do not appreciate unnecessary tests for children who are not able to understand why they are being held down and "tortured." Insurance often will not pay for these "non-mainstream" tests; a full array of diagnostics can be quite expensive, with no guarantee that the results will lead to effective treatments. Still, there are many parents who are willing to invest in such testing and there is a growing amount of clinical lab-test data to help us understand more about dysregulated immunity, impaired detoxification, and seemingly subclinical infections. In addition to the CBC, metabolic panel, and other tests already described, the following are helpful in immunologically evaluating ASD children:

COMPREHENSIVE (HERPES) VIRAL SCREEN

Elevated antibody titers to viruses are often found when ASD children undergo immunological testing. This viral screen differentiates the IgG (indication of past exposure or chronic activation) and the IgM antibodies (indication of very recent infection or recent reactivation) of herpesviruses such as HSV1, HSV2, Varicella Zoster virus (VZV), EBC, Cytomegalovirus (CMV), and HHV6. Impaired immune function along with impaired detoxification and ever increasing environmental toxins may predispose toward chronic viral infections otherwise normally immunosuppressed. I usually also order IgG Rubeola antibodies in addition to the herpes viral screen with this panel.[14]

MYELIN BASIC PROTEIN (MBP) ANTIBODIES

Myelin is a multilamellar membrane surrounding nerve fibers in both the central and peripheral nervous systems, derived from the plasma membrane of the oligodendrocyte in the CNS and the schwann cell in the peripheral nervous system. Antibodies (IgG, IgA, IgM) against MBP have been observed in a high percentage of ASD children. Positive tests are an indication of autoimmunity.

Case History–Suzie

In 1998 I was asked to work with a high-functioning 16-year old autistic girl whose mother thought she might have a "brain virus." I told the mother I had never treated anyone for a brain virus before and suggested she see another doctor in the area known for his work with immune dysregulation and viruses as causes of autism—but she was persistent. I will always be grateful to this parent as well as other devoted parents who have challenged me to learn more in order to help their children. I went back to the textbooks, research articles, and some new sources such as Teresa Binstock's published and informal writings on pathogens, viruses, and autoimmunity. Getting ready to work with Suzie, I began to learn all I could about these complicated issues.

Suzie was (is) a beautiful, petite girl who I would have guessed to be about fourteen rather than sixteen years of age. The mother, a teacher/writer who became a full-time mother when Suzie was born, described a crew of daily tutors (including week-ends), and other enormous efforts made through the years to keep her daughter in public school. Having managed to stay at her grade level, Suzie was a junior primarily by struggling extremely hard to please teachers and parents. However, socially she was isolated, had no friends, and no boys had ever shown interest in her even though she had nice features and an attractive though somewhat immature body. She seemed a bit dreamy and distracted, yet could answer factual questions fairly well. She had strange eating patterns, having refused to eat with her family for years, and liked only a few foods. In taking the medical history, her mother told me that Suzie was normal until around age four when she got roseola, a usually mild and transient childhood disease caused by the HHV6 virus and typically presenting with a widespread rash. After the disease was over, she began behaving differently and, though she never lost speech, did not seem to learn as well as other kids in her classes. The mother showed me pictures of Susie through the years in which occasional breakouts of what looked like brief recurrences of the roseola rash would show on her limbs. (It appeared that she had a chronic low-grade HHV6 infection that occasionally reactivated.)

I conducted routine screening tests which all were within normal limits and put Susie on a nutrient program (to which she agreed) and suggested dietary modifications (with which she had trouble cooperating). It is much easier to get three and four year olds on a GF/CF/SF diet than a teenager! I conferred with Dr. Ari Vojdani, then director of Immunosciences Laboratory in Beverly Hills, (no longer open for testing at this lab) who has been another wonderful resource in helping me begin to understand more about viruses and the immune system. He advised me to order a comprehensive viral panel and a natural killer cytotoxicity test in addition to the CBC,

Chemistry Panel, and Thyroid Panel I had already done. Her tests came back with positive IgG (past or chronic infection) and IgM (current infection or reactivation) of HHV6 (the roseola virus). She also had very low NK (natural killer) cytotoxicity function, meaning that her immune system was impaired in its first line of defense to combat viruses. I was surprised; Susie's mother was not. She is one of the many wise mothers I have met since starting to work with these "special needs" children.

I had already started Susie on a small dose of an SSRI hoping to alleviate some of her social anxiety, which did seem to help her be a bit more outgoing. She had been on the SSRI and the nutrient program for several months by the time I started her on acyclovir (the antiviral useful against many strains of HSV and VZV, and with varying degrees of effectiveness against EBV and HHV6). Soon we moved to a modified acyclovir, called Valtrex, which has a different rate of assimilation and is said to be approximately 6 times more potent. I had used Valtrex for many adult herpes patients through the years and knew it as a very safe drug.

After just a week to ten days of the Valtrex, the change in Suzie was amazing. Her eyes brightened, she was more "present," became wittier and more expressive generally, and was starting to acquire friends. It was as if her classmates had never seen her before. Within three months she was on her way to becoming a normal, rebellious, typical teen-ager, totally mystifying her parents and surprising tutors who had been working with her for years. Soon, she started rebelling against spending so much time with the tutors and, as she let most of them go, pleasantly surprised her parents by maintaining her B and C grades. She started attracting boys for the first time in her life and began the usual dramas of high school "thrills and heart-breaks" so characteristic of neurotypical kids. She still exhibited some learning difficulties, but the positive change in all areas of her life was noticeable to anyone who had known her before the treatment. Her parents were enormously delighted and grateful for her "emergence." The mother felt her "inner certainty" that Suzie had a medical problem had been vindicated in the face of Suzie's physician-father who had steadfastly attributed her traits to learning disabilities that needed to be handled by educational psychologists (as had been done with her older sister).

Suzie stayed on the SSRI's for just a few months and the Valtrex (1500mg per day) for 18 months; her viral titers kept going down while her NK values kept going up. At various times in her course of treatment, she took various immune enhancing agents and also the natural anti-viral Monolaurin (Lauricidin). Even after being stabilized, her mother was reluctant to take her off the Valtrex even though Suzie hated the routine "safety" blood tests we needed in order to make sure her liver was not being affected by the treatment. (It wasn't.) Finally, we did phase her out of all her medicines as she approached graduation. She also became weary of taking so many nutrients as she started to feel better. She still maintained her somewhat eccentric eating habits as she left home to attend a small private fine-arts college a few hours away, but we all gratefully accepted that. Recently, the parents called to inform me that Susie was maintaining a B average in school and had a steady boy friend the parents liked. I consider her free of the diagnosis of autism, even though she retains some of her eating idiosyncracies. Interestingly, I find her erratic diet not terribly different from many young women in her age group who place a greater investment in staying thin than they do on good nutrition.

Anti-Viral and Immune Treatment Issues

Needless to say, the success with Suzie thrilled me and inspired me to obtain viral panels on all the children I evaluated (including Chelsey), starting them on anti-virals with any sign of elevated titers to the herpes family of viruses. However, though some younger children gradually improved, none had the startling and immediate success with the anti-virals that I had experienced with Susie. I was reassured soon after that my results with Suzie were not anomalous when I discovered that other physicians (eg, Michael Goldberg & Sidney Baker) were describing in conferences and on internet websites a subgroup of children for whom anti-virals induced major improvements. I was using anti-virals along with implementing other treatments with the younger kids such as GF/CF/SF diet, secretin, vitamins, nutrients, etc., so the source of any improvement was not so obvious as it was in Suzie's case. Then, in the summer and fall of

2000, I started hearing of the improvement in children undergoing chelation for heavy metal toxicity, particularly mercury, and began actively investigating and using this therapy in my practice, finding more response to chelation than to anti-viral therapy.

The heavy metal issue brought a lot of things together for me. I could understand that mercury impairs the immune system, interferes with certain enzyme systems, and allows yeast, colonizing bacteria, and perhaps even some viruses to get a firm hold on the gut tissues. These factors—along with food hypersensitivity—would interfere with nutrient transport across intestinal membranes and would make it chronically difficult for the child to receive adequate brain nourishment. Furthermore, inadequate availability of nutrients can reduce immunity and make it difficult to heal the opportunistic infestations that are so common in ASD children. I began to see that many ASD children seem to have entered into a vicious cycle of intestinal pathology, suboptimal nutrition, and weakened immunity, all of which needed treatment. Impaired detoxification and the subsequent accumulation of toxic metals seem easier for me to understand and treat than the immune, autoimmune, and viral issues. It seemed reasonable to me—and to other physicians who have subsequently presented evidence to the NIH, the IOM, and the FDA—to try and get the toxic metals out of the child so that other simultaneous or subsequent treatments would be more effective.

Chelation seemed especially important in the light of chronic intestinal pathology since the anti-virals do not affect bacterial or fungal colonizations. In fact, we were all discovering at that time that yeast kept coming back and that gut issues remained a serious problem in some kids no matter what we did. If lab-testing and an initial chelation treatment indicated heavy metal poisoning, my view was—and still is—that healing the gut, optimizing nutritional status, and removing heavy metals may be sufficient for boosting the child's immune system to the point where it can do its job of suppressing viruses and other pathogens wherever they may be. As I have repeatedly emphasized, we know chelation should not be instituted until after the gut healing is well under way, otherwise it may be ineffective or even make the gut situation worse.

If—after gut healing and nutritional restoration—diagnostic studies do not indicate heavy metal poisoning, or after progress in chelation has plateaued with no known explanation before full healing, I proceed to the investigation of the immune system by doing more specific immune and viral studies to detect atypical presence of pathogens as an etiologic factor in the child's disorder.

TREATMENTS TO ENHANCE THE IMMUNE SYSTEM

The immune system is intimately related to the gastrointestinal tract, as I have said repeatedly. In addition to its role in defense, the gut-associated lymphoid tissue prevents systemic immune responses to food antigens and plays an important role in maintaining tolerance to self. More immunoglobulin is synthesized and secreted (secretory IgA antibodies) into the digestive tract each day than is produced anywhere else in the body. Immunoglobulin in the intestinal tract may help protect against autoimmunity and the initiation of autoimmune diseases. It is impossible to know which starts the pathology in these children, the gut injury or the immune impairment, as they are so intertwined. There has been a certain amount of investigation of ways to enhance the weakened immune systems of ASD children. Certainly, removing foods that are toxic because of the child's hypersensitivity is necessary as a first step and providing essential nutrients to counteract the deficiencies comes next. We have already discussed in Chapter Seven the removal of heavy metal and other toxins which are well-known immune suppressors. We can use anti-fungal, anti-bacterial and anti-viral medications to treat the illnesses secondary to the immune impairment, but obviously something that could directly go to the cause of the problem and help the body's immune system would be extremely helpful.

Immunomodulators and Immune Boosters

Certain compounds seem to be beneficial in boosting the function of the immune system. Michael Goldberg MD, founder and director of NIDS (Neuro-Immune Dysfunction Syndromes), states that the mission of his organization is to facilitate the employment of immune-modulating therapies in the treatment of what he calls "acquired autism." He believes immune dysregulation or possibly viral-mediated states link all the multiple etiologies and various clinical manifestations of ASD. Dr. Goldberg is well known for his use of a combination of prescription medications for his patients including anti-virals, anti-fungals, and SSRI's. He also used an older medication called Kutapressin (no longer available), a porcine liver extract previously used as a medication for herpes zoster or shingles, known to inhibit human herpes viruses and reduce inflammation. This needed to be given by IM injection over an extended period of time and produced mixed results (as do many of our treatments) as reported by his clients in autism internet support groups. To my knowledge there is not yet a prescription drug category called immunomodulators and I know of no medication specifically used for that purpose other than Kutapressin and IVIG (discussed below).

Natural immunomodulators that I use in my practice are:

- Larch arabinogalactan, a naturally occurring polysaccharide extracted from the Larch tree and known to provide a number of immunological properties. I obtain this from Thorne as Arabinex; Larch is an almost tasteless water-soluble powder, easy for kids to take, and extremely effective in cutting down the number of infections.

- Moducare, from Thorne Research, is a "plant fat" extracted from the African potato (in the family of sterols and sterolins), and is considered an immune system modulator. Research studies have shown the sterols enhance NK and T-helper cell activity while dampening overactive antibody responses; clinically I have found it to be a very powerful immune enhancer. Its main drawback is that it must be taken on an empty stomach for maximal effectiveness.

- Inositol hexaphosphate (IP-6) has been documented to increase NK cell function and protect cells against damage from toxins. It is a phosphorus compound of plants particularly abundant in seeds, legumes and cereal grains. This is available from Enzymatic Therapy, Vitamin Research Products, JHS Natural Products, and Thorne Research.

- Dimethylglycine (DMG) has been shown in many studies to boost NK cells; it is non-toxic and naturally sweet.

- L-glutamine is the most prevalent amino acid in the bloodstream and is considered "conditionally essential." The gastrointestinal system is by far the greatest user of glutamine in the body; there are a large number of immune cells including fibroblasts, lymphocytes, and macrophages along the walls of the gut. The ability of glutamine to nourish these immune cells may account for its positive impact on immunity. Many ASD children with chronic gut problems test low on glutamine. I recommend 1000-4000 mg/day; it is non-toxic and very beneficial to gut function generally.

- Mushroom compounds contain proteoglycans and polysaccharides, including alpha and beta glucans. Studies have shown these preparations to be potent immune enhancers by increasing tumor necrosis factor alpha, stimulating macrophage phagocytic activity, improving NK cell number and activity, stimulating interleukins 1 and 2, B-lymphocyte stimulation, improvement of T-cell ratios, and gamma interferon stimulation. I use 10-15 drops in pear juice of Thorne's 7-mushroom compound Myco-Immune extract 2-3 times/day to bolster immune function in ASD children.

- Lauricidin, a component found in coconut and breast milk, has been researched by Dr. Jon Kabara, with studies showing effectiveness against certain viral groups. This nutrient comes in two forms: the Monolaurin capsule containing 300mg (obtained from Ecological Formulas), and Lauricidin (obtained from Med-Chem Labs), 8-oz jars of mini-pellets that are pure, highly concentrated and very helpful for prevention of herpes outbreaks. The bad taste of these pellets (long lingering and soapy) prevents me from administering them to some children who I am sure would benefit, but I can't find a way to get them down. The children who can take them usually benefit highly, particularly those children who get repeated herpes lesions on their lips or faces. A child must take 7 (large) Monolaurin capsules (which don't taste very good either) for the equivalent of one scoop of the mini-pellets, daunting enough whether the capsules are swallowed or dissolved in some medium which hopefully can hide the taste. I consider

Lauricidin to be a safe and often effective natural antiviral, particularly against Herpes Simplex 1 & 2 and varicella.

Rosemary Waring, PhD is a well known expert on sulfur metabolic pathways at the University of Birmingham, UK, and parent researcher Susan Owens has studied with her on sulfation issues. In a recent response on our internet biomedical group to parents' posts that Monolaurin had helped their children's bowel function, Ms. Owens reported that Dr. Waring's work on fatty acid effects on the gut has shown that lauric acid enhances an enzyme important for regulation of intestine function known to be low in ASD children (tyrosyl protein sulfotransferase). Dr. Waring's work has shown that the sulfur-transferase system is one of the body's major means of detoxification; many ASD children are deficient in sulfur.

- I am encouraging Dr. Kabara to continue his efforts to find a palatable form for such a valuable agent.

- Epicor: A new immune enhancer/modulator carried by Vitamin Research Products, Epicor is a yeast-derived end product (Saccharomyces cerevisiae) reported to increase Secretory IgA levels.

- Other immune enhancers: **The best is fresh fruits and vegetables (which many of our children will not eat!).** Others are: whey protein (watch for casein), echinacea, elderberry extract, germanium, CoEnzyme Q10, garlic, N-acetyl cysteine (provides sulfur), astragalus root, licorice root, olive leaf extract, grapefruit seed extract, and A-lipoic acid (also provides sulfur), and many others not listed. Parents should educate themselves about any over-the-counter nutrients and heed warnings of dose and safety limitations.

Probiotics as Immunomodulators

There is mounting scientific evidence that probiotics may provide significant health benefits including modulation of the immune system. Probiotics are recognized to function in cell-mediated immunity (Th1) and humoral immunity (Th2) cells, directly interacting with the immune system to help immunological defenses such as down-regulating pro-inflammatory cytokines and up-regulating anti-inflammatory cytokines. Probiotics modulate localized endogenous flora (GALT–gut-associated lymphoid tissue), enhance secretory IgA production, and positively influence the gut immunological barrier.[16]

Oral probiotic supplementation may play a crucial role in severe inflammatory bowel conditions and usually without eliciting harmful inflammatory responses. Use of high potency and multi-spectrum probiotic formulations appear to provide clear safety as well as clinical efficacy in those with autism related gut disorders.

Klaire Labs' new Ther-Biotic[a] line[17] uses their proprietary InTactic[a] technology to deliver far higher functional potency than many other probiotic formulations, and these are the ones I use the most now for children who need a high level of intestinal support. (To order directly from Klaire, call 888-488-2488 to receive a 20% discount on all their products by telling them I (or my book) sent you.

Certain nutrients known to be especially important to the immune system are the minerals zinc and selenium, the anti-oxidants A, C, D and E, and a balanced array of amino acids and fatty acids. (please see discussion in Chapter Six).

Glutathione, or GSH

Glutathione is a tri-peptide produced and stored in the liver that is made from the amino acids glycine, glutamic acid and cysteine. It protects the body against toxic agents such as heavy metals by acting as a powerful antioxidant that prevents formation of free radicals and inhibits cellular damage. The reduced form called L-glutathione is the most active kind and the one recommended for ASD children. It is especially important during chelation, but some children have difficulty tolerating it, and some doctors advise omitting glutathione during the "on" days of chelation. IV glutathione is being used with great benefit by some practitioners. Since oral glutathione is not usually well absorbed, transdermal agents are being produced that may offer a more effective approach to providing this essential nutrient. It is important for the amino acid precursors to be taken in the diet or with supplementation to make sure enough glutathione can be produced to prevent oxidative stress caused by viral infections, environmental toxins including heavy metals, inflammation, and dietary deficiencies of GSH precursors and enzyme cofactors.

IVIG (INTRAVENOUS IMMUNE GLOBULIN [HUMAN])

Immunoglobulins are proteins produced by B-lymphocytes and are the major effector molecules of the humoral immune system. Generally, immunoglobulin molecules are antibodies that react with specific antigens. IVIG therapy is believed to act through inhibition of cytokines and the removal of autoantibodies, although medical literature also describes its antiviral effects. Panglobulin IVIG is an FDA approved drug for the treatment of primary immunodeficiencies made from human plasma collected from more than 16,000 volunteer donors at licensed donor centers in the U.S. This product contains primarily IgG, with a small amount of IgA, and traces of IgM. If tests show your child has immunoglobulin deficiency with recurrent infections, a total IgG deficiency, persistent seizures or some other indicated neurological indication, insurance companies are bound under insurance rules to pay for this very expensive treatment. Autoimmune encephalopathy—which some researchers believe to be a form of autism—is not a reason for insurance companies to pay yet. Only laboratory documented immune disorders and intractable seizure disorders are covered by most insurance companies. There is no anti-measles remedy safe for children except for gamma globulin and Vitamin A.

HIGH-DOSE VITAMIN A PROTOCOL

For children who have had the MMR vaccination, and especially those children who regressed following the MMR, the high-dose Vitamin A protocol is considered to be safe for use once every six months if 3 out of the following 5 conditions are met:

1. History of regression after MMR

2. Persistent gut problems, pain in spite of interventions

3. More than slightly elevated IgG serum rubeola antibodies

4. Elevated anti-MBP & anti-NF antibodies (shows autoimmunity)

5. Endoscopy showing ileal hyperplasia or positive PCR

Recommendation is for use of Klaire's Mycelized Vitamin A drops, 5000iu per drop under the tongue in a bolus in the morning, 200,000iu to 400,000iu, depending upon size of child, for two days running, then wait 6 months before doing it again. Daily maintenance is 10,000iu to 25,000Iu again depending upon the size of the child.

> ** Please see discussion of Vit A and D in Chapter 6 under Recommended Supplements for recent information on these vitamins.

PRESCRIPTION IMMUNE-ENHANCING MEDICATIONS

Two promising new immune-enhancing and modulating agents that are quite popular now are Actos and Low-Dose Naltrexone (LDN). Actos, or Pioglitazone, is being studied by Dr. Marvin Boris and associates for immunity and inflammation. LDN is an opioid antagonist being used for modulating the immune system and to regulate mood, being studied by Penn State University for MS and Crohn's, and by Dr. J. McCandless in autistic children. See descriptions of Actos and LDN in Chapter 10.

ANTI-VIRAL PRESCRIPTION MEDICATIONS

For antiviral medications, I use acyclovir for the younger children and Valtrex, a form of acyclovir that is 6 times more biologically active, for kids over five or over 40 pounds as my first choice. For most children acyclovir is safe and effective against most but not all strains of HSV1, HSV2, and VZV, is ineffective against most cytomegalovirus strains, and has various levels of effectiveness against some strains of EBV and HHV6. In my experience and in reports of several other clinicians with very large autistic practices, acyclovir is estimated to be effective in about 30% of the children who take it. Another antiviral used when acyclovir or Valtrex becomes ineffective is Famvir, (famciclovir) which functions in a similar way to acyclovir. Rotating anti-virals sometimes seems to help maintain responsiveness to the drugs. "Safety" tests for blood count and chemistries are essential for any of these prescription medications since they may stress the liver. I usually perform these tests after the first month in an extended treatment course, and then every two or three months thereafter unless there is some indication clinically that something is not going well.

A Parent's Story

Mr. Stan Kurtz is a former technology executive who founded Children's Corner School in Van Nuys, CA. Mr. Kurtz's school is dedicated to helping families, especially those with children with special needs, including autism and ADHD. The dietary and nutritional principals Mr. Kurtz uses at his school are based on the same philosophies he used to help recover his child with autism.

In 2005 during the semi-annual Spring Defeat Autism Now! Conference, Mr. Kurtz showed a video presentation about his son Ethan's recovery from autism using footage he had taken before during and after Ethan's diagnosis and recovery. Mr. Kurtz attributes the success of Ethan's treatment to a combination of dietary restriction (SCD less IGG Food Sensitivities), and the drugs valtrex and diflucan (alternated with nizoral) administered over a period of 9 months. The notable recovery chronicled in the video roused parental interest about anti-viral therapy for their children, especially in the new parents attending the conference.

Although his son did not have positive tests for viral titers, Mr. Kurtz' observations of Ethan and studying of the literature gave him the strong intuition that his boy was affected by viruses, possibly in conjunction with fungus. This intuition led Mr. Kurtz to find a physician who was willing to prescribe Valtrex and Diflucan without testing.

Though prior to this most doctors (including the author of this book) and many parents preferred to have a battery of immune and viral titer testing before embarking upon prescriptive medications, Mr. Kurtz' success led many parents who felt they could not afford expensive lab testing or who just did not want to have their children veni-punctured to want to try his protocol. Valtrex is known to be a very safe medication so before long quite a few families undertook a course of this anti-viral. Some who could not obtain it began using various natural anti-virals, especially Olive Leaf Extract sometimes combined with a protease inhibitor called Virastop, obtaining some of the same benefits and reactions as the children on Valtrex. Mr. Kurtz says parents using both types of antivirals often reported yeast flare-ups, even in children who previously did not seem to have yeast issues. This led to a combination approach of both antiviral and antifungal therapy which seemed to work more often than just antiviral therapy alone. Mr. Kurtz also reported more than half of the parents posting on his internet group stated that their children got rashes shortly after starting the Valtrex. He also said that some families were reporting a greater amount of metals excretion when using this combination approach.

Mr. Kurtz hypothesized from these reports that the anti-virals helped mercury excretion and that this was a "mercury rash." Some families posted test results in his group that seemingly demonstrated better metals excretion during antiviral therapy combined with metals detoxification compared to just metal detoxification alone. Dr. Syd Baker's work on the metabolite adenosine led to his report that acyclovir modulated adenosine levels in children with autism. Baker stated that high levels of adenosine were lowered, while low levels were raised. Abnormal levels of adenosine can impair methylation by pulling back homocysteine and raising levels of a methylation inhibitor S-adenosyl-homocysteine (SAH).

Mr. Kurtz believed that the reverse is also true, that an active virus can impair mercury excretion; like many ideas, he acknowledges that this would require studies to ascertain the correctness of this belief.

Mr. Kurtz' observations and chronicling of his child's improvement with his particular approach and his persistence in bringing this to the community's attention add him to that special group of parents who, in addition to the 24/7 duties of caring for their children's special needs, help not only other parents but health professionals too to expand their views of therapeutic approaches to the ASD complex.

Parents and professionals interested in Mr. Kurtz' protocols and recovery videos can visit Mr. Kurtz' site www.recoveryvideos.com.

Viral/Immune Treatment Summary

The connection between measles vaccine strain virus and gastrointestinal disease in autistic children described as measles enterocolitis by Dr. Andrew Wakefield has been verified by other noted gastrointestinal specialists. There is no specific treatment for measles enterocolitis other than supportive therapies including anti-inflammatories and treatment with vitamin A, which has been shown to provide immune defense against measles. Analysis of several studies on oral supplementation with large doses (200,000 IU) of Vitamin A shows significant reduction in serious effects of measles, including duration of pneumonia, fever, and diarrhea. Improvement in the immune response of children treated with vitamin A has been demonstrated by higher lymphocyte counts and more robust IgG anti-measles antibody production in treated compared to untreated children. Supportive treatments for measles of the gut consist of dietary restriction to help against inflammation caused by the large peptides and use of enzymes to help digestion and absorption. Treatments that help the general immunity of these children help them to improve and develop more normally, such as good nutrition, methylation strategies, decreasing heavy metal load (detoxification), anti-oxidants, nutrients, gut healing and liver support. Some parents have reported a good response in their children who have been given the high dose vitamin A protocol to help them with their gut problems and peripheral visual issues such as side-ways glancing.

Latent viral infections may remain dormant for years, but from time to time can become activated. It seems clear that subsets of autistic children (as well as other groups of immune-impaired persons) have chronic, low level viral infections that are etiologically related to the child's autism. These children have enough immunity to keep from appearing sick, yet they have an underlying immune impairment that permits an atypical chronic infection to exist. Attempts are regularly made through our Defeat Autism Now! biomedical treatments to try to enhance our children's general immunity. Prescriptives for this purpose are immunoglobulins, given orally, intramuscularly, or intravenously. Other prescriptives currently being studied are Actos, a PPAR for pre-diabetic persons, helpful for ASD children because of its anti-inflammatory effects and its shifting of immunity from T2 or humoral immunity more characteristic of autoimmune disorder to T1 or cellular immunity. A new use of an old medicine in a new form, dosing and timing is Low-Dose Naltrexone (LDN), also noted to shift immunity from T2 towards T1 in a few studies. Studies show that opioids alter both innate and adaptive immune cells – NK cells, macrophages, immature thymocytes, T cells and B cells. LDN is being studied to see what regular use at the very low doses known to elevate beta-endorphins will do to the immune system clinically and by changes in immune panels. (See more about Actos and LDN in Chapter 10).

Specific prescriptives for viral issues are not virucidal, but virusuppressive except for some very strong ones usually reserved for hospital use in severely ill persons. The primary ones I use clinically are acyclovir for the small children and valacyclovir for the larger children when testing shows viral elevations. I sometimes use them when tests are not economically feasible but clinical evidence (frequent infections, cold sores, warts, etc) indicates there may be infection with viruses or when the child does not seem to be responding to usual therapies. Valacyclovir (valtrex) can be rotated with famcyclovir (famvir) when the child's improvement plateaus; the two medications seem equally effective but some children do seem to grow resistant to one or the other after a while, with an upsurge in benefits when switched.

Some immune-enhancing nutrients are: Omega-3 fatty acids, glutathione, methylcobalamin/folinic acid, probiotics, vitamins A, C, D, E,A, and Co-Q-10, zinc, and selenium. There are many natural anti-virals in use by our ASD families: Lauricidin[18] has been studied for many years and found to be useful in enveloped viruses. I have given this nutrient to hundreds of children (and adults) over the years with great benefit. Children (and adults) who have herpes of the lips often stop having these infections on lauricidin. Other nutrients that have been well-studied for their anti-viral effects are: garlic[19], olive leaf extract[20], glutamine[21], probiotics, black elderberry extract[22], oil of oregano[23], IP-6 (inositol hexaphosphate)[24], grape peel extract[25], green tea[26], and others. Parents have been very resourceful in finding combinations of these anti-pathogenic nutrients to keep their children well, often rotating them.

Life style factors are very important in virology. Fatigue, lack of a good diet, prolonged emotional or physical stress, and social isolation have been noted to increase susceptibility to viral infections. Activities that impair the immune system such as smoking and ingesting a lot of sugar in the diet have shown a tendency to create susceptibility for viral infections.

Physicians vary in their treatment priorities; many in the Defeat Autism Now! community including myself have generally felt that getting the toxic metal load down takes first priority, as the impairment that heavy metals and particularly mercury make on the immune system is thought to set our children up for viral invasion in the first place. Recently there has been an upsurge in the use of valtrex according to internet autism e-groups since presentation of a film by the parent discussed above in A Parent's Story showing his son making a good recovery with the use of diet, anti-fungals, and valtrex. A considerable number of these children have not had any immune testing. However, many of the children starting on valtrex are already in the midst of detoxification or have had one or more courses of it already, so the jury is still out how much this therapeutic trio (SCD, diflucan, valtrex) will be effective without specifically also using detoxification strategies to lower metal accumulation that most of our autistic children carry. This therapy as many others needs to be researched to ascertain whether indeed effective detoxification can take place without the use of specific detoxifying agents. There is a great deal we do not know about virology in general and especially in as complex a disease as autism.

The health of the immune system clearly plays a central role in the treatment of ASD. Immunity and autoimmunity are inseparable from the status of the gut, resistance to infections and other viral pathologies. Ultimately the treatment of ASD comes down to helping the children develop strong, self-regulating, infection-resisting and pathogen-suppressing immunity. In the final analysis, I do not believe ASD will persist in many and perhaps most ASD children if the child has recovered a healthy immune system.

References

1   Comi A.M. et al., "Familial clustering of autoimmune disorders and evaluation of medical risk factors in autism." J. Child Neurol 1999 Jun;14(6): 388-94

2   van Gent T. et al., "Autism and the Immune System," J. Child Psychol Psychiatry 1997 Mar;38)3): 337-49

3   Hassen, A.N. et al., "Neuroimmunotoxicology: Humoral assessment of neurotoxicity and autoimmune mechanisms, Environmental Health Perspectives Vol. 107. Sup. 5 Oct. 1999

4   Singh, Vijendra K., "Abnormal Measles Serology and Autoimmunity in Autistic Children." J. of Allergy Clinical Immunology 109(1):S232, Jan 2002, Abstract 702

5   Frith, Uta , p. 79-80, Autism: Explaining the Enigma, 1989, Blackwell Publishers Inc, Malden, MA 02148

6   Kawashima H., et al., "Detection and seqencing of measles virus from peripheral mononuclear cells from patients with inflammatory bowel disease and autism. Dig. Dis. Sci. 2000 Apr;45(4): pp. 723-9

7   Romani L., "Cytokine modulation of specific and nonspecific immunity to Candida albicans. Mycoses, 1999; p. 42 Suppl 2: pp. 45-8. Review. Also, Romani L., Immunity to Candida albicans: Th1, Th2 cells and beyond. Curr Opin Microbiol. 1999 Aug;2(4):363-7. Review

8   Binstock T., Intra-monocyte pathogens delineate autism subgroups. Med Hypotheses. 2001 Apr;56(4): 523-31

9   Gesser R.M., Koo S.C., "Oral inoculation with herpes simplex virus type 1 infects enteric neuron and mucosal nerve fibers within the gastrointestinal tract in mice. J. Virol. 1996 Jun;70(6): 4097-102

10 Binstock T, "Fragile X and the amygdala: cognitive,interpersonal, emotional, and neuroendocrine considerations," Dev Brain Dysfunction 1995 8: pp. 199-217

11 Berkowitz C. et al., "Herpes simplex virus type 1 (HSV-1) UL56 gene is involved in viral intraperitoneal pathogenicity to immunocompetent mice." Arch Virol 1994;134(1-2): 73-83

12 Tomsone V. et al., "Associatioin of human herpesvirus 6 and human herpesvirus 7 with demyelinating diseases of the nervous system." J. Neurovirol 2001 Dec;7(6): 564-9

13 Singh V.K. et al., "Serological association of measles virus and human herpesvirus-6 with brain antoantibodies in autism." Clin Immunol Immunopathol. 1998 Oct;89(1): 105-8

14 Hayney M.S. et al., "Relationship of HLA-DQA1 alleles and humoral antibody following measles vaccination. Int. J. Infect Dis. 1998 Jan-Mar;2(3): 143-6

16 Fukushima Y et al. Effect of a probiotic formula on intestinal immunoglobulin A production in healthy children. Int J Food Microbiol. 1998 30;42(1-2):39-44.

17 Ther-Biotic Complete http://www.protherainc.com/prod/proddetail.asp?id=V775-06

18 Lauricidin: Kabara. J.J, Swieczkowski, D M. Conley. A J and Truant, J P Fatty Acids and Derivatives as Antimicrobial Agents Antimicrobial Agents and Chemotherapy 2(l):23-28 (1972) Kabara. J.J.. Conley. A J.- Swieczkowski. D M. Ismail, I.A . Lie Ken Jie and Gunstone, F D Antimicrobial Action of Isomeric Fatty Acids on Group A Streptococcus J. Med Chem 16:1060-1063 (1973). Conley. A J and Kabara. J.J. An-

timicrobial Action of Esters of Polyhydric Alcohols. Antimicrob. Ag and Chemother 4:501-506 (1973) Kabara. J.J., Vrable, R. and Lie Ken Jie, M.S.F Antimicrobial Lipids: Natural and Synthetic Fatty Acids and Monoglycerides. Lipids 12:753759 (1977). Kabara, JJ Fatty Acids and Derivatives as Antimicrobial Agents-A Review. In: The Pharmacological Effect of Lipids. Jon J. Kabara, ed Champaign, Illinois: The American Oil Chemists' Society (1979),pp. 1-14 In The Hierholzer, J.C. and Kabara, J.J. In Vitro Effects of Monolaurin Compounds on Enveloped RNA and DNA Viruses. J. Of Food

[19] Garlic: Immunomodulatory affect of R10 fraction of garlic extract on natural killer activity International Immunopharmacology, Volume 3, Issues 10-11, October 2003, Pages 1483-1489 Zuhair M. Hassan, Roya Yaraee, Narges Zare, Tooba Ghazanfari, Abul Hassan Sarraf Nejad and Bijhan Nazoric

[20] Olive leaf extract: The olive leaf extract exhibits antiviral activity against viral haemorrhagic septicaemia rhabdovirus (VHSV) Antiviral Research, Volume 66, Issues 2-3, June 2005, Pages 129-136 Vicente Micol, Nuria Caturla, Laura Pérez-Fons, Vicente Más, Luis Pérez and Amparo Estepa

[21] Glutamine: Glutamine Protects Activated Human T Cells from Apoptosis by Up-Regulating Glutathione and Bcl-2 Levels Clinical Immunology, Volume 104, Issue 2, August 2002, Pages 151-160 Wei-Kuo Chang, Kuender D. Yang, Hau Chuang, Jia-Tsong Jan and Men-Fang Shaio

[22] Black Elderberry (Sambucol): Antiviral activity in vitro of Urtica dioica L., Parietaria diffusa M. et K. and Sambucus nigra L. Journal Ethnopharmacology, Volume 98, Issue 3, 26 April 2005, Pages 323-327 R.E. Uncini Manganelli, L. Zaccaro and P.E. Tomei

[23] Oil of Oregano: In Vitro Antioxidant, Antimicrobial, and Antiviral Activities of the Essential Oil and Various Extracts from Herbal Parts and Callus Cultures of Origanum acutidens Münevver Sökmen, Julia Serkedjieva, Dimitra Daferera, Medine Gulluce, Moschos Polissiou, Bektas Tepe, H. Askin Akpulat, Fikrettin Sahin, and Atalay Sokmen J. Agric. Food Chem.; 2004; 52(11) pp 3309 - 3312; (Article) DOI: 10.1021/jf049859g

[24] IP-6 (Inositol hexaphosphate) ISSN 1007-9327 CN 14-1219/R World J Gastroenterol 2005 August 28;11(32):5044-5046 Inositol hexaphosphate-induced enhancement of natural killer cell activity correlates with suppression of colon carcinogenesis in rats Zheng Zhang, Yang Song, Xiu-Li Wang

[25] Grape peel extract (resveratrol): Docherty, John J., Jennifer S. Smith, Ming Ming Fu, Terri Stoner, and Tristan Booth. Effect of topically applied resveratrol on cutaneous herpes simplex virus infections in hairless mice. Journal of Antiviral Research. January 2004, 61(1) p. 19-26.

[26] Green Tea: Antiviral effect of catechins in green tea on influenza virus Antiviral Research, Volume 68, Issue 2, November 2005, Pages 66-74 Jae-Min Song, Kwang-Hee Lee and Baik-Lin Seong

For Further Reading

Autistic disorder and viral infections: Journal of NeuroVirology, ll:1-10,2005

Abnormalities in T cells and T cell subsets, Depressed responses to T cell mitogens, Decreased killer cell function, (Stubbs, et. Al. 1977, Warren, etal. 1990, Yonk, et al. 1990, Warren, et al. 1995, Gupta, et al. 1998)

Comi A.M. et al., "Familial clustering of autoimmune disorders and evaluation of medical risk factors in autism." J.Child Neurol 1999 Jun;14(6): 388-94

Singh, Vijendra K., "Abnormal Measles Serology and Autoimmunity in Autistic Children." J. of Allergy Clinical Immunology 109(1):S232, Jan 2002, Abstract 702

Wakefield, A.J. et al., "Ileal-lymphoid-nodular hyperplasia, non-specific colitis, and pervasive developmental disorder in children." Lancet 1998 Feb. 28;351(9103):637-41.

Coutsoudis A, Kiepiela P, Coovadia HM, Broughton M. Pediatr Infect Dis J 1992 Mar;11(3):203-9 Vitamin A supplementation enhances specific IgG antibody levels and total lymphocyte numbers while improving morbidity in measles.

Binstock T., Intra-monocyte pathogens delineate autism subgroups. Med Hypotheses, 2001 Apr;56(4): 523-31

Annals 1st Super Sanita, 1996;32(3):351-9, Scifo R, Marchetti, et al, "Opioid-immune interactions in autism: behavioural and immunological assessment during a double-blind treatment with naltrexone.

NINE

HBOT-HYPERBARIC OXYGEN THERAPY FOR AUTISM SPECTRUM DISORDERS
(ABBREVIATED VERSION)

Complete version hosted at www.drneubrander.com under the HBOT tab

Written by Jim Neubrander, M.D.
Reviewed by Dan Rossignol, M.D.
Edited by Sharon Waldman, M. Ed., M.SE.

FOREWORD
HISTORY AND DESCRIPTION
BENEFITS
SIDE EFFECTS
MULTIPLE MECHANISMS OF ACTION
BASIC PRINCIPLES AND SAFE PROTOCOLS
QUESTIONS AND CONCERNS
SUMMARY
SELECTED BIBLIOGRAPHY

Foreword

From collective observations following hundreds of thousands of treatment hours by colleagues and myself, the evidence is now irrefutable that hyperbaric oxygen therapy is a valuable treatment option for children with autism. Unfortunately, hyperbaric treatment is expensive and insurance companies are not yet reimbursing for its use. Therefore many parents have not been able to take advantage of the benefits it potentially may offer their children. Fortunately, research studies currently in process are documenting the benefits hyperbaric oxygen therapy provides for children with autism. Once published, they will provide the scientific validation that is required so insurance companies will finally reimburse for this valuable therapy.

History and Description

Hyperbaric oxygen therapy is *classically defined* as the inhalation of 100% oxygen at greater than 1 atmosphere absolute (ATA) in a pressurized chamber. This definition is now *popularly defined* as the inhalation of varying degrees of oxygen at greater than 1 atmosphere absolute (ATA) in a pressurized chamber. You will hear many terms used interchangeably by lay people and professionals alike. However, the most common way the term is used by the autism community is to just say "HBOT".

Conventional wisdom believes that unless one receives HBOT in a hard chamber with 100% oxygen at pressures no less than 1.5 atmospheres, little or no benefit will be seen; if parents use a soft chamber with lower pressures and lower oxygen concentrations, they are just wasting their money and cheating their children of the benefit hyperbaric therapy has to offer. However, as history has shown repeatedly throughout the years, ***convention is only convention until challenged, proven wrong, and then changed*. SUCH IS THE CASE WITH HBOT AND AUTISM TODAY!**

Both high and low pressure treatments may be effective for any given child. Which treatment or treatments to use for that specific child will depend on multiple factors, some practical and some medical. *Practical factors* include, but are not limited to, a family's finances; availability of the type of treatments offered at a clinic (high pressure, low pressure, or both); the cost of those treatments at the clinic; the ease by which a family can receive treatments based on the time required and the distance they must travel to get to a clinic; the number of times per week a family can actually receive treatments in order to see benefits and maintain them; and the ability to continue treatments over time (repeated sets of treatments needing to be done at a clinic vs. owning a home unit). *Medical factors* include, but are also not limited to, the primary and secondary disorders to be treated with any given child, e.g. a child with autism *and* cerebral palsy; the underlying mechanism one wants to focus upon, e.g. inflammatory, vascular, etc.; and the seriousness of the medical condition being treated. *Each of these <u>medical and practical considerations</u> must be evaluated on a <u>case-by-case basis</u> and no broad generalizations should be made when considering which treatment option may be best for your child.*

Benefits

Essentially any of the symptoms common to autism have the potential to be helped by HBOT. However, certain benefits seem to be more common than others, and the intensity of the response is often greater when present. For example, one of the most hoped-for responses parents desire is improvement in their child's *language*. In my practice this is one of the most commonly reported benefits. Parents frequently tell me their child exhibits more conversational language and uses longer sentences with more complete and complex sentence structure that now includes pronouns, prepositions, adjectives, and adverbs. They report an increase in spontaneous speech with initiation of conversation at appropriate times. They report that their child's vocabulary is more complete than ever before and that their child will now *ask* a question, *wait* for their response, and then *respond* appropriately to what they just said. I can report hundreds of improvements in language function in the children whom I have treated with HBOT. Most improve, but do not reach total recovery until their treatment is combined with other major treatments, such as methyl-B$_{12}$, healing the gut, etc. However, I have witnessed incredible results in children of all ages, not just those below the age of six. One eleven-and-a-half-year-old boy came to me in August 2005 with only two to three word occasional utterances. After using one of my advanced protocols, he left my clinic thirty days later speaking in six to nine word sentences that included pronouns, adjectives, and adverbs! Another young man in his early twenties came to me with essentially no functional language. After repeated treatments in my clinic he was able to hold a conversation for more than five minutes! Another four year old child I treated was diagnosed as "profoundly autistic" and had no language other than the ability to label a few nouns. He followed my advanced protocol for ten months, gained complete command of the English language, and has officially lost his diagnosis! Fortunately, these stories are not isolated stories. *The use of HBOT, especially if preceded by my specific protocol for methyl-B$_{12}$, is undoubtedly the best combination of treatments I have to improve spontaneous speech and conversational language!*

Another frequently reported category of benefits includes those that occur within the frontal cortex of the brain where executive functioning originates. In my practice, increased *awareness,* with all of its associated findings, is almost universal in children treated with HBOT. Children become more *"present"*, meaning that they become more involved and *actively engaged* in what they are now *aware* of. They are much more *attuned* to what is happening on a day-to-day basis and now *understand their* relationship to the world and what is happening around them, and how they fit into the scheme of things. With this new level of awareness they become less frustrated, *less fearful* and therefore less rigid, more *flexible*, more *resilient*, and more tolerant to changes that before would upset their world. However, should something now upset them, they are able to bounce back more quickly and recover in a much shorter period of time than they ever would have prior to treatment. Another extremely common occurrence is that the children's *eye contact* becomes markedly improved. They are now very aware that they are being called or spoken to. They respond by looking into their parent's eyes and by holding eye contact for a significant period of time, rather than their usual fleeting glance, as was typical in the past. They are more aware of what they are to do, when to do it, and how to do it to please others. In addition they will sit still and *tend to tasks at hand* for much longer periods of time, often completing them, something they were never able to do before.

Parents frequently report that their child now has a new level of *understanding cause and effect* and they *understand new concepts* and follow through with the appropriate actions. For example, one child who was previously unaware that he could fall and hurt himself whenever he was high up in the air suddenly turned to his mother when he saw her near the edge of a ledge and said, "Mommy, no fall – back!" Parents report that *cognition* becomes more complex, more consistent, and that their children handle *age-appropriate* problem-solving of all types much more accurately and in far less time than ever before. Parents report that their children's *comprehension* becomes greater, that the child understands more complex thoughts and concepts, and that s/he understands them more quickly, allowing parents and teachers to not have to repeat or re-teach as much as they needed to before. The children become far more *inquisitive,* asking, "What's this – what's that?" Parents report that it is as if their children are *seeing the world for the first time* and are finally taking the *initiative* to explore new things that they never would do on their own before.

Another major set of symptom improvements that are commonly seen include the area of socialization and emotion. Very frequently parents report that their child will *initiate play* with a peer or adult, whereas before such an event was uncommon or rare. Parents report that for the first time their child *makes his/her needs known* to family, friends, or playmates and actually expects the family, friends, or playmates to respond. The children frequently become *engaged* or are engaging. Parents often report that for the first time they observe from the corner of their eye that their child is watching them closely, studying everything they are doing, and later they find their child trying to *imitate* their actions. Many parents report that for the first time their child finally *understands facial expressions and body language and the feelings of others.* They are thrilled when they see their child respond to an emotional situation with the appropriate reaction, e.g. when a mother was sad her son said, "No sad, Mommy"; or when a father was angry his daughter responded by taking her father's hand and pulling him out of the yard where he was arguing with a neighbor, saying, "No mad; no mad – go home."

Two other wonderful benefits are frequently reported by parents. The first is that children suddenly have an *increased appetite* and are willing *to try new foods* without putting up a fight. Many parents report that for the first time in over two years their child is finally *gaining weight!* *One of the other most consistent responses in the top 20 most frequently reported benefits* is that a child's *bowel function improves, often remarkably so!* It is not uncommon for a child who has had typical autistic-like loose "mashed potatoey" unformed stools for years, many of whom have even been taking major GI medications, to start HBOT and have their stools become "picture perfect" for the first time in their life! Several parents have reported that their child self-potty trained over a weekend, when prior to HBOT, they had struggled with this issue for years.

Because parents want to know how to obtain the greatest number of improvements in the least amount of time, I am often asked, "Which is better, hard chamber or soft? Does one show better benefits, different benefits, or stronger benefits than the other?" To that I can say that *both hard and soft chamber treatments essentially show the same benefits* and that the number and intensity of benefits are most often *related to the total number of oxygen units, pressure units, time units, and cellular product units.* These benefits will be described in the Protocol Section of the complete version of this chapter you will find on my website. However, it has been my observation that *hard chamber treatments are often superior when motor functions play into the equation*, and symptom improvements like gross and fine motor skills, muscle tone, and apraxia are more quickly affected with hard chamber treatments than with soft.

Side Effects

All is not perfect with HBOT and children who have autism. The HBOT textbooks state that the most common side effects include barotrauma (2%), sinus squeeze (pain in the sinuses from changes in pressure), serous otitis (a watery non-bacterial inflammation of the ear due to irritation of the eardrum), claustrophobia (fears of being confined), reversible myopia (near-sightedness), and seizures (0.01–0.03%). Side effects do exist in my practice. They are most often what I call positive-negative side effects, rather than negative-

negative side effects, and tolerable side effects rather than intolerable side effects. The most common negative-negative but tolerable side effect is hyperactivity, though there are some physicians who consider this a positive-negative side effect. According to Rossignol's study, the hyperactivity diminishes over time, often within fifteen to twenty hours of treatment. Increased stimming is also a fairly common negative-negative, but tolerable side effect. By contrast, most of the behavior problems parents commonly see are *positive-negative responses* and *indicate that HBOT is actually working* and that it is a good thing being manifested in a bad way. Frequently children may become more frustrated, more aggressive, less compliant, tantrum more, become less cooperative, follow directives or commands less, become more irritable, have more mood swings, and show less flexibility. The most common reason for this set of unwanted behavior reactions is that the child's brain is "coming back" and the child is more aware in general. Therefore the child becomes more self-assured, more self-confident, more independent, more opinionated, and becomes a child who wants and expects more control of his/her own situation in life. Therefore, when unchallenged and/or no demands are being placed on the child, the parents see many of "the good things" mentioned above. However, when the parents make a request or put a demand on the child, the child often responds in these negative and unpleasant ways. For example, when a parent tells their child that she will need to take a bath, put the Gameboy away, eat dinner now, or to come inside from playing, the child sees it as a challenge to her right to control her life. She may respond by kicking, crying, screaming, or having a meltdown. Likewise, when a child now becomes aware of what he wants to communicate to his parents but is aware that he can't, because of the language barrier, the same negative reactions may occur because he is either frustrated at himself or frustrated that his parents have a problem—not him—and don't understand what it is he wants. The key to knowing whether an action/reaction is a positive-negative behavior or a negative-negative behavior is to determine whether the unwanted behavior occurs after you make a request or demand that the child does not want to do at the time, or whether the unwanted behavior occurs after the child makes a request or demand to you that you cannot accommodate immediately.

A few rules will usually help parent and clinicians make the best decision how to proceed when deciding to continue or discontinue HBOT when side effects occur to more than a mild or moderate degree. *Rule 1*: Side effects that disrupt the life or safety of the child or others, or that disrupt the child's ability to learn are considered "intolerable" and the treatment should be discontinued or the protocol altered *significantly*. *Rule 2*: If the child's gains are *undeniably* present and the side effects are "tolerable", though very much a nuisance and undesirable, the total number of hours used per treatment and the frequency of treatments may remain the same or be varied *only slightly*. However, the child will usually be able to continue the treatments without protocol changes, and the side effects will typically pass if given enough time.

Multiple Mechanisms of Action

A few of the multiple mechanisms demonstrating how HBOT may work for children with autism are listed below. A more comprehensive discussion of each can be found in the complete version of this chapter on my website.

1. Angioneogenesis from the addition of oxygen.
2. Angioneogenesis from the removal of oxygen.
3. Increases in blood flow independent of new blood vessel formation.
4. Decreasing levels of inflammatory biochemicals.
5. Up-regulation of key antioxidant enzymes and decreasing oxidative stress.
6. Increased oxygenation to functioning mitochondria.
7. Increased production of new mitochondria.
8. Bypassing functionally impaired hemoglobin molecules, the result of abnormal porphyrin production, thereby allowing increased delivery of oxygen directly to cells.
9. mprovement in immune and autoimmune system disorders.
10. Decreases in the bacterial/yeast load found systemically and in the gut.

11. Decreases in the viral load found systemically and possibly decreases in a viral presence that may exist in the intestinal mucosa.
12. Increases in the production of stem cells in the bone marrow with transfer to the CNS.
13. (Theoretical only) Direct production of stem cells by certain areas in the brain.
14. Increased production and utilization of serotonin.
15. (Theoretical but doubtful) The possibility that oxidation may help rid the body of petrochemicals.
16. (Theoretical but doubtful) The possibility that oxidation may help rid the body of mercury and heavy metals.

It is my opinion that the *specific* mechanisms of action are influenced by important *general* mechanisms of action. These general mechanisms of action include: a) *increasing total concentration of oxygen per treatment; b) increasing total time of treatment using lower oxygen concentrations and lower pressures; c) increasing or using pressure independent of oxygen concentration.* Though these three concepts are not new, the way I interpret them and how I apply them are my hypotheses, my opinions, and do not necessarily reflect those of my colleagues.

Basic Principles and Safe Protocols

The amount of oxygen that can be dissolved into body water (plasma, lymph, cerebral spinal fluid, interstitial fluid) is dependent upon two factors, the atmospheric pressure used and the concentration of the oxygen provided. Unfortunately, the higher the concentration of oxygen dissolved into body water, the shorter the treatment time can be before oxidative stress, oxygen toxicity, central nervous system (CNS) toxicity, and pulmonary toxicity become a concern. The opposite is also true, whereby the lower the concentration of oxygen dissolved into body water, the longer one may safely continue treatment, as long as the final concentration of dissolved oxygen is within physiologic ranges. The importance of this for your child is that by adjusting the oxygen-oxidizing concentration and the pressure used, any range of oxygen concentration per unit of body water can be achieved and can vary between slight, moderate, marked, or excessive. With marked or excessive concentrations of dissolved oxygen, or with extended use of even *slight* concentrations of dissolved oxygen, toxicity can occur.

IT IS IMPORTANT TO UNDERSTAND THAT "TOXICITY" IS NOT EQUIVALENT TO "SENSITIVITY". Children on the autism spectrum appear to be much more sensitive to the effects of oxygen concentration relative to the pressures used and the total treatment times to which they are exposed. That is the reason I have developed what I believe to be safer and more effective protocols specific to my patient population. These protocols can be found in the complete version of this chapter on my website. *Included are diagnostic and repeat-use protocols for hard and soft chamber use.* As a general rule, it is wise to *start low and go slow* when it comes to the use of HBOT and children with autism!

The complete version of this chapter, as seen on my website under the HBOT tab, shows five tables. The first table compares "time units, oxygen units, pressure units, and cellular product units" between high pressure and low pressure treatments. The second and third table show the *"diagnostic protocols"* I use to determine soft chamber responders and to determine hard chamber responders. The fourth and fifth table show the protocol I recommend for home chamber users, and the protocol I prescribe for parents who are repeating sets of hard chamber treatments for their child.

Questions and Concerns

The most common concern parents have is that HBOT may not work for their child and therefore will be a costly experiment. I agree that HBOT is one of the most expensive treatments used for children with autism. However, in our clinic we can document HBOT initially works to some degree for more than 80% of our children. If treatments are continued once the child has been determined to be a responder, it has been our experience that many of the benefits gained will continue to increase over time. It has also been our experience that new benefits will often be added. Once made, we have seen many of the positive responses hold. *Unfortunately, several of the gains either diminish or are lost within a few months if treatment is not continued.*

My opinion has definitely changed from the first time I wrote this chapter in 2006. Once I started using my more advanced protocols, my frequency of response rate jumped significantly, as did the intensity of the responses I was seeing. I now have hundreds of responders and a greater number of happy parents than ever before. With my current protocols, parents "prove to themselves" how valuable HBOT is for their child, and don't have to be sold on its value. It is my ever-strengthening bias that the benefits are cumulative, but only if treatments are accompanied by *significant breaks*. Many parents have reported only a few, if any, benefits during the treatment period itself, only to see amazing results begin a week or two after the treatments ended! It is also my bias that if you don't know what you're looking for, you'll never see it. This is why the evaluation form we use, in the way we use it, is so important for parents to know what to expect. When considering the responder group's *initial response*, only 10% of children have exceptional improvements (significantly increased language, normal bowel movements, socialization, cognition, executive functions) within the first 30 days of the diagnostic protocol. An additional 20% would be rated as showing good improvements, (often the same as just mentioned but of a lesser intensity); and the remaining 70% would be rated as mild-to-moderate responders (many but not all of the same improvements and most with a lesser intensity of response). Just as tulip seeds do not grow into beautiful flowers within 30 days, just as tree seeds do not grow tall enough to produce cooling shade within 30 days, and just as children entering school do not learn their ABC's in 30 days, neither do most children completing their first 30 day round of HBOT accomplish everything parents wish for their children to accomplish. However, if parents are taught what to expect during the initial diagnostic phase of treatment, and if they are taught when and how to continue treatments if their child responds, even if only to a mild degree, then there will be less chance of the devastating disappointment that is born from unfulfilled expectations.

With all the good things that I've described—things that every parent wants to hear about for any treatment they hope may work for their child—I must offer a *strong word of caution*! During all the years I have been refining my skills, *no skill has become more important* than helping parents be *patient* with their hopes, while at the same time teaching them how to be *accurate and comprehensive with their observations*. Therefore I tell every parent that the more inconvenient, the more costly, and the more 'hype' that surrounds *any* given treatment, HBOT or anything else, the more parents demand to see bigger changes before saying that that treatment is valuable enough to continue. Because of the high cost of HBOT, because HBOT is not yet paid for by insurance companies, and because HBOT is inconvenient, this demand by parents to "get what they want or call it quits" becomes even more of a problem. Therefore it is more imperative than ever before that parents know what they should be looking for, and for parents and clinicians to be able to compare the results they are seeing in a specific child with the results that other parents are seeing in general. In my practice *the parents* have created *an evaluation tool that tells, in their own words, how they see things*. This *HBOT Parent Designed Report Form* (PDRF) has been able to pick up on small, subtle changes that parents tell me they would have otherwise missed, or did miss, when using other evaluation tools. The PDRF, *their evaluation tool*, not mine, is *more sensitive* and *more specific* for the common symptoms seen when children use HBOT. Its use does not mean that other, more standardized evaluation tools should not be used at the same time. However, it has been the parents' experience that, by documenting in great detail all "*undeniable changes*" observed, allows them to see positive changes sooner than they would if they had not taken the time to do this. Seeing these changes earlier, and comparing them to what other parents "just like them" are seeing, encourages them to continue treatment. They confess they would have otherwise quit HBOT treatment because the intensity or numbers of "obvious responses" were so few in comparison to the "subtle but yet present changes" that were, in reality, quite common.

The second most common concern parents have is that their child will not get into the chamber. To date I have only had a few children who did not like the chamber once they got used to it, so this concern is not usually a problem. In fact, many of the children run down the hallway and cannot wait to get inside, some even banging on the chamber to get the other child out!

The third most common concern parents have is that HBOT may cause problems with their child's ears, because of pain or sound sensitivity. Sound sensitivity is something that can be handled for most of the children by using sound muffling devices, so it is usually not a problem, especially after the child gets used to the chamber. That leaves the issue of pain. Pain is the result of barotrauma. *Baro* means pressure and *trauma* means damage. Therefore barotrauma of the ears is damage to the eardrums (tympanic membranes) due to pressure effects. Barotrauma is the most common side effect of HBOT. It is usually associated with pain in the ears, teeth, or other "closed spaces", and varies in degree from mild to extreme. Well-trained chamber operators know how to avoid causing barotrauma in the first place. Well-trained chamber operators learn how to differentiate the signs and symptoms of barotrauma, sound sensitivity, or the child's anxiety. Well-trained chamber operators also learn how to differentiate primary child anxiety that occurs because the child is scared because HBOT is an unfamiliar new procedure; or secondary anxiety, which is initiated when the child senses a parent is anxious and unsure about things as well! Whenever parents are renting or purchasing a chamber to be used in their home, our clinic teaches them "hands on" how to be "well-trained chamber operators".

The fourth most common concern parents have is that HBOT will not be covered by their insurance company. Unfortunately, hyperbaric oxygen therapy is only approved for reimbursement by insurance companies or Medicare for the following conditions: a) Blood loss, extensive, including *severe* anemia; b) burns, thermal; c) carbon monoxide poisoning; d) compartment syndrome; e) crush injury; f) decompression sickness; g) embolism, air/gas; h) gangrene, gas; i) infections, necrotizing soft tissue; j) ischemia, acute traumatic (some, not all); k) osteomyelitis, refractory; l) osteoradionecrosis; m) skin grafts and flaps (compromised); n) smoke inhalation, severe, acute; o) wounds, problem type (not all). All other diagnoses including autism, PDD-NOS, and encephalopathy are called "off-label" and do not qualify for insurance reimbursement. Rarely, some insurance companies may pay for hyperbaric oxygen therapy for off-label reasons. Since we started doing this in our clinic in 2005, this has only happened twice. The second person was audited and the ruling was then reversed. Several other leading physicians who do a significant amount of HBOT report the same lack of insurance reimbursement for off-label use.

Summary

In summary, I can emphatically state that HBOT—hard or soft—is one of the most valuable tools I have added to my tool chest to treat children with autism. ***HBOT is not the magic bullet that we are all looking for.*** Such a bullet does not exist. ***However, HBOT has the potential to be a powerful adjunct to all the other therapies that a child is using.*** When done consistently and with realistic expectations, and when parents use the Parent Designed Report Form evaluation tool that they themselves have created, more than 80% of them will be able to say that HBOT works for their child, too!

Selected Bibliography

1. Collet JP, Vanasse M, Marois P, et al. Hyperbaric oxygen for children with cerebral palsy: a randomised multicentre trial. Lancet 2001;357(9256):582-6.

2. Golden ZL, Neubauer R, Golden CJ, Greene L, Marsh J, Mleko A. Improvement in cerebral metabolism in chronic brain injury after hyperbaric oxygen therapy. Int J Neurosci 2002;112(2):119-31.

3. Granowitz EV, Skulsky EJ, Benson RM, et al. Exposure to increased pressure or hyperbaric oxygen suppresses interferon- secretion in whole blood cultures of health humans. Undersea Hyperb Med 2002;29(3):216-25.

4. Gutsaeva DR, Suliman HB, Carraway MS, Demchenko IT, Piantadosi CA. Oxygen-induced mitochondrial biogenesis in the rat hippocampus. Neuroscience 2006;137(2):493-504.

5. Harch, PG, McCullough, V. The Oxygen Revolution. Hatherleigh Press, April 2007.

6. Heuser G, Heuser SA, Rodelander D, Aguilera O, Uszler M. Treatment of neurologically impaired adults and children with "mild" hyperbaric oxygenation (1.3 ATM and 24% oxygen). In Hyperbaric oxygenation for cerebral palsy and the brain-injured child. Edited by Joiner JT. Flagstaff Arizona: Best Publications; 2002:109-15.

7. James SJ, Cutler P, Melnyk S, et al. Metabolic biomarkers of increased oxidative stress and impaired methylation capacity in children with autism. Am J Clin Nutr 2004;80(6):1611-7.

8. Knighton DR, Halliday B, Hunt TK. Oxygen as an antibiotic. The effect of inspired oxygen on infection. Arch Surg 1984;119(2):199-204.

9. Lavy A, Weisz G, Adir Y, Ramon Y, Melamed Y, Eidelman S. Hyperbaric oxygen for perianal Crohn's disease. J Clin Gastroenterol 1994;19(3):202-5.

10. Mukherjee, Arun. New Dehli, India. Presentation at the Neuro-HBOT Training Course, Pittsburg, PA., October 2008.

11. Nie H, Xiong L, et al. Hyperbaric oxygen preconditioning induces tolerance against spinal cord ischemia by upregulation of antioxidant enzymes in rabbits. J Cereb Blood Flow Metab 2006;26(5):666-74.

12. Rossignol DA, Rossignol LW. Hyperbaric oxygen therapy may improve symptoms in autistic children. Med Hypotheses 2006;67(2):216-28.

13. Rossignol DA, Rossignol LW, James SJ, Melnyk S, Mumper E. The effects of hyperbaric oxygen therapy on oxidative stress, inflammation, and symptoms in children with autism: an open-label pilot study. BMC Pediatr 2007: Nov 16;7-16.

14. Rossignol DA. Hyperbaric oxygen therapy might improve certain pathophysiological findings in autism. Med Hypotheses 2007;68(6):1208-27.

15. Rossignol DA. The results of a six center collaborative study for children with autism using low pressure with a low oxygen concentration has been submitted for publication, November 2008.

16. Stoller KP. Quantification of neurocognitive changes before, during, and after hyperbaric oxygen therapy in a case of fetal alcohol syndrome. Pediatrics 2005;116(4):e586-91.

17. Thom SR, Bhopale VM, Velazquez OC, Goldstein LJ, Thom LH, Buerk DG. Stem cell mobilization by hyperbaric oxygen. Am J Physiol Heart Circ Physiol 2006;290(4):H1378-86.

18. Vargas DL, Nascimbene C, Krishnan C, Zimmerman AW, Pardo CA. Neuroglial activation and neuroinflammation in the brain of patients with autism. Ann Neurol 2005;57(1):67-81.

19. Vlodavsky E, Palzur E, Soustiel JF. Hyperbaric oxygen therapy reduces neuroinflammation and expression of matrix meralloproteinase-9 in the rat model of traumatic brain injury. Neuropathol Appl Neurobiol 2006;32(1):40-50.

20. Wilson HD, Wilson JR, Fuchs PN. Hyperbaric oxygen treatment decreases inflammation and mechanical hypersensitivity in an animal model of inflammatory pain. Brain Res 2006;1098(1):126-8.

TEN

LATEST DEVELOPMENTS

A. METHYLATION

Introduction

I.   Methylation General

II. Methylation Science
R. Deth, PhD

III. Methylation Clinical
J. McCandless MD

B. GENETIC TESTING FOR METHYLATON DEFECTS
C. Schneider, MD

C. ACTOS
M. Elice, MD

D. LOW-DOSE NALTREXONE (LDN)
J. McCandless, MD

E. LOW OXALATE DIET (LOD)
S. Costen Owens

A. METHYLATION

INTRODUCTION

A general introduction to methylation is followed by the latest information on the science behind methylation by Richard Deth, PhD , neuropharmacologist and professor of pharmacology at Northeastern University in Boston, Massachusetts; Dr. Deth Is on the scientific advisory board of the National Autism Association. and clinical aspects of methylation by Jaquelyn McCandless, MD.

Cynthia Schneider, MD, private practitioner specializing in autism, has been studying genomics and describes how this new science relates to autism currently.

Marvin Boris, MD and his assistants Allan Goldblatt, PA, and Michael Elice, MD have continued their investigation of Actos as an anti-inflammatory and immune enhancer, and Dr. Elice will write on this topic as it relates to autism.

Jaquelyn McCandless, MD will describe her work with Low-Dose Naltrexone (LDN) for mood and immunomodulation in autistic children and autoimmunity.

Susan Costen Owens, Autism Researcher, will introduce her studies and latest information on the Low Oxalate Diet.

I. METHYLATION GENERAL

We have known for a long time that Vitamin B12, folate, and thiamine are important players in the body's metabolic cycles. Methylcobalamin is a key factor in the transference of methyl groups (transmethylaton) of folate to methionine. Vitamin B12 in its coenzyme form as methylcobalamin together with folinic acid participates in methionine synthesis and affects the metabolism of sulfur-containing substances. Since every cell in the body expresses the folate/methionine cycle, defects in transmethylation can affect vital biochemical reactions at many places in intermediary metabolism. We are finding more every day about how sulfhydryl (SH) reactive metals such as mercury, lead, arsenic and cadmium appear to be "triggers" for multiple disease symptoms in ASD.

The evidence for transmethylation defects in autism disorders is accruing thanks to talented researchers helping us to understand the basic science behind our clinical observation that certain treatments help these children. Since 2003 we have heard Jill James, PhD from University of Arkansas for Medical Sciences discuss the impairment in transulfuration and the resulting oxidative stress that occurs in ASD from depletion of glutathione, the major intracellular antioxidant essential for detoxification in the body. Her studies using intervention with folinic acid and betaine showed a highly significant increase in plasma methionine, cysteine, and glutathione after only three weeks. When 8 of the 20 children in her original group continued on this dietary schedule for 3-4 months adding injectable Methyl-B12, results were even more positive, suggesting that methylation capacity and antioxidant potential can be increased with obvious clinical benefits in ASD children. The dietary nutrients Dr. James showed as supportive of methionine synthesis were: Zinc, folinic acid, betaine (TMG), methyl-B12, and choline. Most of the children receiving the methyl-B12 injections were on folic acid, as it has been known for some time that B-12 needs folate to be given along with it for effective utilization in the body. Dr. James indicated that folinic acid (5-formylTHF) enters the folate pathway in a reduced form which is more easily asimulated into folate metabolism than the synthetic vitamin form, folic acid.

In the same year we heard Richard Deth, PhD from Northeast University describe his research showing the effects of thimerosal on methionine synthase and emphasized the devastating role this neurotoxin can have in the disordered methylation in our afflicted children. His studies showed how thimerosal alters methionine synthesis activity with the potential to disrupt normal development via its neurotoxic effect on DNA methylation and gene expression. Dr. Deth will help us understand the latest information on methylation science.

II. METHYLATION SCIENCE
RICHARD DETH, PHD

The Latest on Methylation Science and
Its Relationship to Autism

Methylation is the biochemical process by which a carbon atom (a methyl group) is added to a molecule, typically for the purpose of altering its activity. For example, methylation of the neurotransmitters dopamine epinephrine renders them inactive. Perhaps the most important role for methylation is the epigenetic regulation of gene expression by methylation of specific DNA locations known as CpG sites[1]. Upon methylation of the C in such a CpG site, a sequence of events ensues that ultimately causes the adjacent DNA to tightly wind around the protein histone, effectively silencing the gene. Since all cells in an individual contain the same DNA, specific cell types reflect distinctive patterns in DNA methylation that sustain their unique activities (e.g. making a liver cell different from a neuron or a muscle cell). Indeed, human development, starting from a fertilized egg, is driven by progressive shifts in DNA methylation that is most remarkable during fetal development and early years of postnatal growth, but continues throughout the lifespan. No wonder it can be said that to understand life, you must first understand methylation.

Methylation is carried out as a part of sulfur metabolism. The sulfur-containing essential amino acid methionine is the source for almost all of the methyl groups used by cells. Methionine must be first activated to be a methyl donor by ATP (i.e. by adenosylation) to form S-adenosylmethionine (SAM or SAMe)[2]. The methyl group of SAM is transferred to a wide array of molecules (dopamine, DNA etc.) by methyltransferase enzymes, leaving behind S-adenosylmethionine (SAH). If levels of SAH build up for any reason, as is the case in most autistic children, it blocks SAM from binding to methyltransferase enzymes, thereby reducing methylation. Thus SAH is an important regulator of methylation. SAH is broken down into adenosine (leftover from ATP) and homocysteine (HCY), which is methionine without a methyl group. Importantly, the breakdown of SAH to HCY and adenosine is reversible, and SAH is kept at a low level by the further metabolism of HCY and adenosine. Some HCY is converted back to methionine to complete the so-called methionine cycle, and some is sent toward the synthesis of cysteine and the anti-oxidant glutathione (GSH) via the transsulfuration pathway. Regulation of this critical metabolic intersection, where HCY can be used either to support methylation or to reduce oxidative stress, is not only fundamental for cell survival, but it is also for controlling many cellular functions via methylation. This intersection is at the very heart of autism.

Relative activities of the two enzymes that metabolize HCY, methionine synthase and cystathionine-beta-synthase (CBS), determine HCY and SAH levels and they are both targets of regulation that is responsive to the oxidative status of the cell[3]. Inhibition of either enzyme causes HCY to accumulate, causing increased SAH levels resulting in impaired methylation. In the case of CBS, oxidative stress brings about cleavage of an inhibitory portion of the enzyme, releasing higher activity and promoting GSH synthesis. Mutations in CBS are associated with neurological disorders, including autism.

Methionine synthase (MS) utilizes cobalamin (vitamin B12) to remove a methyl group from methylfolate and then transfer it to HCY, creating methionine. In doing so it limits the need for dietary methionine in supporting the methionine cycle and also limits transsulfuration. Conversely, any reduction in MS activity will increase utilization of dietary methionine for methylation and will augment cysteine and GSH synthesis. During evolution, a number of molecular strategies for limiting MS activity in response to oxidative challenges have arisen. Indeed, biosynthesis of cobalamin apparently arose as a metabolic response to an oxygenated environment. Since children with autism exhibit signs of severe oxidative stress[4], we can assume that a number of these adaptive strategies, as well as others not involving MS, have been activated and the various symptoms of autism reflect the consequences of this metabolic disruption. There is now very strong evidence that autism is caused by oxidative stress, and that children with autism represent a genetically vulnerable subpopulation more susceptible to factors capable of inducing oxidative stress, including exposure to heavy metals and xenobiotics (foreign compounds). These ìenvironmentalî factors trigger the disorder, in which impaired methylation plays a major role.

The cobalamin cobalt atom in MS, which is the essence of its activity, exists in several different oxidation states during the enzymatic cycle. Cbl(I) is its empty state and, after the folate-derived methyl group has been attached, the cobalt is Cbl(III), more commonly known as methylcobalamin or methylB12. Cbl(I) is the most highly reactive and consequently the most easily oxidized material in biological systems, and it readily oxidizes to Cbl(II), depending upon whether it encounters an oxidizing molecule (e.g. ROS or xenobiotic metabolite) in its local environment. As such, Cbl(I) serves as an exquisitely sensitive sensor of the cellular redox environment, and when it does oxidize, MS activity is temporarily turned off, leading to increased GSH synthesis. Thus inactivation of vitamin B12 is an elegantly simple mechanism to maintain cellular redox balance. MS can be reactivated after Cbl(I) oxidation by converting the Cbl(II) to methylcobalamin. In the brain, methylB12 to be synthesized via a two-step mechanism that requires GSH, and if GSH levels are lower than normal, which they commonly are in autism, the enzyme remains inactive.

A number of neurodevelopmental toxins inhibit MS activity by lowering GSH and interfering with methylB12 synthesis[5,9]. This is not really a surprise, since changes in methylation activity are critical for turning genes off and on during development. Mercury and other heavy metals remain primary suspects for causing oxidative stress and impaired methylation in autism, although there is room for important contributions from other environmental toxins as well. Recently, I summarized the relationships linking the effects of environmental exposures to the metabolic pathways involved in supporting antioxidant and methylation activities, and formulated a "Redox/Methylation Hypothesis of Autism"[9].

The neurological symptoms of autism are rooted in dysfunction of dopamine-stimulated phospholipid methylation (PLM), a unique activity of the D4 dopamine receptor which was discovered by our laboratory[6]. In this mechanism, dopamine activates the D4 receptor to carry out the methionine cycle using a methionine that is an integral part of the receptor itself. This methionine, found only in the D4 type of receptor, donates a methyl group to nearby phospholipid molecules that surround the receptor on the surface of neurons, causing a localized increase in the fluidity of the membrane. The change in membrane fluid properties can alter the activity of ion channels located in the receptorís microenvironment, with the net result of changing the rate of nerve firing to a higher frequency[7,8]. By modulating the frequency of firing, dopamine can select certain information for attention. When different brain regions are firing at the same frequency (i.e. in synchrony) they can interact and work together for complex tasks. Failure of the D4 receptor PLM mechanism may underlie the impaired synchronization that is a feature of autism.

MS activity is absolutely critical for dopamine-stimulated PLM to work properly. Indeed, while increased utilization of dietary methionine can at least partially offset the effect of oxidative stress on the ìnormalî methylation cycle, MS is the exclusive source of methyl groups for D4 receptor PLM. As a result, when oxidative stress turns off MS, it will have a negative impact on its physiological role in neuronal synchronization and attention. Genetic variations in the D4 receptor are linked to ADHD risk, as well as the personality trait of novelty seeking, and recent studies indicate that these same variations give rise to differences in gamma frequency synchronized oscillations in cortical networks during attention.

In summary, impaired neuronal synchrony is an important feature of autism, and it seems very likely that reduced activity of dopamine-induced PLM, secondary to oxidative stress, underlies this reduction. This highly unifying hypothesis of autism is strongly supported by the symptomatic improvement in many autistic children upon administration of methylB12.

References

[1] Rodenhiser D, Mann M. Epigenetics and human disease: translating basic biology into clinical applications. CMAJ. 2006 Jan 31;174(3):341-8.

[2] Loenen WA. S-adenosylmethionine: jack of all trades and master of everything? Biochem Soc Trans. 2006 Apr;34(Pt 2):330-3.

[3] Banerjee R, Evande R, Kabil O, Ojha S, Taoka S. Reaction mechanism and regulation of cystathionine beta-synthase. Biochim Biophys Acta. 2003 Apr 11;1647(1-2):30-5.

[4] James SJ, Melnyk S, Jernigan S, Cleves MA, Halsted CH, Wong DH, Cutler P, Bock K, Boris M, Bradstreet JJ, Baker SM, Gaylor DW. Metabolic endophenotype and related genotypes are associated with oxidative stress in children with autism. Am J Med Genet B Neuropsychiatr Genet. 2006 Aug 17; [Epub ahead of print]

[5] Waly M, Olteanu H, Banerjee R, Choi SW, Mason JB, Parker BS, Sukumar S, Shim S, Sharma A, Benzecry JM, Power-Charnitsky VA, Deth RC. Activation of methionine synthase by insulin-like growth factor-1 and dopamine: a target for neurodevelopmental toxins and thimerosal. Mol Psychiatry. 2004 Apr;9(4):358-70.

6   Sharma A, Kramer ML, Wick PF, Liu D, Chari S, Shim S, Tan W, Ouellette D, Nagata M, DuRand CJ, Kotb M, Deth RC. D4 dopamine receptor-mediated phospholipid methylation and its implications for mental illnesses such as schizophrenia. Mol Psychiatry. 1999 May;4(3):235-46.

7   Deth RC, Kuznetsova A, Waly M. ìAttention-related signaling activities of the D4 dopamine receptorî in *Cognitive Neuroscience of Attention*, Michael Posner Ed., Guilford Publications Inc., New York, 2004.

8   Demiralp T, Herrmann CS, Erdal ME, Ergenoglu T, Keskin YH, Ergen M, Beydagi H. DRD4 and DAT1 Polymorphisms Modulate Human Gamma Band Responses. Cereb Cortex. 2006 Jun; 17(5): 1007-119.

9   Deth R, Muratore C, Benzecry J, Power-Charnitsky VA, Waly M. How environmental and genetic factors combine to cause autism: A redox/methylation hypothesis. Neurotox. 2008 Jan;29(1):190-201.

III. METHYLATION CLINICAL ASPECTS
JAQUELYN MCCANDLESS, MD

Current Clinical Use of Methyl-B$_{12}$ in Autism

One of the most important treatment modalities to come out of the strong focus on biomedical and metabolic aspects in autism in recent years is the use of injectable methylcobalamin, or methyl-B$_{12}$. The evidence for transmethylation defects in autism disorders was already starting to accrue thanks to talented researchers Jill James and Richard Deth (mentioned above) helping us to understand the basic science behind our clinical observation that certain nutrients help these children.

In May 2002 my Defeat Autism Now! colleague and friend Dr. James Neubrander made the "accidental" discovery that showed him methyl-B$_{12}$'s profound effect on autism. Experimenting with different members of the cobalamin family, Dr. Neubrander was able to ascertain that the benefits of methylcobalamin far surpassed the cyanocobalamin and hydroxycobalmin forms used for autism prior to 2002. Since every cell in the body expresses the folate/methionine cycle, defects in transmethylation can affect vital biochemical reactions at many places in intermediary metabolism.

Because of Dr. Neubrander's work, methyl-B$_{12}$ was provided for 8 of the 20 children in Dr. James' group. These 8 children continued on their dietary schedule for 3-4 months with the added injectable methyl-B$_{12}$ and results were even more positive, suggesting that methylation capacity and antioxidant potential can be increased with obvious clinical benefits in ASD children. The dietary nutrients Dr. James showed as supportive of methionine synthesis were: Zinc, folinic acid, methyl-B_{12}, choline, and betaine (TMG), later seen as part of an alternate pathway and only helpful for a small percentage of children. His studies lent tremendous credence to the importance of methylation disorders and their treatment in autism. Prior to a Defeat Autism Now! presentation in Spring 2005 I queried three of the more popular compounding pharmacies for the number of autistic children for whom they were providing the methyl-B_{12} injectables, and the total was 4500 children being given injections two or three times per week at that time. By now it is being used all over the United States and in many countries all over the world by both adults and children.

Methyl-B_{12} is estimated to be active and effective to some degree in 80-90% of ASD children. Dr. Neubrander has an elegant Parent Designed Report Form which helps parents assess whether their child is a responder, downloadable for free from his website www.drneubrander.com. He advises parents to make no changes in their child's nutrient program when adding the methyl-B_{12} for a period of five weeks to see how responses show its effect. Then he adds folinic acid and any other nutrients that testing has shown the child needs, as he agrees with the Defeat Autism Now! principle that these children need a broad-spectrum treatment approach. Though the parent form looks for many possible responses, the primary ones for methyl-B_{12} are executive function, speech, language, socialization, and emotion. However, Dr. Neubrander fears that if parents only look for these signs, they may give up before adequately utilizing this treatment, and feels that if given in the right dosage, timing, and form that up to 94% will show benefit.

Besides the myths that methyl-B_{12} only works in 30-40% of ASD children, other myths Dr. Neubrander would like to dispel is:

1. That this nutrient works better for younger children.

2. That oral, sublingual, transdermal, or intramuscular routes are just as effective as the subcutaneous injections. (At the present time, a nasal spray has been introduced which has become popular with parents who do not want to

give their children injections; many of us have tested to compare this with the tried and true subcutaneous route, and Dr. Neubrander (and I) experiencee the subcutaneous route as superior, but nasal route (for those children who can and will sniff strongly enough and high enough) superior to sublingual whichh is superior to oral.

3. That the concentration of the methyl-B$_{12}$ solution does not matter as long as the total dose remains the same. (Many tests have shown that the 25mg/ml injections at 64.5 mcg/kg every three days is the optimal dose, volume, and frequency for the majority of children though there are exceptions.) Currently, 40% of those treated by Dr. Neubrander are shwing better results with daily injections (same dose).

4. That the fat in the arm, abdomen, or thigh produce the same results as from the fatty part of the buttocks.

In general lowering the dose until side effects disappear is a mistake—often the children with the most side effects who stay with the course are the ones who make the most recovery. The most common side effects are hyperactivity with or without increased "stimming," changes in sleep patterns, and increased mouthing (not pica, or eating of non-food item) of objects. Dr. Neubrander agrees that certain side effects are an indication to stop this nutrient, such as an older child becoming uncontrollable and potentially dangerous to others or side effects that are so disruptive that a child can no longer function or learn. However, he encourages parents to continue as long as a child can learn, attend to tasks, and stay focused in a controlled situation no matter how much increased activity there may be at home when the child can just let loose. Mouthing objects is a sign that previously inactivated peripheral nerves are waking up and this represents a "positive negative" and a sign that the methyl-B$_{12}$ is working. Within two to six months the majority of side effects diminish or disappear completely while the child continues to improve.

Other caveats: Use a good compounding pharmacy that knows how to make the proper dose as recommended by Dr. Neubrander. Do not pinch the fat for the injection. Inject as narrow an angle as possible to avoid hitting any muscle; pink urine *always* means you injected too deeply. The shots if given correctly are seldom painful. There is no way if proper needles (BD 3/10 cc insulin syringe with an 8 mm, 31-gauge needle, item #328438 only) and injection technique are used that the sciatic nerve could possibly be injured, even in the smallest baby. There is no way to test who will or will not be a responder to methyl-B$_{12}$. Blood B$_{12}$ levels are high-normal to high in almost all children documented to be responders. Though there may be a high level in the blood, it is in an oxidized form that cannot be reduced and recycled. Genomic testing is not yet advanced enough to reliably predict response, as these tests may miss the majority of children that clinically respond and should be treated.

Mr. Stan Kurtz, the parent discussed in Chapter 8 with his use of anti-virals in the recovering of his son, also has contributed to our methylation therapy by introducing Nasal Spray MB-12. Dr. Jim Neubrander, the leading health worker in the emphasis on the usefulness of methylcobalamin for autistic children, ran an informal test comparing the MB12 nasal spray with the subcutaneous injections and stated that although the shots were overall preferable, the nasal spray was effective and certainly a better option for those families averse to injecting their children. Some, in fact, felt the nasal spray was equal to or superior to the injections, whereas other families (including the kids!) preferred to stay with the injections, which they knew were helping them, and to which they had become accustomed. In the nasal form, the MB-12 can be combined with folinic acid, and some children as well as adults have started using the Nasal Spray instead of the subcutaneous injections. Like the injections it does have to be prescribed and created by a compounding pharmacy.

The only way to know if your child (or you!) is one of the majority of autistic children (or adults) that will benefit from this important treatment with methyl-B$_{12}$ is to use it, as there are no good lab tests for MB-12. Methylation is one of the more important biomedical interventions that Defeat Autism Now! has pioneered in the last few years along with dietary restriction, nutrients, healing the gut, detoxification (formerly called chelation), anti-viral/ immune enhancing strategies, anti-inflammatory strategies, and HBOT that are improving and recovering more and more autistic children every day.

B. GENETIC TESTING FOR METHYLATON DEFECTS

CYNTHIA SCHNEIDER, MD

It has become increasingly evident that individuals with autism have impairments in their capacity to methylate. Methylation reactions are those reactions in our metabolism that involve the transfer of a methyl group (a carbon with three hydrogens attached) from one compound to another. These reactions are required for many of the most vital pathways in our metabolism. The building or repair of every cell in our bodies requires methylation. The silencing of viral genes involves methylation. We must be able to methylate the dopamine receptor in order for it to bind with dopamine, transform lipid membranes, change the frequency of brain waves, and increase our attention. The coffee addict craves caffeine, a methyl donor, because it causes a burst in focus and attention. An alarmingly large percentage of our pediatric population has been placed on Ritalin (methylphenidate), a methyl donor, for the same reason. Messages are not transmitted along neurons accurately and efficiently unless the nerve is insulated with a substance called myelin, which cannot be produced without methylation. The most commonly known defect in myelination (the protection of nerves with myelin) is multiple sclerosis, a condition in which anti-myelin antibodies are made. Anti-myelin antibodies are frequently found in children with autism as well, and levels of these anti-myelin antibodies correlate with their levels of anti-measles antibodies, raising speculation that a chronic measles infection of the nervous system may be one cause of autism. The success of methylcobalamin (methyl B12) injections in the treatment of multiple sclerosis led Dr. James Neubrander to explore methylcobalamin as a treatment for autism, which has proven to be highly effective.

A person who is less able to methylate may present with inflammatory conditions such as eczema, colitis, asthma, or arthritis, as methylation is also required to produce glutathione, our body's primary antioxidant. Chronic inflammation and the associated tissue damage can lead to an autoimmune disease, a condition in which a person's immune system begins to make antibodies against his or her own tissue. Diabetes, Crohn's disease, lupus, and multiple sclerosis are examples of autoimmune conditions and are commonly seen in the families of individuals with autism. Anxiety and obsessive-compulsive tendencies are also common, as the production of serotonin, our anti-anxiety neurotransmitter, requires properly functioning methylation pathways. Serotonin then goes through a series of reactions including methylation and is converted to melatonin, the compound that allows us to fall asleep. The association between sleep disorders and autism is well known to most parents of these individuals and to even their least enlightened physicians. A person with impairments in methylation is likely to be more susceptible to viral infection and to adverse reactions to live viral vaccines. Chronic viral infections are common and viruses such as measles that attack the gut and nervous system are of most concern.

Although millions of dollars have been spent on genetic research, no autism gene has been identified. There are many genes of interest that are found more frequently in individuals with autism, but none of these genes cause the condition and most people who carry the genes do not have autism. Autism has all the characteristics of a multifactorial disorder, meaning that both environmental and genetic risk factors interact to cause the condition. A person with several genetic weaknesses in his or her ability to methylate, for example, might be perfectly healthy in an ideal environment, but easily become ill in a less than perfect environment. Certain metabolic weaknesses have no impact if exposure to toxins such as mercury or pesticides does not occur, but may lead to rapid deterioration in health and function under conditions of exposure to these and other toxins. Nutritional status is also very important. Many genes have catalysts or cofactors that allow them to operate more efficiently. Without these cofactors, which are often vitamins and minerals, they do not function well. With them, even a weaker enzyme may operate within the normal range. It is for this reason that many functional medicine practitioners utilize higher than average levels of targeted nutritional supplements. Those practitioners that understand the biochemistry behind these supplements can use them to treat the core problem rather than simply reduce the symptom. For example, a serotonin reuptake inhibitor such as Prozac might rapidly increase the amount of time that serotonin remains in the synapse and available to neurons and thereby alleviate some of the symptoms of a serotonin deficiency such as anxiety or depression. A more holistic viewpoint would be that a person with those symptoms might suffer from a methylation defect, making him or her susceptible to a whole range of health problems which result when methylation is impaired. Correcting the serotonin issue with Prozac, even if successful, has only solved one of potentially many related problems, whereas enhancing methylation in general would have widespread beneficial effects.

Rather than thinking in terms of an autism gene, we would be wise to think in terms of autism pathways. Methylation pathways are the best candidates, as permutations in these reactions could lead to any of the deficits and symptoms described in autism and the biomedical treatments that have met with success are ultimately impacting these pathways.

Genetic testing is available through various laboratories and in research protocols. The most intriguing genes to date include catecholamine-O-methyltransferase (COMT), methylenetetrahydrofolate reductase (MTHFR), methionine synthase (MS), methionine synthase reductase (MSR), dihydropteridine reductase (DHPR), cystathione beta synthase (CBS), S-adenosylhomocysteine hydroxylase (SAHH), adenosine deaminase (ADA), Paraoxonase (PON1) and reelin. The interplay between these genes determines many aspects of our personality due to their effect on neurotransmitter levels. They also work in concert to allow us to build and repair cells, a process that continues even after growth has ceased. A person undergoing chemotherapy is taking drugs that diminish the capacity for cells to replicate. The most common side effects of chemotherapy are nausea, vomiting, and diarrhea, largely because the cells that line the bowel are unable to replicate. The thin lining of our bowel wall is ordinarily replaced gradually day by day with a complete turnover of cells occurring every three days. Other areas of the body in which cells do not turn over so rapidly are less affected by these drugs and likewise less affected by methylation defects. One could liken a child with autism who has methylation defects to a person on chemotherapy. Such a person would be likely to have gastrointestinal symptoms, be more susceptible to infection, be less able to focus, and may decline cognitively.

The question is then how to enhance methylation in those who have methylation defects. A wide range of methyl donors are available and the optimal combination of compounds is a matter of trial and error. In those who can obtain genetic testing, errors are less frequent because more information is available. The most commonly beneficial supplements include methylcobalamin, the active form of folic acid called 5-methyltetrahydrofolate, and coenzyme Q10. Many, but not all individuals tolerate vitamin B6 or its more active form, pyridoxyl-5-phosphate (P5P), magnesium, and zinc with considerable benefit, as these enhance the function of critical enzymes. Some do well with dimethylglycine (DMG) or trimethylglycine (TMG), as they influence the direction of traffic along certain methylation pathways. It is not unusual for irritability, hyperactivity, or insomnia to develop if the wrong supplement is given or if the right supplement is given at the wrong time. When side effects occur, the guidance of a qualified health professional should allow identification of the problem. Some adverse effects are simply evidence of detoxification. In these cases, symptoms resolve and areas such as language and attention improve after toxins have cleared. When in doubt, urinary tests for toxic metals should be obtained to investigate the possibility of toxic metal excretion. Some of these same supplements have the capacity to increase ammonia levels, which would cause irritability, lack of focus, and/or an increase in self-stimulatory behaviors. Accurate ammonia measurements are difficult to obtain outside of a hospital setting, but the possibility of ammonia toxicity should be considered when these behaviors are present. Many genetic variants, such as the more active CBS allele, the less active MTHFR allele (A1298C), and weaker variants of nitric oxide synthase (NOS) may predispose an individual to high ammonia levels. When these genes are present, ammonia levels must be managed in a variety of ways. Certain gut bacteria produce high levels of ammonia. Improving bowel health and digestion through various means such as aggressive management of constipation, the administration of probiotics, the reduction of simple carbohydrates in the diet, and the provision of digestive enzymes when tolerated will significantly decrease bacterial ammonia production. Limiting protein intake and dividing this intake between meals rather than allowing a protein load at one meal will place less demand on the pathways that clear ammonia. In those who tolerate it, 5-methyltetrahydrofolate will often decrease ammonia levels by increasing tetrahydrobopterin (BH4) levels. BH4 may also be given toward this end, although pharmaceutical grade BH4 is difficult to obtain and not yet FDA approved. A less pure source of BH4 is available by the trade name Bio Thyro and has been effective in many cases. Some practitioners advocate the use of activated charcoal to decrease ammonia levels, but frequent use of charcoal is not practical because it interferes with the absorption of nutrients and is highly constipating. The administration of charcoal must be followed by high dose magnesium or other means to induce a bowel movement for this reason.

Paraoxonase (PON1) is an enzyme required for the metabolism of organophosphate pesticides. Many forms of this gene exist, some allowing organophosphate pesticides to be cleared 40 times more rapidly than others. The PON1 gene is located in 7q21.3-22.1, a region showing strong genetic linkage with autism. Persico *et al* assessed three functional genetic variants called C-108T, L55M, and Q192R in 177 Italian and 107 Caucasian-American families with one or more affected children. Caucasian-Americans displayed a significant association between autism and the PON1 variant marked by L55 and R192 (P<0.025 with patients vs normal controls, transmission/disequilibrium test, family-based association test, and haplotype-based association test). No trend was found in Italian children with autism. This was the predicted finding, as organophosphate pesticide use is much higher in the United States than in Italy and the predominant form of autism in America does not seem to be the same as that most frequently seen in Italy. Caucasian-American children with autism carrying at least one copy of the R192 (weaker) variant had significantly lower serotonin blood levels, but Italian children with this gene did not. This may be explained by the impact of paraoxonase on an enzyme called dipeptidyl peptidase IV (DPPIV). When paraxonase activity is impaired through either the inheritance of a weaker version of the gene or by pesticide exposure, this in turn affects the activity of an enzyme called adenosine deaminase (ADA). When ADA does not function properly, levels of its substrate adenosine rise. This becomes a roadblock to methylation, potentially leading to any or all of the complications previously described. DPPIV and ADA function may be increased by the avoidance of two of the substrates for DPPIV, gliadomorphin and casomorphin. It is by this and other mechanisms that avoidance of gluten and casein lead to enhanced cognitive function, decreased inflammation, and improved attention.

Bibliography

D'Amelio M, Ricci I, Sacco R, Liu X, D'Agruma L, Muscarella LA, Guarnierei V, Militerni R, Braccio C, Elia M, Schneider CK, Melmed RD, Trillo S, Pascucci R, Puglisi-Allegra S, Reichelt K-L, Macciardi F, Holden JJA, and Persico AM. Paraoxonase Gene Variants are associated with Autism in North America, but not in Italy: Possible Regional Specificity in Gene-Environment Interactions. Molecular Psychiatry, 10: 1006-1016, 2005.

Persico AM, D'Agruma L, Zelante L, Militerni R, Bravaccio C, Schneider C, Melmed R, Trillo S, Montecchi F, et. al. Enhanced APOE2 Transmission Rates in Families with Autistic Probands. Psychiatric Genetics, 14(2): 73-82, Jun 2004.

Conciatori M, Stodgell CJ, Hyman SL, O'Bara M, Militerni R, Bravaccio C, Trillo S, ontecchi F, Schneider C, Melmed R, Elia M, et. al. Association between the HOXA1 A218G Polymorphism and Increased Head Circumference in Patients with Autism. Biological Psychiatry, 55(4): 413-419, 2004.

Persico AM, D'Agruma L, Maiorano N, Totaro A, Militerni R, Bravaccio C, Wassink TH, Schneider C, Melmed R, Trillo S, Montecchi F, Palermo M, Pascucci T, Puglisi-Allegra S, Reichelt KL, Conciatori M, Marino R, Baldi A, Zelante L, Gasparini P, and Keller F. Reelin Gene Alleles and Haplotypes as a Factor Predisposing to Autistic Disorder. Molecular Psychiatry, 6: 150-159, 2000.

Persico AM, Militerni R, Bravaccio C, Schneider CK, Melmed RD, Trillo S, Montecchi F, Palermo M, Pascucci T, Puglisi-Allegra S, Reichelt K, Conciatori M, Baldi A, and Keller F. Adenosine Deaminase (ADA) Alleles and Autistic Disorder: Case-Control and Family Based Association Studies. American Journal of Medical Genetics (Neuropsychiatric Genetics), 96:784-790, 2000.

Persico AM, Militerni R, Bravaccio C, Schneider CK, Melmed RD, Conciatori M, Damiani V, Baldi A, and Keller F. Lack of Association between Serotonin Transporter Gene Promotor Variants and Autistic Disorder in Two Ethnically Distinct Samples. Americal Journal of Medical Genetics, 96:123-127, 2000.

C. ACTOS
MICHAEL ELICE, MD

It is becoming more and more accepted every day that autism is a complex neurodevelopmental disorder. Although all the specific causes remain to be determined, there is strong evidence that genetic, environmental, inflammatory, immunological and metabolic factors all play a prominent role in this disease.

Cytokines are small proteins that direct the movement of circulating white blood cells to sites of inflammation or injury. Originally studied because of their role in inflammation, cytokines and their receptors are now known to play a crucial part in a wide range of diseases with prominent inflammatory components. For example, elevated levels of cytokines in the joints of patients with rheumatoid arthritis coincide with movement of monocytes and T cells into the synovial tissues. Inflammation is also a key factor in asthma, in which cytokines recruit eosinophils, or white blood cells that respond to allergies, to the lung. Psoriasis is another example of cytokine-mediated cell recruitment and inflammation. Multiple sclerosis is an example of how cytokines can influence the progression and severity of an auto-immune disease.

Altered immune responses in children with Autistic Spectrum Disorders (ASD) have been well documented. In 1976, Stubbs published that 5 of 13 autistic children had no detectable rubella antibodies despite prior immunization. (1). An additional study by Stubbs showed that certain white blood cells known as monocytes and T lymphocytes were functioning abnormally. (2) In children with ASD, there is a preponderance of Helper 2 – (Th2) T- cells over the Helper 1 (Th1) T- cells. This finding was confirmed at the Cincinnati Children's Hospital Medical Center. (3) In 2005 the study of children with ASD had their cytokines compared to control patients. In all, the Th2 cytokines were significantly higher than the Th1, demonstrating an abnormal autoimmune and /or inflammatory response.

Peroxisome proliferators-activated receptors (PPARs) are a class of nuclear transcription factors that are activated by fatty acids and their derivatives. They were discovered by early electron microscopists in the 1950's. Christian de Duve, in Brussels, Belgium, subsequently isolated these structures, demonstrated hydrogen peroxide generation and renamed them peroxisomes.(4) By the 1990's PPARs were identified and shown to be transcription factors. They were found to control a number of genes, most of which have little or nothing to do with peroxisomes. PPAR gamma is important both in fat cell metabolism and modulating cellular responsiveness to insulin. Hence, the connection with diabetes. They were subsequently found to regulate T-cell responsiveness and to suppress macrophage and microglia activation. Both of these actions are relevant to multiple sclerosis and other neurodegenerative diseases as well.

The discovery that insulin sensitizing thiazolidinediones (TZD's), specific(PPAR-g) agonists, have antiproliferative, anti-inflammatory and immunomodulatory effects has led to the evaluation of their potential use in the treatment of diabetic complications and inflammatory, proliferative diseases in non-insulin-resistant, normal glycemic individuals (5). In addition to improving insulin resistance, currently approved TZD's have been shown to improve psoriasis, ulcerative colitis, other autoimmune, atopic, inflammatory and neurodegenerative diseases (e.g. asthma, atopic dermatitis and multiple sclerosis, Alzheimer's disease, Parkinson's Disease.) These discoveries pave the way for the development of drugs for treating metabolic diseases for which therapy is presently insufficient or non-existent.

The anti-inflammatory effects on neural cells include suppression of cytokines and enzymes involved in free radical production including NOS and COX2. (6) Some PPAR agonists have been proven to be blood brain barrier permeable suggesting direct effects on brain physiology. Pioglitazone, known as Actos and rosiglitazone, known as Avandia, activate PPAR gamma which suppresses T-cell, macrophage and microglial immune responses. If the suppression of these immune responses is of potential benefit for inflammatory diseases of the brain, then pioglitazone should provide therapeutic benefit in multiple sclerosis and other autoimmune disease entities. These drugs were originally designed as anti-diabetic drugs due to their insulin sensitizing effects and have been in clinical use for many years. The clinical safety of Actos has been established by clinical studies worldwide, in which over 4500 subjects have been treated. Since FDA approval, Actos has been widely prescribed to several million patients. The adverse effects associated with PPARg agonists are generally mild and transient. Those effects returned to their baseline upon withdrawal from, or completion of the studies. (7). Since the recent studies with PPARg drugs in animal models of neurological conditions and diseases have led to clinical testing of these drugs in Alzheimer's disease and multiple sclerosis, they make promising candidates for a therapeutic approach to influence the clinical course of Autism and Autistic Spectrum Disorders.

In a clinical practice dedicated to treating children on the autistic spectrum with over 3000 patients, Marvin Boris, M.D. and Michael Elice, M.D. have been treating patients with Actos in the attempt to improve their immune status. Ages of patients range from 2 years and older. The diagnosis of autism was established by pediatric neurologists, developmental pediatricians and /or psychiatrists meeting the DSM IV criteria prior to being seen in their practice.(8) All the children had been receiving behavioral and educational therapies. These included speech, occupational and physical therapy, applied behavioral analysis (ABA) and auditory integration therapy (AIT). The children also received biomedical interventions for at least one year from the group.

The main hypothesis is that treatment of autistic children with Actos that is currently FDA approved for treatment of type 2 diabetes, but which also shows important anti-inflammatory and cytoprotective effects on neural cells, will provide clinical benefit associated with a change in serum cytokine levels. Since June 2007, Actos and Avandia will carry "black box" warning that the drugs may trigger heart failure. This class of drugs may increase a person's risk of congestive heart failure, secondary to retention of fluid in a minority of individuals. This warning has nothing to do with heart attacks. In order to determine if Actos is safe and tolerable to autistic children, monthly exams, measurements of blood for liver enzymes, standard chemistries, glucose and insulin levels have been performed. If there is any concern about the child's cardiac status, a pediatric cardiologist is consulted prior to administration of Actos. Patients are always cautioned about the development of excessive weight gain or periorbital edema, indicators of fluid retention in the body.

Effects on disease are assessed by evaluation of the aberrant behavior checklist (ABC) as recommended by the American Society of Psychiatry. Modification of inflammatory markers in the autistic patients was accomplished by measurement of serum cytokine levels and reactive oxygen species, and by isolation and characterization of serum T-cells.

In over 1000 patients prescribed Actos conducted in this private practice setting, Boris and Elice have shown improved cognitive function and improved receptive and expressive language as well as increased spontaneous language, decreased hyperactivity, decreased lethargy, decreased stereotypical behavior (stimming), better eye contact and socialization. In follow-up lab testing, there have been no alterations in blood glucose or insulin levels.

Blood plasma samples from autistic children treated off-label with Actos for up to 6 months were analyzed for 9 different cytokine levels by ELISA assay and compared to values from non-treated patients. For 8 or 9 cytokines, Actos reduced plasma levels. An additional observation has been the consistent elevation of platelet counts on routine CBC's in the autistic population. This thrombocytosis is a known marker for inflammation. After administration of Actos, 76% of patients had reduction of platelet counts to normal ranges. Patients showed improved behavior described by treating physicians and parents with no adverse effects. This suggests the safety of Actos in autistic children and can influence inflammatory responses which could moderate clinical symptoms.

Drs. Boris and Elice are currently treating and evaluating children on the autism spectrum using Actos in conjunction with Celecoxib (Celebrex), vitamin A and Montelukast (Singulair). Celecoxib belongs to a class of non-steroidal anti-inflammatory drugs (NSAIDs) known as COX -2 inhibitors. Celecoxib is effective in treating pain and inflammation but is less likely to cause serious gastric side effects than other NSAIDs such as Ibuprofen and Naproxen. Celecoxib has been routinely used in children with rheumatoid arthritis without cardiac problems. The dose of Celecoxib is 50 mg BID for 10-25kg body weight; 100mg BID for 25kg or more. Vitamin A, a retinoid, is given in higher doses of 10,000 to 25,000 units daily. Montelukast, a leukotriene antagonist is given as a single dose of 10 mg/day, regardless of the age of the child.

Since February 2007, the FDA has granted approval for the administration of Actos for this "off-label" use. When using Actos in conjunction with Celebrex,

Vitamin A and Singulair, Boris and Elice have found a 62% benefit to the autistic children. Adverse effects of this therapy have been a 6% increase in aggressive behavior, 8% increase in sleep problems, 12% had GI disturbances, 5% experienced weight gain and/or periorbital swelling, and one child had transient elevation in liver enzymes which returned to normal levels after the discontinuance of therapy.

References

[1] Stubbs EG, Autistic children exhibit undetectable hem agglutination-inhibition antibody titers despite previous rubella vaccination, J> Autism child Schizophrenia. 1976; 6:269-274

[2] Stubbs, EG and Crawford ML, Depressed   lymphocyte responsiveness in autistic children, J.Autism Child Schizophr. 1977;749-55

[3] Molloy CA, Morrow AL, etal. Elevated cytokine levels in children with autism spectrum disorder. J. Neuroimmunology. 2005 Dec 14

[4] Pershadsingh HA, Peroxisome proliferators-activated receptor-g: therapeutic target for diseases beyond diabetes:quo vadis? Expert Opinion on Investigational Drugs. 2004;13:3

[5] Mrak, RE and Landreth, GE. PPAR-g, neuroinflammation, and disease. J. of Neuroinflammation. 2004,1:5

[6] Roberts-Thomson SJ. Peroxisome proliferator-activated receptors in tumorigenesis: targets of tumour promotion and treatment: Immunol Cell Biol 2000; 78:436-41

[7] Gelman, L,Fruchart JC, Auwerx J. an update on the mechanisms of action of the peroxisome proliferators-activated receptors (PPARs) and their roles in inflammation and cancer. Cell Mol Life Sci 1999;55:932-43

[8] Baba, S, Pioglitazone: a review of Japanese clinical studies. Curr Med Res Opin, 2001. 17(3): 166-89

[9] Diagnostic and Statistical Manual of the American Psychiatric Association 4th ed. (DSM-IV) *American Psychiatric Association, 1994*

D. LOW-DOSE NALTREXONE (LDN) FOR IMMUNE ENHANCEMENT AND MOOD IN AUTISM, CANCER AND AUTOIMMUNE DISORDERS

JAQUELYN MCCANDLESS, M.D.

What is naltrexone? And what is the difference between naltrexone and low-dose naltrexone (LDN)?

Naltrexone is a medication used for exogenous opiate antagonism for treating opiate drug and alcohol addiction since the 1970s. It has been FDA-approved since 1984 and has been available since 1998 in generic form as well as in the brand name ReVia, both only in 50mg tablets. At regular dosing to treat addiction, usually 50 to 150mg a day, this drug blocks the euphoric response to opiates such as heroin or morphine as well as alcohol. Low-dose naltrexone (LDN) usually ranges between 1.5 and 4.5mg, less than 1/10th of regularly manufactured naltrexone, (standard is 50mg tablets) and must be compounded in capsules or a transdermal cream to get the tiny doses.

Endogenous opioids operating as cytokines create immunomodulatory effects through opioid receptors on all immune cells. A popular immune classification method is referred to as the Th1/Th2 balance: Th1 cells promote cell-mediated or innate immunity, while Th2 cells induce humoral or acquired immunity. Simplistically, the inability to respond adequately with a Th1 response can result in chronic infection and cancer; an overactive Th2 response can contribute to allergies and various syndromes and play a role in autoimmune disease, which most autism spectrum children show on immune testing. The November 13, 2003 issue of the New England Journal of Medicine (1a) notes: "Preclinical evidence indicates overwhelmingly that opioids alter the development, differentiation, and function of immune cells and that both innate and adaptive systems are affected."

Since the 1970ís, studies have consistently shown a variety of immune system disorders in autistic children.[1b] Infectious agents, toxic chemicals (such as adjuvants in vaccines) and dietary peptides have been shown to be triggers for immune dysregulation and autoimmunity.[2] The hypersensitivity reactions to the large peptides found in casein and gluten (and often soy) products by autistic children inspired research into the opioid antagonist naltrexone in hopes of avoiding restrictive diets to prevent caseo-opioid and gluteo-opioid compounds in the brain from creating deleterious effects cognitively and behaviorally.[3a, 3b, 3c] An Italian study done in 1996 with varying naltrexone dosing showed significant reduction of autistic behaviors in 7 out of 12 children.[4] Behavioral improvement was accompanied by alterations in the distribution of the major lymphocyte subsets with increase in normalization of the CD4/CD8 (T/1) ratio.[5] No similar immune studies have since been reported on the use of naltrexone in autism, while a large body of research has pointed repeatedly to endogenous opioid secretions as playing the central role in the beneficial orchestration of the immune system.[6] Opioids are endorphins and operate as cytokines, the principal communication signalers or neurotransmitters of the immune system.[7] Studies at UC Davis Mind Institute show that cytokine responses elicited by the T-cells, B-cells, and macrophage cell populations following their activation differ markedly in children with autism compared to age-matched neurotypical children in the general population.[8]

History of LDN

Bernard Bihari, MD, a New York physician studying the immune responses in HIV+ AIDs patients in 1985,[9a, 9b] discovered that an ultra-low dose of naltrexone, approximately one-tenth or less than the usual dosage, boosts the immune system and helps fight diseases characterized by inadequate immune function. These diseases include autism, cancer, and autoimmune disorders. The temporary inhibition of brain endorphins when patients are given a very tiny dose of naltrexone apparently results in a reactive increase in the production of endorphins, tending to normalize/optimize the immune system with this elevation, accomplishing its results with virtually no side effects or toxicity. Naltrexone is considered very safe and has never been reported as being addicting. When LDN is given between 9 p.m. and 2 a.m., the pituitary is alerted and the body attempts to overcome the opioid block with an endorphin elevation, staying elevated throughout the next 18 hours. Studies in human cancer patients show that LDN acts to increase natural killer cells and other healthy immune defenses, and many hundreds of multiple sclerosis patients have totally halted progression of their disease for up to 8-10 years or more so far with regular use of this medication. Restoration of the bodyís normal production of endorphins in those with cancer or autoimmune diseases is the major therapeutic action of LDN, which needs to be given only once a day between 9pm and 1-2am.

LDN In Autism

The use of LDN for children with autism spectrum disorders was previously studied in the 1990s, with researchers using from 5 to 50mg daily or every other day. In these early trials, researchers were looking for opioid antagonism because of these childrenís hypersensitivity reactions to the large peptides found in casein and gluten products. The enzyme needed to break down these peptides (DPP-IV) is defective in most autistic children, and they are believed to form caseo-opioid and gluteo-opioid compounds in the brain creating deleterious effects cognitively and behaviorally. Researchers were hoping to counteract these opioid effects with the opioid antagonism offered by naltrexone rather than subjecting the children to dietary restriction (GF/CF) for these very common foods. Panksepp, Shattock and other early researchers noted variably better results with low doses; studies on higher doses were more equivocal in children, and non-compliance due to the bitterness of the drug posed a problem for autistic children most of whom could not swallow capsules.

For private clinical studies in response to my request for a suitable transdermal form of LDN, molecular pharmacologist Dr. Tyrus Smith then (2005) at Coastal Compounding Pharmacy in Savannah GA created a very effective transdermal cream compounded with emu oil. This allowed easy adjustment of dosing (some of the smaller kids did better with only 1.5mg), the bitter taste was no problem, and the cream could be put on the childrenís bodies while they slept. The cream is put into syringes, with 0.5 ml providing 3mg for children or 4.5mg for adults; most adults prefer capsules; both are equally effective. Many Crohn's patients are now coming to prefer the transdermal form where absorption does not have to depend on a well-functioning gut mucosa.

I completed a preliminary eight-week informal study on 15 of my autism patients May-June 2005 applying 3mg of LDN transdermally between 9 and 12 p.m. Several adults participated also, one with Crohn's disease (CD) and one with chronic fatigue syndrome (CFS) using 4.5mg nightly. Parents and participating adults reported weekly on the results of the treatment.

Eight of the 15 children in this study had positive responses, with five of these eight having results considered quite phenomenal according to their parents. The primary positive responses are in the area of mood regulation, cognition, language, and socialization. Two small children responded better when changed to 1.5mg dosing. No allergic reactions were noted, and the primary negative side effect was insomnia and earlier awakening, usually fairly short-lived. The two adults in the study had very positive responses, with the Crohn's participant still reporting that she has been in remission since starting LDN (over several years at this writing).

All of the children in my study were on well-controlled dietary restriction, a standard part of the biomedical treatment of children with autism as practiced and taught by the (Defeat Autism Now!) Defeat Autism Now! branch of the Autism Reseach Institute. I have received reports from the LDN-Autism e-list I monitor (over 1500 participants now) of about 5-10% of other children (not my patients) having side effects such as irritability, agitation, and restlessness, subsiding as soon as the drug is withdrawn. I queried parents about gluten/casein/soy in the children's diets, as this response is likely indicative of withdrawal symptoms of opioid block even though brief. I suspect that children on a strict GF/CF/SF diet are less apt to show this response, and I personally see this negative reaction as a diagnostic clue that the child would benefit from dietary restriction; this has yet to be tested.

The immediate positive mood/cognitive/social effects seen in many children starting this intervention is unlikely to be from immune enhancement showing up so quickly, sometimes within a few days. For other autoimmune studies on adults using LDN, the evidence is that the optimum immune response can take up to four to six months. In private correspondence with earlier autism researchers Drs. Panksepp and Shattock, they postulated that the LDN therapeutic effect with the rebound of endogenous opioids in the brain ìloosens upî the opioid social-reward systems so children who were not connecting to the many known opioid based social rewards in the environment begin to respond to those rewards. (Endorphins are considered a source of our sense of well-being). Even traumatized animals (canines and primates) show new socialization behavior on LDN that had been previously missing. Both these researchers emphasized the importance of positive social reactions being reinforced and enhanced substantially by social support and encouragement, helping the new behavior become part of positive behavior modification. A certain proportion (estimate 15%) of children upon starting LDN show not only some increased hyperactivity and sleep changes, but a bout of what seems like ìinfection activationî in the form of a cold, fever blister, yeast flare-up and other reactions. These do not seem to be contagious and are usually short-lived, often followed by a burst of improved language, cognition, and socially seeking behavior. More recent input about this transition effect indicates that it is probably a ìperturbationî of the immune status to another level of functioning, and some pathogen levels previously immunosuppressed may be disturbed while immune elements are changing. Those children whose parents state ìthey never get sickî may now be moving from their reactive hyperimmune state to one where they are responding as most neurotypical children do to exposure to a new pathogen, giving the immune system an opportunity to develop antigens which will be in place to fight this organism when it reappears in their environment. Now, instead of immediately lowering the dose, I ask parents to use the full dosage quite soon, which seems to cut down this time of adjustment for most of the children, not all. Some need to go down in dosage, but I urge parents to try to stay the course if possible as I suspect the maximum immune benefits occur with full dose, whereas the immediate social-reward and cheerfulness effects occur on ultra-tiny doses perhaps without maximizing immune benefits for long-term healing.

LDN For HIV+AIDS

My second clinical study in 2006 with 20 ASD children and 38 adults, mostly parents of ASD children, showed that 80% of the children had an increase in their CD4+ cell count on 16 weeks of LDN and 70% of the adults studied showed an increase. We (the author and her husband Jack Zimmerman PhD) are working now with a health team in Mali Africa conducting a study for HIV+ adults to formally determine whether this medication can enhance/modulate the immune system to prevent progression to full-blown AIDS (See www.LDNAfricaAIDS.org). As opposed to the current standard AIDS medications which aim at disabling or killing the HIV virus, LDN is directly used to enhance one's own endogenous immune system so it can ably fight the loss of cells essential to proper immune functioning and oppose any pathogen invasion or immune dysregulation.

Recent and Proposed New Research

As of this writing (early 2009) two more studies by Dr. Jill Smith on Crohn's disease have been approved at Penn State, one a Phase 2 study for adult Crohn's disease, and her Phase I study for children with Crohn's is seeking participants. A study has been approved for a behavioral/cognitive study in Israel on autistic children, and LDN studies on MS and fibromyalgia at first-rate universities are on-going. In recent correspondence with neuropharmocology researcher Richard Deth, PhD, he reports that a new connection between opiate receptors such as naltrexone and redox (reduction-oxidation reactions) has emerged. This study shows that morphine treatment causes a sizable down-regulation of the transporter that brings cysteine into neurons. This transporter is known as EAAT3, named after its ability to also transport glutamate, and it is essentially the sole source of cysteine to neurons.(10) As such, it regulates neuronal redox status, especially in human neurons where the supply of cysteine from homocysteine transulfuration is very limited. The finding that morphine down-regulates this transporter raises the intriguing possibility that low-dose naltrexone may serve to up regulate cysteine uptake, with beneficial redox (detoxification) consequences.

Other studies have shown acute down-regulation of glutathione in cerebrospinal fluid after morphine.(11) Dr. Deth believes this finding deserves further investigation. He believes that some of the effects of opiates can be considered as a decrease in the mechanism of attention caused by interference with dopamine-stimulated phospholipid methylation by lowering glutathione levels. This recent research pointing toward the possibility that LDN could play a role in brain redox by creating more cysteine and therefore more glutathione to neurons is very exciting and can be tested. Dr. Deth says, "Redox is at the heart of all cells, so it's not surprising to think that agents affecting redox will exert broad benefits." Research along these lines is being considered by Dr. Deth and his colleagues, and if successful and positive could markedly enlarge the understanding behind benefit being seen in so many people with so many different illnesses taking LDN for immune enhancement.   (A common comment upon hearing about LDN is, "It sounds too good to be true.")

Summary

As an effective, non-toxic, non-addicting, and inexpensive behavioral and immuno-enhancing/modulating intervention, LDN is joining our biomedical arsenal to help more and more children recover from autism as well as helping many persons both adult and children with autoimmune diseases including HIV+ AIDS, MS, Crohn's, and cancer or any disease that is caused by immune/autoimmune impairment or endorphin deficiency. Currently used in these ultra small doses as an "off-label" FDA approved medication, it must be prescribed and also compounded for the tiny dosing required. The filler medium carrying the medication is very important - it should be hypoallergenic and immediate-release to get the "jumpstart" for the brain to send the message out to the adrenal and pituitary glands to tell them to make endorphins. As to the carrier, I personally prefer emu oil for transdermal, avicel for capsule preparations.

For more information on LDN, see www.lowdosenaltrexone. org, join Autism_LDN@yahoogroups.com, and see www.LDNAfricaAIDS.org.

References

1a NEJM 349:1943-1953 Nov 13 2003 #20, Ballantyne J, Mao J,"Opioid Therapy for Chronic Pain"

1b Cohly HH, Panja A., ìImmunological findings in autism.î Int Rev Neurobiol 2005;71:317-41

2   A Vojdani, JB Pangborn, E Vojdani, EL Cooper: ìInfections, toxic chemicals and dietary peptides binding to lymphocyte receptors and tissue enzymes are major instigators of autoimmunity in autism," International Journal of Immunopathology and pharmacology, Vol. 16, #3, 189-199 (2003)

3a Paul Shattock, Alan Kennedy, Frederick Rowell, Thomas Berney, ìRole of Neuropeptides in Autism and Their Relationships with Classical Neurotransmitters," Brain Dysfunct 1990;3:328-345

3b Jaak Panksepp, Patrick Lensing, Marion Leboyer, Manuel P. Bouvard, "Naltrexone and Other Potential New Pharmacological Treatments of Autism", Brain Dysfunct 1991:4:281-300

3c Paul Shattock, Paul Whiteley, ìBridging the Gap—Opioid Peptides and Executive Function," Paper presented at the Durham Conf 1998, Univ of Sunderland, UK

4   Scifo R, Cioni M, Nicolosi A, Batticane N, Tirolo C. Testa N, Quattropani MC, Morale MC, Gallo F, Marchetti B, ìOpioid-immune interactions in autism: Behavioral and immunological assessment during a double-blind treatment with naltrexone," Ann 1st Super Sanita. 1996;32(3):351-9

5   MP Bouvard, Marion Leboyer, JM Launay, C Recasens, MH Plumet, D Waller-Perotte, F. Tabuteau, D Bondouz, M Dugas, P Lensing, J Panksepp, "Low-dose naltrexone effects on plasma chemistries and clinical symptoms in autism: a double-blind, placebo-controlled study", Psychiatry Research 58 (1995) 191-201

6   Lois McCarthy, Michele Wetzel, Judith Sliker, Toby Eisenstein, Thomas Rogers, ìOpioids, opioid receptors, and the immune response," Drug and Alcohol Dependence 62 (2001) 111-123 (Review)

7a Jean M. Bidlack, (Minireview), ìDetection and Function of Opioid Receptors on Cells from the Immune System,î Clinical and Diagnostic Laboratory Immunology, Sept 2000, p 719-723

7b Michel Salzet, Didier Vieau, Robert Day, ìCrosstalk between nervous and immune systems through the animal kingdom: focus on opioids,î Trends Neurosci (2000) 23, 550-555

8   UCDavis Health System, ìChildren with autism have distinctly different immune system reactions compared to typical children,î News release from UC Dvis M.I.N.D. Institute, 5/2006

9a www.lowdosenaltrexone.org: LDN and HIV/AIDS—"Low Dose Naltrexone in the Treatment of Acquired Immune Deficiency Syndrome,î a paper presented in 1988 to the International AIDS Conference in Stockholm, Sweden, describing in detail the 1986 LDN HIV/AIDS clinical study.

9b www.lowdosenaltrexone.org: LDN and HIV/AIDS—"Low Dose Naltrexone in the Treatment of HIV Infection," an informal description of the results in Dr. Bernard Bihari's private practice through Sept 1996

10 Liling Yang, Shuxing Wang, Backil Sung, Grewo Lim, and Jianren Mao1 From the MGH Center for Translational Pain Research, Department of Anesthesia and Critical Care, Massachusetts General Hospital, Harvard Medical School, Boston, Mas-

sachusetts 02114 "Morphine Induces Ubiquitin-Proteasome Activity and Glutamate Transporter Degradation," Received for publication, January 30, 2008, and in revised form, May 16, 2008 Published, JBC Papers in Press, June 6, 2008, DOI 10.1074/jbc. M800809200

[11] Leonidas C. Goudas, MD, PhD*, Agnes Langlade, MD, PhD‡, Alain Serrie, MD, PhD‡,Wayne Matson§, Paul Milbury§, Claude Thurel, MD‡, Pierre Sandouk, MD\ , and Daniel B. Carr, MD, FABPM*†-Depts of *Anesthesia & †Medicine, New England Med Ctr & Tufts University School of Medicine, Boston, Massachusetts; ‡Centre de Traitement de la Douleur, Hopital Lariboisiere, Paris, France; §ESA Corporation, Chelmsford, Massachusetts; and \INSERM, Paris, France, "Acute Decreases in CBS Fluic Glutathioe Levels after Intracerebroventricular Morphine for Cancer Pain"

E. LOW OXALATE DIET
SUSAN COSTEN OWENS, Autism Researcher

A new diet began to be investigated in autism in spring of 2005. This diet, called the Low Oxalate Diet, has been used for many years by patients with kidney stones and other conditions where oxalate crystals were forming or where oxalate in soluble form was entering cells and further inflaming damaged tissues. The diet restricts the quantity eaten of a substance called oxalate.

Oxalate is present in varying amounts in plants, but it is especially high in nuts and seeds and in certain specific vegetables and fruits. This simple compound is made of carbon and oxygen and is very reactive. It likes to bind positively charged ions, especially calcium, but it also forms highly insoluble complexes with lead and mercury.

Scientists have found that whenever oxalate is present in excess, it tends to find and bind to injured tissues where it may cause pain and inflict oxidative damage, causing lipid peroxidation in the membrane, depleting the cell of glutathione, and turning on inflammatory factors like NFKappa B, arachidonic acid and Cox2.[1] Oxalate has also been found to impair key processes in the energy metabolism in the mitochondrion of cells because it inserts itself in biotin-dependent carboxylase enzymes and selected other enzymes, impairing their function. This inhibition of energy involves glycolysis, gluconeogenesis, the citric acid cycle and the electron transport chain.[2,3,4]

Kidney doctors discovered many years ago that people with gut inflammation absorb about seven times as much oxalate as does someone with a healthy gut. Because so many people with autism have gut inflammation, poor fat digestion, diarrhea, constipation, or a leaky gut, it made sense that this could be leading to an excess absorption of oxalate, with consequences that were unknown.[5]

A small pilot study conducted in May of 2005 revealed that the children we tested on the autism spectrum did have periodic hyperoxaluria. This means that the levels of oxalate in their urine rose far above normal at particular times of day, but not necessarily all day long. These children began a low oxalate diet.

What followed was a surprising constellation of physiological and neurological improvements which led to the hypothesis that oxalates might be crossing the blood brain barrier and affecting the brain. Significant improvements in these children and in the ones who followed took place in areas of gross and fine motor skills, motor planning, expressive speech, cognition and executive function.... all suggesting that something positive was happening with brain function, especially in the cerebellum. Improvements were being reported in gastrointestinal areas that had not improved sufficiently in the same children on either the gluten and casein-free diet, or the Specific Carbohydrate Diet. Many other improvements in other physical areas were observed such as a resolution of persistent skin lesions and rashes, and catch-up growth. One child went from having multiple seizures a day to having no seizures at all. Many other areas of improvement reported by parents are noted on the website given in the last paragraph of this section.

At the beginning of the Autism Oxalate Project, we had no way to predict where excess oxalate might have gone in the body or what it might be doing if it had been absorbed in excess. The work of oxalate researchers in the last few years helped us understand that oxalate will cross cell membranes by using specific transporters that are designed to move other compounds that are normal to the body. They learned that oxalate will exchange for sulfate, or bicarbonate or chloride and experimentally, it would exchange with salicylate.[6] This may explain why all of these substances have been either craved by children with autism, have caused problems, or they have been efficacious in therapy.

Since one of these compounds, sulfate, tends to be low in plasma in autism, and is not functioning normally in most cases of autism[7], this suggested that excess oxalate might be trafficked to different places in the body in autism. That might explain why oxalate would cause different issues in autism compared to its effects in kidney patients.

The task of characterizing why there could be differences in transport is underway currently by Daniel Markovich at the University of Queensland, in Brisbane, Australia, and by others who reported their results at the NIH's meeting in December of 2008 entitled "Anion Transporters and Oxalate Homeostasis: From Genes to Diseases." Dr. Markovich's genetically modified Nas1 knockout mouse is an appropriate model for autism because it has low plasma sulfate and high urinary excretion of sulfate. This Nas1 mouse, as you might expect, over expresses SAT1 sulfate transporters in the liver.[8] In other places in the body, if cells over expressed SAT1 trying to increase their intake of sulfate, those cells might instead take in inappropriate levels of oxalate whenever oxalate became elevated outside those cells.

Sulfate and other sulfur related issues in people with autism were characterized more than a decade ago by Rosemary Waring at the University of Birmingham, in England.[7] The abnormalities she found might change the way excess oxalate is trafficked to the kidney and might affect other sites of excretion, like the bowels, the lungs, and the skin. Sulfur deficiencies she found in autism would additionally affect how the body's chemistry would handle metabolites or precursors to oxalate, changing the enzyme activity of molecules like glycolate oxidase and lactate dehydrogenase.[9,10] These differences in the sulfur chemistry are why the ratio of oxalate in the blood to oxalate in the urine would be expected to be different in autism compared to those without similar sulfur issues. For this reason, a study is being prepared for publication that looks at the variability of both urinary and plasma levels of oxalate in autism.

The body seems to be able to secrete oxalate to skin, lungs, feces and urine. As of today, scientists do not yet fully understand how or when the body chooses these alternative routes, or how to tell when certain routes are not working properly. This makes urinary tests of oxalate difficult to interpret. As an example, recent clinical and laboratory data sent from Dr. Maria Jesus Clavera in Spain found that pre-diet levels of oxalic acid on the organic acid test of Great Plains Laboratory did not predict which patients did and did not respond to the low oxalate diet. Some patients who initially had low normal values on that test ended up being some of the best responders. Their urine levels of oxalate may have been low initially because they were experiencing impaired kidney secretion, which may have meant that atheir tissue levels of oxalate compared to someone with good secretion. Additionally, Dr. Clavera found that beginning urinary levels of oxalic acid were ineffective in predicting the eventual level of improvement on the diet in behavior and cognition. Because of the issues raised by this clinician's data, our project is working with oxalate scientists who can help us determine which tests outside of urinary oxalate testing will be most effective in predicting the best candidates for this diet. At this point, genetic tests and tests for the oxalate degrading capacity of the stool may end up being the most successful tests in predicting risk from dietary oxalate.

Oxalate scientists only recently discovered that the gut serves as a secretory organ for excess oxalate much like the kidneys. In the gut, the body's excess oxalate is secreted from intestinal cells into the stool. The regulation for this process uses molecules that also regulate thirst, urinary output, and appetite for salt, so this regulation may account for some frequency of excess urination or drinking in certain individuals with autism. It makes sense for oxalate to be routed to the gut because the gut contains microbes that can utilize oxalate as food so that the oxalate is not absorbed. The most important microbe with this job is *oxalobacter formigenes*, but it is easily killed by commonly used antibiotics. Once gone, it is very hard to get *oxalobacter* to populate the gut again.[5] Even so, a probiotic for this bacterium is under development and expected to come on the market for genetic hyperoxaluria in early 2009.[11] Some strains of *Lactobacillus* and *bifidus* bacteria also can utilize oxalates as food, but they are not nearly as capable as *oxalobacter*, and they may die back if there is too much oxalate in their environment.[5] Scientists have not yet determined the identity of the very sandy stools that sometimes contain black specks. These very grainy stools seem to occur more frequently on this diet, and appear at the same time as other "dumping" symptoms that are usually rapidly followed by new improvements.

Other microbes, including candida, may actually make oxalate or its immediate precursor out of substances as ordinary as sugar. Candida can metabolize the sugar arabinose into a precursor of oxalate.[5] Arabinose has been found to be frequently high through organic acid testing in children with autism.[12] This sugar may derive from hyaluronic acid, which gets elevated during gut inflammation, and especially when gamma delta T cells are elevated in the gut.[5] Elevations of gamma delta T cells were found in autism by investigators at the Royal Free Hospital years ago.[13]

Relatively new research is now suggesting that human beings may have another way of detoxing oxalate through the use of an energy cycle that previously was thought to exist only in microbes or in plants. This cycle, called the glyoxylate cycle, is intimately tied to the process of metabolizing long-chain fatty acids in the peroxisome. [14] This organelle is also where oxalate is detoxified inside our cells. This cycle is activated after fuel from glucose is scarce or unusable at the cellular level. The induction of this cycle occurs when a lack of carbohydrate forces the cell to shift into using fat as fuel, and is tied to the beta oxidation of long chain fatty acids.

It is well known that these fatty acid reserves for energy also become important during infection. In fact, gene defects in fatty acid metabolism in the peroxisome are often discovered only after a child with this sort of genetic weakness becomes ill for the first time in his life. Glyoxylate is the key intermediate in this alternative energy cycle, which is actually an abbreviated version of the citric acid cycle. The citric acid cycle takes place in the mitochondrion, whereas the glyoxylate cycle takes place in the peroxisome

Recent work from France has strongly suggested that glyoxylate will also form as an intermediate when the body is presented with a load of oxalate that is introduced from outside the body. [15] Since glyoxylate from either source ends up in the peroxisome, the enzyme, malate synthase, which is induced when the glyoxylate cycle is active, may detoxify glyoxylate. Of course, if that enzyme is not available, then the glyoxylate formed in this cycle may form oxalate anew, or else another enzyme in the peroxisome called AGT, which needs B6 to work, will convert glyoxylate to glycine. The efficiency of these enzymes is where we may find a great diversity in the autism population which could explain differences in response to exposures to oxalate

It is possible that the induction of the glyoxylate cycle could be involved in explaining why certain people on the Specific Carbohydrate Diet are able to handle its higher levels of oxalate.without developing problems. The lowered complex carbohydrates on SCD may limit carbohydrate fuel to intestinal cells and to microbial metabolism sufficiently to activate the glyoxylate cycle in either as an alternative energy source. If that does happen, the induction of malate synthase may help detoxify the glyoxylate formed from the excess oxalate in that diet. However, people with weaknesses in malate synthase, or weaknesses in AGT may be at additional risk from the formation of glyoxyate from isocitrate in this cycle. Laboratory research will be needed to clarify the role of genetics and this alternative energy cycle in adding to or reducing risks from oxalate in different circumstances. For an illustration of this cycle and its steps, please see: http://www.chembio.uoguelph.ca/educmat/chm452/gif%5Cglycycle.gif.

A small percentage of children with autism do have kidney stones and another small percentage seem to have urinary problems. We were glad to see urinary issues improve with the low oxalate diet in those who had those problems, including pain in the genital area and/or excess or overly frequent urination. Similar urinary improvements were reported as a benefit of the low oxalate diet when it was used to treat women with vulvodynia and urinary issues.[16]

Kidney patients who get calcium oxalate kidney stones have specific problems with protective molecules that are specialized in the kidney and are the reason they are at risk for developing kidney stones, because their urinary levels of oxalate may be in similar ranges to patients without stones. In fact, these kidney risk factors may be inapplicable to most children with autism, and this may spare them from kidney stones or other noticeable urinary problems in spite of their absorbing excess oxalate from the gut. The tendency to detoxify oxalate through the stool may also protect their kidneys.

Oxalate scientists know that oxalates can collect in the brain and in its blood vessels[17,] but studies have not made clear what circumstances besides poisoning with antifreeze might lead to oxalate accessing the brain. Most people with kidney oxalate problems are not known to develop serious neurological problems, but this issue has not been studied in patients with neurological disease who do not already have kidney disease to raise suspicions. Even so, cancer patients given platinum oxalate through an IV in chemotherapy had a high rate of neurotoxicity with no evidence of increased problems in the kidney.[15] The vulnerability of the brain might be related to a weakened blood brain barrier, or could have a different explanation related to the trafficking of molecules that oxalate can imitate in transporters. Daniel Markovich at the University of Queensland in Brisbane, for instance, discovered that the transporter molecule that exchanges sulfate for oxalate in the kidney is also very important to two areas of the brain: the cerebellum and the hippocampus.[6] If a low oxalate diet helps the bodyís organs shed excess oxalates, then oxalates collecting in the brain but leaving with the diet may account for the improvements in these brain functions that we have seen in the children on the spectrum who have lowered their exposure to oxalate from food.[5] Our burden now is to understand WHY the changes occur that parents have reported.

Oxalates may also become high in the body in someone who does not have gut inflammation, and in some diseases, gene defects expressed in the colon may increase gut permeability to oxalate. In some cases, an elevation of oxalate could be caused by the body making oxalate all by itself. This might happen when particular enzymes lose function because they need vitamins and minerals like Vitamin B6 (pyridoxine), magnesium, thiamine and pantothenic acid. These nutrients that have an excellent track record for helping children with autism are able to help these enzymes process the normal metabolic products of oxalate (glycolic acid and glyoxylate) to harmless things instead of to oxalate. Excesses of glycine and megadoses of Vitamin C can also lead to elevations in oxalate.[5]

Negative symptoms were no surprise to our project because many of the same symptoms have been described in kidney patients in the months or years after a defective liver was replaced that had been producing dangerous amounts of oxalate. Scientists found stored oxalates all over the body in these patients on autopsy. Later research showed that after a liver transplant removed their source of new oxalate, the oxalate that had been stored in the body (termed oxalosis) gradually left the cells where it had impaired cellular chemistry all over the body. This process of detoxification was noted to take months to years to be complete. The evidence that this was happening was suddenly INCREASED oxalate levels in both blood plasma and urine. Doctors noted that this long detox process eventually restored organ function in organs that were known to have been previously damaged by their excess oxalate.[18]

This liver transplant model has been our only precedent for understanding why many children and adults on the low oxalate diet actually have periods of time when their symptoms are worse (which we have called "dumping"), but these periods tend to be followed by big improvements after each round is over. These rounds come in cycles, and generally get farther apart and last a shorter time the longer someone has been on the diet.

Now that our project is four years old, we have found that some with autism, like some reported liver transplant patients[18], still have occasional "dumping" symptoms even two years into the diet or after the transplant. So far, the big improvements in executive function have generally appeared after the first year on the diet, with some earlier exceptions. Students with attention deficit disorders, and students in college with Aspergers have mentioned that the diet has been very helpful in improving their higher level academics and their organizational ability. Even adults with decades of severe autism have seen changes big enough to change their lives. This brings in a lot of hope that autism will be similar to kidney disease in that damage from oxalate may not produce irreversible damage if the exposure can be stopped and the body can detoxify. At the date of this publication, none of these cognitive improvements that parents reported have been studied formally in partnership with educational and neuroscience professionals, but that is on the project's agenda.

Our experience so far in this project has shown us that lowering dietary oxalate in someone who before this was eating a very high oxalate diet for a long time while their gut was inflamed or leaky may make the early diet's detox process much more intense with excess negative symptoms. When this happens at the beginning of the low oxalate diet, it may discourage some people from continuing, but our experience has been that these dieters are likely to be the ones who see the most improvements if they stay on the diet, and follow the instructions that are listed on our website about how to reduce symptoms. The observation of worsened early symptoms in those who previously increased the oxalates in their diet when they began gf/cf or SCD has by no means been excluded to autism. As our listserve became populated by people with many conditions seeking help with the low oxalate diet, some of the worst negative symptoms were described in adults with bowel disease who had been for years on a high oxalate version of the other diets. These adults who had been pleased with the benefits on their previous diet still wanted to try the low oxalate diet to see improvements in areas that were still problems. They said new improvements on the low oxalate diet encouraged them to continue keeping oxalates lowered.

As more testing becomes available to evaluate what is happening during these "dumping" times, we will have more tools to help us diminish or prevent the negative symptoms. Strategies we have learned so far are enumerated on the internet list that was set up by our group in July of 2005 called Trying_Low_Oxalates @yahoogroups.com.

In that group, people can receive the most current information on how to effectively implement this diet and they can network with those with multiple other conditions that improve after use of this diet. So far, that has included people with celiac disease, cystic fibrosis, vulvodynia, interstitial cystitis, fibromyalgia, arthritis, carpal tunnel syndrome, inflammatory bowel disease, Rett Syndrome, Angelman syndrome and more. A recent paper has also found that oxalate is an issue in Down syndrome, a genetic condition that has a high comorbidity with autism.[19]

On the listserve for the low oxalate diet, parents and professionals will be advised of developments in the research side of the project with continued insights on how this diet is working in multiple conditions. A website named www.lowoxalate.info is now available to keep the public informed of developments in this research, and will continue to be updated as more discoveries are made by oxalate scientists, and as more foods have been tested. We are very excited to have accomplished the testing of many gluten-free grains, so that those with gluten sensitivities do not have to guess at the oxalate status of alternative grains and those on casein-free diets can learn the oxalate status of alternative milks.

The low oxalate diet, for most people, will not be a "forever" diet, but will provide a time when the body can clear of this stored toxin, and can perhaps heal the gut sufficiently that oxalates in food no longer pose an excessive risk. Already many who had success on LOD have phased out of this diet and moved on to a diet only restricted in the highest oxalate foods. We look forward to learning along with the rest of the autism community how to fit this diet into other healing strategies.

(Written by Susan Costen Owens, Defeat Autism Now! thinktank member, and Head of the Autism Oxalate Project)

References

1 Toblli JE, Cao G, Casas G, Stella I, Inserra F, Angerosa M. Urol Res. 2005 Nov;33(5):358-67. NF-kappaB and chemokine-cytokine expression in renal tubu-lointerstitium in experimental hyperoxaluria. Role of the renin-angiotensin system.

2 Ozawa S, Ozawa K, Nakanishi N. Meikai Daigaku Shigaku Zasshi. 1990;19(2):185-96. Inhibition of pyruvate kinase --glycolysis and gluconeogenesis. [Article in Japanese]

3 Yount EA, Harris RA. Biochim Biophys Acta. 1980 Nov 17;633(1):122-33. Studies on the inhibition of gluconeogenesis by oxalate.

4 Kugler P, Wrobel KH. Histochemistry. 1978 Aug 15;57(1):47-60. Studies on the optimalisation and standardisation of the light microscopical succinate dehydrogenase histochemistry.

5 Owens, SC. The Low Oxalate Diet: Science and Success. AutismOne Conference, May 26, 2006 Chicago, IL http://www.autismone.org/uploads/Owens%20Susan%20 Powerpoint%20USE.ppt

6 Regeer RR, Lee A, Markovich D. DNA Cell Biol. 2003 Feb;22(2):107-17. Characterization of the human sulfate anion transporter (hsat-1) protein and gene (SAT1; SLC26A1).

7 Waring, R. H., & Klovrza, L. V. Journal of Nutritional and Environmental Medicine 2000 (10): 25-32. Sulphur metabolism in autism.

8 Dawson PA, Gardiner B, Grimmond S, Markovich D. *Physiological Genomics* 26:116-124 (2006) Transcriptional profile reveals altered hepatic lipid and cholesterol metabolism in hyposulfatemic NaS1 null mice.

9 Baker PW, Bais R, Rofe AM, Biochemical Journal 1994 Sep 15;302 (Pt 3):753-7. Formation of the L-cysteine-glyoxylate adduct is the mechanism by which L-cysteine decreases oxalate production from glycollate in rat hepatocytes.

10 Sharma V, Schwille PO. Biochem Int. 1992 Jul;27(3):431-8. Oxalate production from glyoxylate by lactate dehydrogenase in vitro: inhibition by reduced glutathione, cysteine, cysteamine.

11 Hatch M, Cornelius J, Allison M, Sidhu H, Peck A, Freel RW. Kidney Int. 2006 Feb;69(4):691-8. Oxalobacter sp. reduces urinary oxalate excretion by promoting enteric oxalate secretion.

12 Shaw W, Kassen E, Chaves E.Clin Chem. 1995 Aug;41(8 Pt 1):1094-104. Increased urinary excretion of analogs of Krebs cycle metabolites and arabinose in two brothers with autistic features.

13 Furlano RI, Anthony A, Day R, Brown A, McGarvey L, Thomson MA, Davies SE, Berelowitz M, Forbes A, Wakefield AJ, Walker-Smith JA, Murch SH. J Pediatr. 2001 Mar;138(3):366-72. Colonic CD8 and gamma delta T-cell infiltration with epithelial damage in children with autism.

14 http://en.wikipedia.org/wiki/Glyoxylate_cycle

15 Gamelin L, Capitain O, Morel A, Dumont A, Traore S, Anne le B, Gilles S. Boisdron-Celle M, Gamelin E. Clin Cancer Res. 2007 Nov 1;13(21):6359-68. Predictive factors of oxaliplatin neurotoxicity: the involvement of the oxalate outcome pathway.

16 Solomons CC, Melmed MH, Heitler SM. J Reprod Med. 1991 Dec;36(12):879-82. Calcium Citrate for vulvar vestibulitis. A case report.

[17] Froberg K, Dorion RP, McMartin KE. Clin Toxicol (Phila). 2006;44(3):315-8. The role of calcium oxalate crystal deposition in cerebral vessels during ethylene glycol poisoning.

[18] Cochat P, Gaulier JM, Koch Nogueira PC, Feber J, Jamieson NV, Rolland MO, Divry P, Bozon D, Dubourg, L Eur J Pediatr. 1999 Dec;158 Suppl 2:S75-80.Combined liver-kidney transplantation in primary hyperoxaluria type 1.

[19] Baggot PJ, Eliseo AJY, DeNicola NG, Kalamarides JA, Shoemaker JD Fetal diagnosis and therapy.2008;23:254-257, Pyridoxine-Related Metabolite Concentrations in Normal and Down Syndrome Amniotic Fluid

ELEVEN

MITOCHONDRIAL DYSFUNCTION & TREATMENTS

A. INTRODUCTION

My first memory of hearing about mitochondria in autism was at the fall 2001 Defeat Autism Now! conference at a Think Tank presentation by Dr. Sudhir Gupta. The noted researcher said, "Genes load the gun, environment pulls the trigger." We were all endeavoring to understand the effects of mercury in vaccines on our children with autism in our research and treatment efforts at that time, and "Autism: A novel form of mercury poisoning" had already been published in Medical Hypothesis (see Appendix B). Dr. Gupta explained that sulfhydryl groups are present in cellular mitochondria, that mercury binds these groups, necrotizing DNA, altering cell membrane permeability, and affecting calcium transport. He went on to tell our group that mercury causes a shift from Th1 to Th2 immunity, dysregulates signaling mechanisms, and induces autoimmunity; he stated: **"Thimerosal is a mitochondrial poison and autism is a disorder of mitochondria."** Gupta then produced a graph from studies showing an increase in cell death rising in direct proportion to the amount of thimerosal present. What was very exciting then was the evidence that we were on the right track about thimerosal and our use of chelating agents in our treatments to lower the mercury load in our children with autism along with our attempts to get the mercury out of our children's vaccines.

Mitochondria are biological power plants within cells that generate the fuel needed for cell function. Symptoms of defects in mitochondria can range from muscle weakness and gastrointestinal or cardiovascular problems to neurodevelopment and neurodegenerative disorders. Though a great deal of research on mitochondrial disorder had been conducted for many years, not a lot of emphasis was given to its role in autism until fairly recently. Interest heightened considerably when the U.S. government through the Department of Justice conceded in late 2007 that Hannah Pohling, a young autistic child with an attorney mother and a neurologist father, had her autism triggered by nine childhood vaccinations when she was 19 months of age. Hannah was awarded a large monetary settlement by the Vaccine Court, though the court officials claimed that this was an isolated case due to her "rare" mitochondrial disorder. Hannah's neurologist father disagreed that this decision was relevant to very few other children with autism.[1]

In an excellent recent review article in the American Journal of Biochemistry & Biotechnology, Defeat Autism Now! Drs. Daniel Rossignol and Jeffrey Bradstreet outline evidence that mitochondrial dysfunction is a common feature of autism, and that toxins, including the mercury in thimerosal-containing vaccines might play a role in the problem.[2] Rossignol and Bradstreet contend that although classical mitochondrial diseases are rare, affecting about 2 in 10,000 children, mitochondrial dysfunction is likely to be much more common. Mitochondrial dysfunction is less severe than classical mitochondrial disease and cannot be diagnosed by the usual test of muscle biopsies but can be inferred from laboratory tests. In their article, they state: "Although biomarkers for mitochondrial deficiency have been identified, it appears that mitochondrial dysfunction is significantly under-recognized in autism, and a widespread under-prescribing of potentially beneficial therapies often occurs."

Since 1997 when I first began learning and then writing and teaching about autism, I called my method a "broad spectrum approach," basing the admittedly somewhat vague expression upon our increasing new knowledge of the causes and effective treatments of this challenging and multifactorial disorder. As the list of research and treatments has grown longer through the years, I found myself impressed recently when starting to explore mitochondrial issues related to autism with the discovery that almost every treatment that has been useful for our children appears in the literature (thanks to researcher Teresa Binstock's great sleuthing efforts, see Appendix D) as important and effective interventions in mitochondrial disorders. However, many of the articles I found about treatments for mitochondrial insufficiencies or injuries have been in the neurodegenerative or anti-aging literature (another strong personal interest of mine). A decade ago, J. Lombard published a paper in Medical Hypotheses entitled: **Autism: A Mitochondrial Disorder?** At that time, Dr. Lombard wrote: *Autism is a developmental disorder characterized by disturbance in language, perception and socialization. A variety of biochemical, anatomical, neuroradiographical studies imply a disturbance of brain energy metabolism in autistic patients. The underlying etiology of a disturbed bioenergetic metabolism in autism is unknown. A likely etiological possibility may involve mitochondrial dysfunction with concomitant defects in neuronal oxidative phosphorylation within the central nervous system. This hypothesis is supported by a frequent association of lactic acidosis and carnitine deficiency in autistic patients. Mitochondria are vulnerable to a wide array of endogenous and exogenous factors which appear to be linked by excessive nitric oxide production. Strategies to augment mitochondrial function, either by decreasing production of endogenous toxic metabolites, reducing nitric oxide production, or stimulating mitochondrial enzyme activity may be beneficial in the treatment of autism.*[3]

Since the early 60's when mitochondrial disease was first described, mitochondrial dysfunction has been implicated in nearly all pathologic and toxicologic conditions.[4] In a paper from Experimental and Molecular Pathology by Steve Pieczenik and John Neustadt written in late 2006, these researchers write: "A wide range of seemingly unrelated disorders such as schizophrenia, bipolar disease, dementia, Alzheimer's disease, epilepsy, migraine headaches, strokes, neuropathic pain, Parkinson's disease, ataxia, transient ischemic attack, cardiomyopathy, coronary artery disease, chronic fatigue syndrome, fibromyalgia, retinitis pigmentosa, diabetes, hepatitis C, and primary biliary cirrhosis have underlying pathophysiological mechanisms in common, namely reactive oxygen species (ROS) production, the accumulation of mitochondrial DNA damage, resulting in mitochondrial dysfunction."[5]

Rossignol and Bradstreet's belief that environmental toxins might be the triggers for mitochondrial dysfunction in autism based on evidence of inhibition of mitochondrial function by heavy metals, pesticides, and industrial chemicals tie together Dr. Gupta's observations in 2001 and Dr. Lombard's hypothesis of a decade ago that autism might be a mitochondrial disorder. Deleterious effects by toxic metals (especially mercury) through the formation of free radicals, resulting in DNA damage, lipid peroxidation and depletion of protein sulfhydryls (eg glutathione) were described by Valko in 2005.[6] Their work on these effects of depleted levels of the active form of glutathione on mitochondrial function connects to the research work of Dr. Jill James whose findings have been so helpful in our methylation treatment protocols for autism. James' studies on biomarkers of increased oxidative stress showed autistics were shy of adequate levels of this all-important antioxidant compared to neurotypical children.[7]

As more and more evidence points to mitochondrial dysfunction as a common cause of autism, and according to Rossignol and Bradstreet, possibly the most common metabolic cause of autism, interest in testing our children for this disorder is increasing. Various biomarkers are: Pyruvate level (may only be available at teaching hospitals), plasma alanine-to-lysine ratio, a surrogate marker for pyruvate, lactate level, and levels of urinary organic acids, such as carnitine, ammonia, and oxidative stress markers. According to Drs. Pieczenik and Neustadt, the most important test for mitochondrial dysfunction is urinary organic acid testing. They consider Drs. Richard S. Lord and J. Alexander Bralley of Metametrix Institute and Laboratory as two of the world's leading organic acid researchers. I have used the Organix (urinary organic acid test) from Metametrix for many years now as my most useful and favorite evaluative test for autism patients. I recognize many of the therapeutic interventions recommended by Metametrix Lab for the abnormal values on this test as nutritional recommendations frequently described as helpful for mitochondrial disorder in the general mitochondrial literature. While indicating the presence of functional nutrient deficiencies, the

Organix also shows presence of toxins that adversely affect detoxification pathways. I highly recommend that any health care worker who uses the biomedical approach to autism and can order testing own and use Lord and Bralley's excellent new laboratory book.[8]

It is very exciting to think that there may be effective treatment protocols for mitochondrial dysfunction, particularly learning that mitochondrial damage is cumulative and that supplementation of certain nutrients in animal studies increases proliferation of intact mitochondria and reduces the density of damaged ones.[9] However, much work has to be done to assess types, doses, ratios and combinations of these nutrients for the many diseases now known to be affected by less than optimal mitochondrial function. In the following section of this chapter are descriptions of therapeutic interventions well-known to be beneficial for mitochondrial injury or insufficiency.

References for Part A—Introduction

1 Pohling, Jon S, Father: Child's case shifts autism debate. Atlanta Journal-Constitution 4/11/08.
   http://www.ajc.com/opinion/content/opinion/stories/2008/04/11/polinged0411.html

2 Rossignol DA, Bradstreet JJ. Evidence of Mitochondrial Dysfunction in Autism and Implications for Treatment. Am J Biochem Biotech 2008 4(2):208-17.

3 Lombard, J., 1998, Autism: a mitochondrial disorder? Med. Hypotheses, 50:497-500.

4 Aw, T.Y, Jones, D.P., 1989, Nutrient supply and mitochondrial function. Annu. Rev. Nutr. 9, 229-251.

5 Pieczenik, Steve R., Neustadt, John, Mitochondrial dysfunction and molecular pathways of disease, Experimental and Molecular Pathology 83 (2007) 84-92.

6 Valko, M., Morris, H, Cronin, M.T., 2005. Metals, toxicity and oxidative stress. Curr. Med. Chem. 12 (10), 1161-1208.

7 James, S.J., P. Cutler et al. Metabolic biomarkers of increased oxidative stress and impaired methylation capacity in children with autism. Am. J. Clin. Nutr., 80:1611-1617.

8 Lord, R.S & Bralley, J. Alexander, Editors: Laboratory Evaluations for Integrative & Functional Medicine, 2nd Edition, 2008, Metametrix Institute.

9 Aliev, G, Liu, J, Shenk, et al, "Neuronal mitochondrial amelioration by feeding acetyl-L-carnitine and lipoic acid to aged rats", J of Cellular & Molecular Medicine, Mar 28 2008.

MITOCHONDRIAL DYSFUNCTION & TREATMENTS

B. TREATMENT ISSUES

1. DRUGS AND MEDICAL STATES THAT NEGATIVELY AFFECT MITOCHONDRIA

2. TESTING FOR MITOCHONDRIAL DYSFUNCTION

3. CURRENT MAINSTREAM MEDICAL TREATMENT STRATEGIES

4. MITOCHONDRIALLY TARGETED NUTRIENTS TO TREAT ASD

1. Drugs and Medical States That Negatively Affect Mitochondria

Many drugs interfere with mitochondrial metabolism and should be avoided in patients with mitochondrial disorders, such as valproic acid, salicylic acid, nucleoside analogs, amiodarone, tetracycline, barbiturates, chloramphenicol, chemical toxins such as iron, ethanol, cyanide, antimycin A, and rotenone. Seizure control should not include phenobarbital because it can inhibit OXPHOS. (OXPHOS is oxidative phosphorylation, the process by which ATP is formed as electrons transferred from NADH OR $FADH_2$ to molecular oxygen (O_2) by a series of electron carriers. The ultimate acceptor of these electrons is O_2. The ultimate acceptor of these electrons is O_2. The electron-transport chain, also known as respiratory chain, is a series of linked electron carriers that transfer electrons from NADH and $FADH_2$ to molecular oxygen (O_2). Valproic acid should likewise be used with caution because of its effects on respiration and fatty acid metabolism. Several nonsteroidal anti-inflammatory drugs

(NSAIDs) inhibit or uncouple OXPHOS, and may result in clinical deterioration. Aminoglycoside antibiotics must be avoided in patients with mitochondrial mutations because of the significant risk for aminoglycoside-induced ototoxicity.[1]

2. Testing for Mitochondrial Dysfunction

Mitochondrial damage is poorly diagnosed and symptoms can range from mild to severe and even life threatening. I use the organic acid test (OAT) as my primary way to assess general mitochondrial dysfunction for evaluating ASD children.[2] The OAT on almost every testing indicates the child's need for L-Carnitine, Riboflavin, CoEnzymeQ10, B vitamins, particularly Thiamine, Nicotinic Acid, and pyridoxine along with riboflavin as lacking in these children. On the OAT (urine or blood) elevated adipic and suberic acids can mean that mitochondrial ability to extract energy from fat molecules is hindered. Organic acid tests assess levels of substances that are part of the energy-transfer mechanism of the mitochondria. (Citric, malic, fumaric and alpha-ketoglutaric acids are some of these.) Pyruvic acid is important too, because it's part of the chemical doorway into this energy-transfer chemistry. When that doorway is blocked (by mercury, arsenic, or not enough thiamin), lactic acid or lactate may accumulate, along with pyruvic acid, so these factors are typically included when organic acids are assayed. Lactate is produced normally by muscle during exercise, or when brain regions are activated, but elevated lactate levels at rest may indicate that glycolysis is compensating for impaired energy production by mitochondria. However, spurious elevations in blood lactate can also occur with tourniquet use to draw blood or in a struggling child, so this is not an easy or sure test in an ordinary lab setting. Lactic acid levels in the blood should be measured without a tourniquet after the child has been resting for at least 5 minutes and has refrained from especially vigorous activity for 24 hours (not easy unless the child is ill!) Other biochemical abnormalities which can raise suspicion of a mitochondrial disorder include elevated levels of the amino acid alanine in fasting blood (or spinal fluid samples), an increased ratio of lactate to pyruvate in blood and spinal fluid, elevated organic acids in urine, or an elevated ratio of acyl-carnitine to free carnitine in blood. It is important to note that biochemical abnormalities may not be present during periods when the mitochondrial disease is quiescent, which is of course a further complicating factor in making a proper diagnosis. There is also a urine test for a substance called methylmalonic acid (MMA) and it is also a regular part of the Organix. Urine MMA is one of the most important telltale signs for mitochondrial dysfunction; clinicians have informally reported between 30% and 60% occurrence of elevated MMA on urine organic acid tests of patients with ASD. I regard high MMA value as evidence of a methylcobalamin (methyl vitamint B12) blockage and always consider this an indication for either the methylcobalamin subcutaneous injections with folinic acid 800mcg orally or nasal spray methylcobabalamin often combined with folinic acid in the spray.

3. Current Mainstream Medical Treatment Strategies for Mitochondrial Disorder

Current mainstream treatment strategies for mitochondrial disorder are generally supportive. Management includes the empiric supplementation with various "mitochondrial cocktails," supportive therapies, and avoidance of drugs and conditions known to have a detrimental effect on the respiratory chain. Examples of symptomatic medical therapies include: sodium bicarbonate for acute and chronic metabolic acidosis; transfusions for anemia and thrombocytopenia; exogenous pancreatic enzyme replacement for chronic pancreatic insufficiency; and electrolyte replacement to compensate for renal losses. Dietary measures, such as avoidance of fasting, have also been advocated, but have not been subjected to clinical trials. Hypermetabolic states, such as exhaustive exercise or fever, should also be avoided. Infections can precipitate rapid metabolic deterioration, and require prompt attention and treatment. Interestingly, sustained aerobic exercise may ameliorate symptoms of exercise intolerance caused by mitochondrial dysfunction.[3]

4. Mitochondrially Targeted Nutrients to Treat ASD

As I mentioned in Part A of this chapter, most of the biomedical therapies I have been using for many years to help ASD children are treatments I'm finding in the mitochondrial literature as being helpful for disorders in this group generally; these have all been discussed in the preceding chapters. Three of the most-discussed and studied nutrients in studying mitochondrial treatments which I have found to be helpful are the carnitines (in the form of L-carnitine, Acetyl-L-Carnitine, Acetyl-L-Carnitine Arginate, and/or Glycine Propionyl-l-Carnitine), CoEnzymeQ10 in its various forms, and Lipoic Acid now usually discussed and used in its most efficient and absorbable form, reduced or (R) Lipoic Acid. A decade ago studies reported by Proceedings of Natl. Acad. Sci., USA on old rats for oxidative stress showed that Acetyl-L-Carnitine restored partial mitochondrial function and muscle activity; even better results were obtained when ALCAR was combined with Lipoic Acid in Moreira's study.[4] N-Acetyl-Cysteine, Riboflavin, Alpha Keto Glutarate, N-Acetyl-L-Carnosine and Uridine (Triacetyluridine) are appearing frequently now in "cocktail" studies and may be familiar to parents treating abnormalities noted in their children's amino acid panels and their organic acid tests.

In an attempt to test the synergy of putting some of the most frequently studied and used nutrients together, many nutrient companies are creating Mitochondrial Cocktail Formulas now: Thorne (Neurochondria), VRP (Neuron Growth Formula), Life Extension Foundation (Mitochondrial Energy Optimizer), Prothera (Mitothera), and Ecological Formulas (Mitochondrial Catalysts). Ecological calls this a "Bioenergetic Formula," consisting of very small doses of Thiamin (as TTFD), Riboflavin, Alpha Keto-Glutarate, Inosine, Gycine Propionyl-L-Carnitine, N-Acetyl-L-Carnosine, and Triacetyluridine. In a private conversation with Dr. Jonathan Rothschild, the director of Ecological Formulas, I mentioned that according to my reading there is evidence that an older child or adult might need as much as 300mg of uridine a day for a beneficial effect, whereas there is only 10mg in this cocktail, and discussed with him the prohibitive cost of a cocktail that would have optimum doses. It is clear that a lot of testing on differing nutrient groups for optimum doses of synergistic cocktails may be very different from what we know are ideal doses using individual components. I created a mixed protocol from several nutrient companies in late 2008 for 12 of my more treatment resistant patients and assessed response, which was quite varied. Interestingly, one adult and two of the adult-sized children were the best responders; however, one older child had no response, and one of the smaller children had a bit of a regression, with the rest of the group in-between, so needless to say the results were quite inconclusive. I am continuing to vary the doses for certain members of this group to seek optimum responses – this is a work still in progress.

Much of the literature about mitochondrial support nutrients appears in studies on the anti-aging and neurodegenerative group of diseases, particularly Alzheimer patients. In 2005 Dr. Parris Kidd wrote an extensive monograph for the Alternative Medicine Review on Mitochondrial Insufficiency (subtitle: "Neurodegeneration from Mitochondrial Insufficiency: Nutrients, Stem Cells, Growth Factors, and Prospects for Brain Rebuilding Using Integrative Management") that is available on the Thorne website. This excellent review offers practical recommendations for integrating safe and well-tolerated nutrients into a supplementation protocol for brain vitality[5]. Again, testing for synergies between these important nutrients is still needed, and the cost may be prohibitive to put many of them together in any one formula. For my own personal anti-aging regiment, I find myself alternating the use of these nutrients, as the list is so long now that I can neither stand to take so many nutrients nor would taking all that are considered important now be generally affordable for me or most of us unless one would get a specific response indicating that a particular nutrient seemed clearly beneficial. If one is generally healthy and taking these nutrients for prophylaxis (e.g. anti-aging) this kind of response may not be forthcoming as it might be from someone who is already very deficient and showing disease evidence.

Important Nutrients for Supporting Mitochondrial Health

I will be discussing below only some of the most studied and currently considered more important nutrients helpful for the ASD population. As we find out more about mitochondrial dysfunction, the nutrient list grows daily; more information regarding specific products is generally available on the internet by the sellers and in the professional literature under mitochondrial support/nutrition. As I have said before, almost every beneficial nutrient treatment I have been learning about for autism is on the list for benefiting the mitochondria, along with certain exercise (resistance and endurance exercise training) programs and HBOT.[21] Some of the important nutrients for optimal mitochondrial function but not included on this short list below are: N-Acetyl-Cysteine (important precursor to glutathione), Lithium Orotate, Inosine, Creatine Monohydrate, NADH, Hydroxylamine, Green Tea Catechins, Taurine, Idebenone, Pyridoxal 5' Phosphate, Curcumin, Estrogen and Progesterone, Glycerophosphocholine, Riboflavin, Thiamine, Methyl Vitamin B12 and other B Vitamins, Vitamin K, Vitamin C, D, & E, Ribose, N-Acetyl-L-Tyrosine, Biopterin, Huperzine, Luteolin, and Magnesium.

A) THE CARNITINES

Acetyl L-Carnitine (ALCAR) is integral to mitochondrial function, boosting the conversion of fats into energy in the mitochondria, helping to ensure that a plentiful energy supply is available for biochemical processes throughout the body. ALCAR and L-carnitine, its non-acetylated derivative, facilitate the transport of fatty acids into the mitochondria to become OXPHOS substrates. Experimental evidence suggests ALCAR boosts mitochondrial ATP production and helps protect mitochondria against oxidative attack.[5] Acetyl-L-carnitine arginate is a patented form of acetyl-L-carnitine that has been shown to protect brain cells against the toxic effects of beta-amyloid, the protein implicated in Alzheimer's disease[7]. It works by stimulating the growth of neurites, which are long, branchlike fibers that connect the brain cells and allow them to communicate, by as much as 19.5 percent[8] in animal studies. I have very seldom evaluated a child with autism whose organic acid test does not indicate a need for L-carnitine to help with fatty acid metabolism. Children do not usually show a reaction to L-carnitine, whereas I sometimes get a hyperactive reaction from the acetylated forms; lately I have been giving these more activating nutrients along with herbals such as Ashwaganda and Bacopa for enhanced benefit and less hyperness.

B) CO-ENZYME Q10

Coenzyme Q10 (ubiquinone, ubiquinol) is a potent antioxidant and is a bioenergetic enzyme co-factor similar to (R) - Lipoic Acid (see below). CoQ10 is incorporated into the mitochondria of cells throughout the body, facilitating and regulating the oxidation of fats and sugars into energy. Unfortunately, levels of CoQ10 decrease with aging. CoQ10 levels in older individuals are only 50 percent of those present in young adults. A National Academy of Sciences study has shown that CoQ10 enhances metabolic energy levels of the brain.[9] This orthomolecule is central to mitochondrial oxidative phosphorylation, shuttling electrons between complexes while providing potent antioxidant protection for the inner membrane OXPHOS complex of the mitochondria. Deficiencies are invariably associated with subnormal or pathological mitochondrial performance.[5] This nutrient is so valuable across all disease lines that I have almost every one of my patients both adults and children on this as ubiquinol, the new highly absorbable form. I order this from VRP, Life Extension Foundation, and others, giving children 50mg 1-2 daily and most adults 100mg or more daily.

C) (R) LIPOIC ACID

A-Lipoic acid is a highly effective antioxidant, readily crossing the blood-brain barrier, capable of conserving and regenerating reduced glutathione (GSH), the central cellular antioxidant, and playing a fundamental role in mitochondrial metabolism. Biologically, it exists in proteins, where it is linked covalently to a lysyl residue as a lipoamide. In recent years, lipoic acid has gained considerable attention, particularly as the reduced form of lipoic acid, (R) Lipoic Acid, which reacts with oxidants such as superoxide radicals, hydroxyl radicals, hypochlorous acid, peroxyl radicals, and singlet oxygen. It protects membranes by reducing oxidized vitamin C and glutathione, which may in turn recycle vitamin E. Administration of alpha-lipoic acid is beneficial to a number of oxidative stress models such as diabetes, cataract, neurodegeneration, and HIV activation. Lipoic acid functions as a redox regulator of proteins such as myoglobin, prolactin, thioredoxin, and NF-kappa B transcription factor, and has shown neuroprotective effects in neuronal cells. One possible mechanism for the antioxidant effect of lipoic acid is its metal chelating activity.[6] Lipoic acid has a longstanding experimental and clinical record of antioxidant, anti-inflammatory and anti-excitotoxic support for the brain.[5]. I use 100 to 300mg of (R) Lipoic Acid daily starting low and building up slowly to find optimum dosing; available at multiple nutrient companies.

D) ESSENTIAL FATTY ACIDS (ESPECIALLY DHA)

Essential fatty acids are required for many biological functions, including protection from the oxidative effects of free radicals. They are also known to be important for good overall brain and cardiac health, and a recent study demonstrated in animal models that supplementation with omega-3 fatty acids actually switched on brain cell genes that contribute to enhanced functioning.[10] These biochemical details may help us understand why diets rich in fish oils and other sources of omega-3 fatty acids are associated with better memory and improved cognition.[11] One of the omega-3 fatty acids in particular, docosahexaenoic acid (DHA), has attracted significant attention for its ability to boost brain function. DHA is found in very high concentrations in cell membranes and is required by developing infant brains. A lack of DHA in a developing brain results in cognitive and learning deficiencies.[12] Studies have shown that DHA helps protect brain cells by suppressing a neurotoxic substance called amyloid-beta and supplementation with DHA can reverse the cognitive effects of DHA deficiencies.[11]. DHA is so valuable to healthy brain function that some experts believe infant formula should be supplemented with it.[13] In my work with ASD children I have found this nutrient to be highly effective in promoting better cognition and speech, especially in conjunction with Uridine (see below), with which it is synergistic. I give from 450mg twice daily to small children and up to 900 twice daily to older children; this is often given along with EPA in equal or slightly less amounts.

E) CARNOSINE

Carnosine is a dipeptide (two linked amino acids alanine and histadine) that occurs naturally in our cells and is a potent antioxidant and free radical scavenger, an invaluable weapon in fighting glycation. Glycation reduces functionality and efficiency of mitochondrial proteins, and occurs when proteins or DNA molecules throughout the body bond chemically with sugar molecules. These sugars are further modified to form advanced glycation end products (AGEs), which cross-link with adjacent proteins, rendering tissues increasingly stiff and inflexible. In appearance, this is what causes collagen and elastin in the skin to lose its suppleness, causing wrinkles to develop. Glycation reduces protein flexibility and functionality, is the culprit behind cataracts, and plays a role in numerous other degenerative processes such as arthritis and atherosclerosis.[14] AGEs also trigger inflammatory reactions throughout the body; in the brain they have been shown to prompt certain cells to pump out free radicals and immune system factors such as cytokines and adhesion molecules toxic to neurons.

Augmenting carnosine with oral supplementation slows down or even reverses some of glycation's effects. Carnosine also scavenges free radicals while inactivating reactive chemicals such as aldehydes and lipid peroxidatiion products. I suggest one capsule of Life Extension Foundation's Super Carnosine twice daily.

E) BENFOTIAMINE, THIAMINE

Rising glucose levels in the body as we age can lead to life-threatening diseases such as metabolic syndrome, diabetes, and cardiovascular disease. High glucose levels are responsible for increased mitochondrial free radical production and other complications of aging. One of the body's proteins, an enzyme called transketolase, is critical in the metabolism of sugar. But like many enzymes, transketolase requires a co-factor, namely, thiamine (Vitamin B1). Thiamine is water soluble which makes it less available to the interior of the cell. Benfotiamine is a slightly altered form of thiamine; its alteration renders it fat soluble, allowing it to enter areas of the body where water-soluble thiamine cannot penetrate; it can increase transketolase activity in cell cultures by 300%.[15] Benfotiamine's robust activation of transketolase was shown to be able to block three out of the four major metabolic pathways leading to blood vessel damage. Benfotiamine also blocked activation of the pro-inflammatory transcription factor, nuclear factor-kappa beta (NF-kB), which has been implicated in inflammation, tumor formation, and the age-related disorder macular degeneration, as well as retinal disease in diabetics. I suggest this to all my adult patients and some of the larger ASD children – it is available as Mega-Benfotiamine 250mg at Life Extension Foundation and at 150mg at Prothera, once or twice daily is advised.

F) PHOSPHATIDYLSERINE

Phosphatidylserine is an essential phospholipid in nerve cell membranes, and has also been found to affect nerve growth factor by enhancing NGF-receptor density. Phosphatidylserine enhances mitochondrial function because it is a precursor to phosphatidylethanolamine, a major phospholipid in mitochondrial cell membranes; it facilitates the efficient transport of glucose into brain cells and boosts the production of acetylcholine. It is sold in Europe and Japan as a prescription drug but is available in the United States as a dietary supplement. European studies have shown enhancement in cognitive function when phosphatidylserine is administered to patients in various stages of dementia. Phosphatidylserine has also been shown to attenuate many neuronal effects of aging and to restore normal memory in a variety of tasks in animal models.[7] In one study, 15 healthy elderly volunteers were given 100 mg of phosphatidylserine three times daily. They were evaluated at baseline, after 6 weeks of treatment, and at the end of the 12-week trial. All but two outcome measures showed significant improvements in cognitive function. Phosphatidylserine has been proven after 21 double-blind trials to be effective for improvement of memory, learning, mood, and alleviation of stress.[16] I usually recommend children over 60# take 100mg of phosphatidylserine daily for memory and cognition; elders benefit by one twice daily.

G) URIDINE (TRIACETYLURIDINE)

Uridine, or its most common salt, uridine-5-monophosphate, UMP, is a building block of RNA and DNA and, like acetyl carnitine arginate and acetyl carnitine, it is important to brain health. Uridine-5-monophosphate is the usual dietary source of uridine, found in the milk of mammals. Recent research is increasingly showing that uridine is essential for growth and development throughout life. It was once thought that only infants needed uridine during early developmental stages since mature mammals are capable of synthesizing their own uridine. Uridine monophosphate is still routinely added to all infant and most parenteral formulas. In the 1960s, it was discovered that uridine is an essential ingredient for adult brain functioning, and in 1968, one researcher found that uridine is the real dietary source of cytidine, a building block of the cell membrane component and signaling agent, phosphatidylcholine, which is necessary for memory and is a major component of cell membranes. Phosphatidylcholine levels decline with age in all mammals and these declining levels appear to play a major role in memory loss.

In 2000 it was shown that human brain cells when exposed to uridine for 4 days had increased neurite outgrowth and neurofilament expression.[17] A variety of chemicals that prevented incorporation of nucleotides into brain cells all prevented the neurite outgrowth in the brain cells caused by uridine, showing that uridine was responsible for the neural regeneration. In 2005, a study confirmed that uridine added to brain cell cultures stimulated neurite outgrowth branching and increased the number of new neurites per cell. The researchers found that uridine stimulated neurite outgrowth and branching by two different pathways—it enhanced phosphatidylcholine synthesis, as was previously shown in the earlier studies, but it also blocked receptors that stopped neurites from growing.

In the same year, a study showed that orally administered uridine-5-monphosphate given to aged rats increased the release of dopamine in the right striatum of their brains to a level of 341 compared to a control group level of 221, a 35 percent increase.[18] Biomarkers of neurite outgrowth, neurofilament-70 and neurofilament-M protein levels increased to 182 percent and 221 percent higher than in the control rats. The study demonstrated that even in old rats, oral uridine intake increases neurotransmitter release and neurite outgrowth in vivo. Ecological Formulas make Uridine (Triacetyluridine), 25mg capsules; I give small children 1 or two a day, older children 2 twice or more daily, usually along with DHA, with which it is synergistic.

H) HERBAL/NATURAL NUTRIENTS FOR MITOCHONDRIAL SUPPORT

(Note: Herbs are often not standardized– follow directions by the manufacturer.)

Ashwagandha. Derived from an Indian herb, ashwagandha has been studied for its ability to rebuild damaged neural networks and restore memory in amnesiac mice. Several lab and animal studies have shown that ashwagandha can increase the growth of dendrites in the brain. In mice, large doses of ashwagandha (50, 100, and 200 mg/kg) were shown to exert a dose-dependent improvement in memory after administration of electroconvulsive shock. After one week of therapy with ashwagandha, the mice exhibited significantly improved memory, leading the authors to suggest that ashwagandha exhibited a brain enhancing-effect on the animals.

Ginkgo (Ginkgo biloba). Ginkgo extracts act as free-radical scavengers, preventing induced lipid peroxidation in neural tissue. Ginkgo has also been shown to relax blood vessel walls, inhibit platelet-activating factor, enhance microcirculation, and stimulate neurotransmitters. Several trials show cognitive benefits with the use of ginkgo. For example, a year-long study of more than 300 participants with dementia who received 120 mg of an extract of ginkgo showed stabilized or even improved cognitive performance during the study.

Bacopa. Bacopa monniera is an Ayurvedic medicinal herb that has been used clinically for enhancing memory and ameliorating epilepsy and insomnia and as a mild sedative. The antioxidant role of Bacopa may help explain its reported antistress, immunomodulatory, cognition-facilitating, anti-inflammatory, and antiaging effects. A study measured bacopa's ability to enhance memory and reduce anxiety in 76 adults between 40 and 65 years of age. A significant effect of Bacopa was shown in the retention of new information.

Another trial examined the chronic effects of Bacopa on cognitive function in healthy human participants. The participants were randomly assigned to receive either 300 mg bacopa or placebo. The results showed significant improvement in speed of visual information processing, learning rate, memory consolidation, and anxiety compared with the placebo group. Maximal effects were evident after 12 weeks. Bacopa may also have the potential to increase T4 levels. The importance of Bacopa (200 mg/kg) in the regulation of thyroid hormone concentrations in male mice was investigated. Bacopa had a thyroid-stimulating effect and increased T4 concentrations by 41 percent. It did not affect levels of T3. Patients under the care of a physician for hypothyroidism should not take bacopa without the consent of their doctor.

Vinpocetine: Vinpocetine, derived from the periwinkle plant, has been shown to enhance circulation and oxygen utilization in the brain, increase the brain's tolerance for diminished blood flow, and inhibit abnormal platelet aggregation that can interfere with circulation or cause a stroke. The effects of vinpocetine on memory function were studied in 50 patients with disturbances of cerebral circulation. Improvement of cerebral circulation was observed after vinpocetine was administered, and after one month of vinpocetine treatment, psychological tests showed an improvement in memory. In a clinical trial, vinpocetine produced a significant cognitive improvement in older patients with chronic cerebral dysfunction. In a study to determine how vinpocetine boosts cognition, scientists measured the electrical firing rate in the neurons of anesthetized rats. The administration of vinpocetine produced a significant increase in the firing rate of neurons, and the dose of vinpocetine used to increase electrical firing corresponded to the dose range that produced memory-enhancing effects. Additionally, vinpocetine has been shown to protect against oxidative damage. One study suggests that the antioxidant effect of vinpocetine might contribute to reducing neuronal damage.

Rhodiola Rosea: Rhodiola rosea, called an adaptogen by Russian scientists who have studied it, is one of the best herbs for enhancing mitochondrial energy production. This herb is noted for increasing resistance to chemical, physical, and biological stressors, including strenuous exertion, mental strain, and toxic chemicals. A recent study in animals trained to exhaustion found that rhodiola significantly boosted the synthesis and resynthesis of ATP in the mitochondria. Besides reducing fatigue under stressful conditions it also exerts an anti-inflammatory effect.[19] It is believed that rhodiola's beneficial properties stem in part from its ability to influence the activities and levels of brain chemicals such as serotonin and norepinephrine and natural "feel good" opioids such as beta-endorphins.[20]

Micronutrients Important to Mitochondrial Health: Iron, Zinc, Copper, Thiamine, Riboflavin, Nicotinamide, Pantothenic Acid, Pyridoxine, Biotin, Glycine.

Antioxidants Besides ALA, CoQ10, and ALCAR for Mitochondrial Health: Vitamin E, Vitamin C

Note on Stem Cells and Mitochondria: In Dr. Parris Kidd's review article on Mitochondrial Insufficiency (see ref #5) he discusses Stem Cells and Mitochondrial Health. Three nutrients have been found in experimental animals to enhance brain growth factor receptors for Nerve Growth Factor (NGF): Acetyl-L-Carnitine (ALCAR), PhosphatidylSerine (PS), and Glycerophosphocholine (GPC). The first two have already been discussed; GPC is a phospholipid clinically validated in 21 clinical trials for attention, immediate recall, and other cognitive functions as well as for dementia and recovery from brain trauma. Coupled with DHA, GPC can be directly incorporated into cell membranes; rat studies have shown GPC treatment maintains brain cell populations significantly higher than in age-matched controls. Exciting further research is forthcoming to ascertain to what degree brain restoration is possible from the use of these three dietary supplements. Suggested dosages of premier brain nutrients by Dr. Kidd are high and costly; GPC 600-1200mg daily, PS 100-500mg daily, and ALCAR 1-3 grams daily, ALA 300-2,400mg, CEQ10 360-2400mg, DHA + EPA 800-3000mg in 1:1 ratio. New nutrient formulations that are better absorbed may help lower both the amounts and costs of these vital nutrients.

For further insights, readers are invited to explore the literatures linking oxidative stress with autism[24-26] and with mitochondria.[27-28]

References for Part B—Treatment Issues

[1] Gillis, L.A., Sokol, R.J.; Gastrointestinal manifestations of mitochondrial disease, Gastroenterol Clin N Am 32 (2003) 1–29.

[2] Rossignal DA, Bradstreet JJ. Evidence of Mitochondrial Dysfunction in Autism and Implications for Treatment. Am J Biochem Biotech 2008 4(2):208-17.

[3] Reddy, Hemachandra; Mitochondrial Medicine for Aging and Neurodegenerative Diseases, Neuromol Med DOI 10.1007/s12017-008-8044-z (original paper).

[4] Moreira PI et al., Lipoic acid and N-acetyl cysteine decrease mitochondrial-related oxidative stress in Alzheimer disease patient fibroblasts, J Alzheimers Dis. 2007 Sep;12(2):195-206.

[5] Kidd, Parris M., Mitochondrial Insuffiency Review: "Neurodegeneration from Mitochondrial Insufficiency: Nutrients, Stem Cells, Growth Factors, and Prospects for Brain Rebuilding Using Integrative Management", Alternative Medicien Review, Vol 10 #4 2005.

[6] Ames, Bruce N, Liu, J., Atamna, H., Kuratsune, H., Delaying Brain Mitochondrial Decay and Aging with Mitochondrial Antioxidants and Metabolites, 133 Ann. N.Y. Acad. Sci. 959: 133–166 (2002). © 2002 New York Academy of Sciences.

[7] McDaniel MA, Maier SF, Einstein GO: "Brain-specific" nutrients; a memory cure? Nutrition, 2003 Nov; 19(11-12):957-75.

[8] Taglialatela G, Navarra D, Olivi A, et al. Neurite outgrowth in PC12 cells stimulated by acetyl-L-carnitine arginine amide. Neurochem Res. 1995 Jan; 20(1):1-9.

[9] Matthews, RT, Yang, L, Browne, S et al. Coenzyme Q10 administration increases brain mitochondrial concentrations and exerts neuroprotective effects. 1998. Proc. Natl. Acad. Sci. USA, 95:8892-8897.

[10] Kitajka K, Puskas LG, Zvara A, et al. The role of omega-3 polyunsaturated fatty acids in brain: modulation of rat brain gene expression by dietary omega-3 fatty acids. Proc Natl Acad Sci USA. 2002 Mar 5;99(5):2619-24.

[11] Kalmijn S, Launer LJ, Ott A, Witteman JC et al. Dietary fat intake and the risk of incident demential in the Rotterdam Study. Ann Neurol. 1997 Nov;42(5):776-82.

[12] Turner N, Else PL, Hulbert AJ. Docoshexaenoic acid (DHA) content of membranes determines milecular activity of the sodium pump: implications for disease states and meteabolism. Naturwissenschaftern. 2003 Nov;90(11):521-3.

[13] McCann JC, Ames BN. Is docosahexaenoic acid, an omega-3 long-chain polyunsaturated fatty acid, required for development of normal brain functin? An Overview of evidence from cognitive and behavioral tests in humans and animals. Am J Clin Nutr. 2005 Aug;82(2):281-95.

[14] Alikhani Z, Alikhani M, Boyd CM et al. Advanced glycation end productgs enhance expression of pro-apoptotic genes and stimulate fibroblast apoptosis through cytoplasmic and mitochondrial pathways. J Biol Chem. 2005 Apr 1;280(13):12087-95.

[15] Hammes HP, Du X, Edelstein D et al. Benfotiamine blocks three major pathways of hyperglycemic damage and prevents experimental diabetic retinopathy. Nat Med. 2003 Mar;9(3):294-9.

[16] Kidd PM. PS (PhosphatidylSerine), Nature's Brain Booster. St. George, UT: Total Health Publications; 2005.

[17] Saydoff J, et al. Oral uridine decreases neurodegeneration, behaviora impairment, weight loss and mortality in the 3-intropropionic acid mitochondrial modelof Huntington's disease. Brain Res. 994)1):44-54, 2003.

[18] Wurtman R. et.al. Synaptic proteins and phospholipids are increased in gerbil brain by administering uridine plus DHA orally. Brain Res. 19:254-58, 2006.

[19] Abidov M, Grachev S, et al Extract of rhodiola rosea radix reduces the level of C-reactive protein and creatinine kinase in the Blood. Bull Exp Biol Med. 2004 Jul;138(1):63-4.

[20] Brown RP, Gerbarg PL, Graham B. The Rhodiola Revolution: Transform Your Health with the Herbal Breaktrhough of the 21st Century. Emmaus, PA: Rodale Books, 2004.

[21] Gutsaeva DR, Suliman HB, et al. Oxygen induced mitochondrial biogenesis in the rat hippocampus. 2006, Neuroscience, 137:493-504.

22 Rossignol, DA, Hyperbaric oxygen therapy may improve symptoms in autistic children. Med Hypotheses. 2007;68(6):1208-27.

23 Rossignol DA et al. The effects of hyperbaric oxygen therapy on oxidative stress, inflammation, and symptoms in children with autism: an open-label pilot study. BMC Pediatr. 2007 Nov 16;7:36. http://www.biomedcentral.com/1471-2431/7/36.

[24] James SJ et al. Metabolic endophenotype and related genotypes are as-sociated with oxidative stress in children with autism. Am J Med Genet B Neuropsychiatr Genet. 2006 Dec 5;141B(8):947-56. http://www.ajcn.org/cgi/content/full/80/6/1611

[25] Yao Y et al. Altered vascular phenotype in autism: correlation with oxidative stress. Arch Neurol. 2006 Aug;63(8):1161-4. http://tinyurl.com/9wj25d

[26] James SJ et al. Metabolic biomarkers of increased oxidative stress and impaired methylation capacity in children with autism. Am J Clin Nutr. 2004 Dec;80(6):1611-7. http://tinyurl.com/a5llvo

[27] Fariss MW et al. Role of mitochondria in toxic oxidative stress. Mol Interv. 2005 Apr;5(2):94-111. http://molinterv.aspetjournals.org/cgi/content/full/5/2/94

[28] Lenaz G et al. Mitochondria, oxidative stress, and antioxidant de-fences. Acta Biochim Pol. 1999;46(1):1-21. http://www.actabp.pl/pdf/1_1999/1.pdf

TWELVE

STARVING BRAINS, STARVING HEARTS, WHAT DOES IT ALL MEAN?

By Jack Zimmerman, PhD

Messages

Why are there so many ASD and other special needs children now and what are we to make of the recent astounding growth in their ranks? Is there a message here for our culture beyond such obvious ones as cleaning up the environment of heavy metals, pesticides and other pollutants; improving the safety of vaccination and dental protocols; eating more wisely; and improving the health of our children's immune systems? Are there other levels of meaning in the ASD epidemic that we should be exploring? Is there a message all these children are trying to bring to us?

Have you found yourself asking questions like these?

Jaquelyn and I have been "living these questions" on our journey with Chelsey and the other special needs children who have come into our life during the past twelve years. It seems fitting that we end the book with a few of our own speculations about the meanings and messages these remarkable children are bringing into our lives.

We have come to believe that the special children are here in increasing numbers to change our fundamental cultural paradigm—to change the way we look at the world and, practice medicine, educate our children, relate to each other and the environment—and, ultimately, the way we learn to become *more alive.*

On the personal level the children with starving brains challenge our capacity to love—particularly in regard to the qualities of patience and perseverance, devotion beyond the usual parental call of duty and the capacity to think and act creatively "out of the box." Often, it is only after a profound challenge to our capacity to love, such as the rearing of an ASD child, that we come to realize how much more there is to discover about loving.

Jaquelyn and I have always seen our relationship as a path of awakening and the primary inspiration for our service to others, yet the love for our compelling, beautiful, mysterious granddaughter has added an entirely new dimension to our marriage. Chelsey upped the ante in the game of love, without ever asking us directly if we wanted to play!

When we looked around at other families struggling with their Chelseys, we saw that virtually everyone was living out their own unique version of the same experience. As we read and heard stories of families transformed by attempts to heal their ASD children, we began to see how the rapid growth in the ASD population had the potential to deepen and expand the ways we all love each other. It was not a huge step to see that the growing presence of all these special children was an opportunity for major personal and cultural transformation.

The children with starving brains are here to help us heal our starving hearts.

This realization began to dawn on us as we struggled to find effective biomedical treatment for Chelsey, while her parents searched for adequate schooling and tried to adjust to a new and sometimes overwhelming family life together. Our search for meaning in the epidemic of autism soon implicated the critical state of the environment, lack of sufficient vision and courage in the way we educate our children, limitations in the established allopathic approach of medicine and abounding unconsciousness in our understanding of family dynamics and intimate relationship.

Exploring such questions truly honors the "specialness" of these children because they embody these big issues in the most personal way possible. The special children have truly become "canaries in the mines of our culture;" they are compelling, not only because we come to love them so much for who they are individually, but also because they are here to catalyze the expanded awareness needed to change our culture—and sooner rather than later.

The vast and increasing numbers of ASD children are messengers reflecting critical unbalances in the ways we live our lives. In their silences and explosions of feeling, in the disruption of their biochemical makeup, in their obvious incompatibility with our established educational system and traditional medical paradigm, they are literally asking us to see how out of balance we have become, collectively and individually. They are a wake-up message, a desperate eleventh-hour call for us to realize the insanity of our priorities and the many dangers in our present courses of action.

In this chapter we will explore what these children are teaching us about family life. Their message in regard to the future of medicine, way we educate our children and a few thoughts about the environmental implications of their growing presence appear in Appendix D.

Most important, we feel that *exploring these larger issues increases our capacity to heal the children.* Understanding why they are here in such numbers, on **both** the biomedical and cultural levels, increases our ability to help them find a fulfilling life. In short, we have come to see :

If we truly hear the whole message, we are more likely to heal the messenger.

We heard the message first through Chelsey so, before we explore issues, I want to tell you a little about these past twelve years with Jaquelyn, Chelsey and her mother, Elizabeth, as a way of inviting you to share the messages you have heard during the adventure of raising and healing your special child. To tell these stories is to honor the children, better understand who they really are and, in this important way, support their healing.

Jaquelyn, Chelsey and Elizabeth

I began to realize that Chelsey might play a major role in our lives when Jaquelyn became convinced that something was not quite right about her developmental progress. For several months we danced around Liz's assurances that her first two kids were slow to develop (true), so not to worry because Chelsey would finally catch up as they had. However, Jaquelyn's agitation grew as she became convinced that Chelsey's behavior was way beyond a case of late blooming. Jaquelyn began to pore through written material on autism and visit the Internet every day. I saw a missionary fire in her eyes that I hadn't seen for quite a while. Our first challenge was to penetrate Liz's denial and bring the increasingly obvious reality about Chelsey to her and her husband, Jim's, attention. Those few months were extremely painful.

What happened was a burst of powerful maternal energy in Liz— along with fear, confusion and self-judgment, and an awakening of Jaquelyn's energy that was awesome to watch. Liz had always held a mysterious, primal place in Jaquelyn's heart, and Chelsey's plight added an entirely new dimension to their already profound connection. Much later on we realized that a part of this strong mother/ daughter bond had to do with Liz's own touch of autistic behavior, particularly when she was a child. Chelsey fanned Jaquelyn's mother-love into a combined mother/grandmother/doctor's passion for making sure Chelsey got better so Liz would not be burdened by intense care-giving for the rest of her life. We were off and running: tests, evaluations by experts, behavior modification programs and a full plunge into the Internet.

By the time Chelsey was three-and-a-half, Jaquelyn was fully immersed in her healing, driven by curiosity and a growing attraction to this mysteriously compelling creature. Every ounce of her medical acumen became activated to make Chelsey better. I became an Internet widower. Our main private conversational theme shifted from the mystery of our own intimate relationship, our work with couples and other clients to the mystery of ASD and Chelsey's healing. I began to see the handwriting on the wall. As the saying goes, "If you can't lick 'em, you'd better join 'em!"

I began to fall in love with my step-granddaughter while follow-ing her around for two hours in Ojai's Libby Park several months before her fourth birthday. She made no eye contact with me at all while she wandered through the bushes and allowed me to push her on the swings. She said nothing to me, even though she had already developed the ability to use single word communication as a result of her behavioral modification training. At one point she stopped a moment under a tree and let me sit next to her for a minute or two. I was amazed at my reaction. I actually felt elated as if some extraor-dinary princess had given me hope that I might gain her favor.

My fate was sealed at the following Christmas family reunion.

I was stretched out (uncharacteristically) on the sofa in our small living room, dominated by a six-foot Christmas tree. Chelsey ran into the room, past the tree, swept by me on the sofa and disap-peared back down the hall. This loop was repeated quite a few times before I realized that she was coming a little closer to the sofa on each successive pass around the room. I felt strangely stirred and put out a silent message that it was safe for her to come closer. Although she made no eye contact or other overt sign of recognition, *it became absolutely clear that Chelsey was relating to me, however indirectly, and, in fact, was subtly inviting me to pay attention to her.* I grabbed the op-portunity, sending her a stronger silent message to approach the sofa more closely. When, on the next loop, she began to sing a line from a Christmas carol (perfectly in tune), she might as well have been a Siren or Circe herself. I was clearly no match for this goddess.

I moved a chair close to the sofa and sent her a silent message to sit in it a moment the next time around. It took four or five more passes through the living room before Chelsey accepted my invita-tion, sitting on the chair's edge for just two seconds at first. Several rounds later she was sitting in the chair (now pulled quite close to the sofa) for almost a minute. After a few more loops I was allowed to touch her arm. That hooked me completely. This little creature entered my inner world and took hold of some tender part previ-ously hidden there. I became determined in that moment to find a way to relate to her as part of the healing process that had begun. I remember also having a feeling then (repeated often since) that some part of Chelsey knew perfectly well what was going on and was in a way "toying" with me. I kept such blasphemies to myself in those days.

By her fourth birthday Jaquelyn and Liz were deeply into the biomedical adventure that Chelsey inspired and, although they both were pleased that "I was taking a special interest in her," I felt on the fringe of the intense activity that had begun to dominate our life. Jaquelyn's photographic mind and amazing retentive capacity blew me away. Our dinners were filled with medical theories, lab test results, heart-breaking stories from the Internet and a growing rage that there was something very wrong about certain vaccinations.

There followed in fairly rapid sequence (considering she lived 360 miles away) a number of encounters with Chelsey that stoked my missionary fire. I would help to "regain" this princess and break the spell she was under in my own way through the relationship route while Jaquelyn was experimenting with secretin, nutritional supplements, transfer factors and the GF/CF diet. By that time Liz had engineered an expanded home schooling program with specially trained behavioral specialists and was already noticing how Chelsey had brought forth in her previously hidden organizational talents, not to mention patience and physical stamina.

A major break-though occurred one afternoon in the summer after Chelsey's fourth birthday when I urged Jaquelyn and Liz to leave her with me while they went out to have some time alone. (The two older kids, Andrea and Alisha, were with Jim, their father, visiting his parents.) . We lived in a little suburban house then whose back yard was almost completely filled with a small swimming pool. Chelsey had shown interest in the pool before, but after the ladies left us alone, she could hardly wait to put on her bathing suit. In fact, if she had had her way she would have gone in without being encumbered by something so civilized.

Water has always been my second home and swimming my favorite form of exercise, so I looked forward to being in the pool with my new friend. There's no way I could have anticipated what happened during the next four hours. After splashing about in the shallow end for a little while, Chelsey very deliberately made up a game. I was to stand waist deep in the water, while she jumped in and swam towards me. I was not to reach out to her or touch her in any way. All contact was to be left in her hands alone. After approaching within a few feet of me, she would turn around, dog paddle back to the steps and climb out. The sequence was repeated many times. The game challenged my restraint capability profoundly; although I found it extremely difficult to keep my hands from reaching out as she came near, I managed to resist.

Then she added sound to our scenario. First, she shouted "AN-ARGY" as she jumped off the side of the pool. A few minutes later, in a more gentle voice, she said "Mabatu" and "Pabatu," alternately as she approached me in the water. I slowly moved further towards the deep end of the pool until only my shoulders were above water and let my hands float in front of me, all the while trying to figure out what she meant by these precisely repeated and obviously significant exclamations. "Anargy" was clearly a call to courage for the leap into the pool—a warrior's cry before the plunge. I finally concluded that Mabatu and Pabatu named figures of importance that somehow related to Chelsey's delight in being in the water. It was as if she had finally found her true home after a long and dry detour (living in Arizona!) of more than four years.

We had been playing this way for almost an hour when she reached out her arms spontaneously and embraced my shoulders after approaching me in the water. I felt a surge of excitement but resisted hugging her back. She repeated the gesture on several successive plunges, each time coming a little closer to me in the water. Finally, after several more passes, Chelsey embraced me with arms slightly outstretched and looked deeply into my eyes. It seemed like an eternity that probably lasted three or four seconds. It was the first time I was privileged to look into what Liz came to call her "Big Browns." I saw a profound being in those eyes. I hadn't a shred of doubt of that. Then she said "Pabatu" and swam back to the shallow end of the pool.

I decided then that she was a dolphin child and immediately understood why some ASD children have been so drawn to make contact with these highly conscious allies of ours. I decided that Mabatu and Pabatu were the female and male names of dolphin gods and anargy was Chelsey's warrior's cry as she plunged into the water to greet them. I took the risk of asking Chelsey out loud whether my conjectures were correct. She didn't answer me directly, of course, but on the next plunge she made even longer eye contact. Then, abruptly, a few rounds later, she said, "Bath time." We filled the tub and Chelsey surrendered her slightly chilled body to the warm water for half an hour. We played with water toys while she made up songs in her clear, perfectly pitched voice and allowed me to soap her back and legs. After a while she said, "Pool," and we repeated the whole cycle.

I could hardly wait to tell Jaquelyn and Liz about my adventure. Naturally, they were delighted, although not quite sure what to make of my interpretation of what had happened. The next day I tried to repeat the ceremony in the pool while they were about, but naturally Chelsey didn't cooperate. I wondered if I had embellished my experience of the day before. When they left the following day, Chelsey did not show any visible feelings, yet Liz told us on the phone that night that Chelsey had started sobbing uncontrollably as they drove off. It was the first time she had ever shown sadness separating from anyone. Although it broke Liz's heart to hear her cry, she was pleased to see such an outpouring of feeling.

That experience started Chelsey and me on a strong practice of water interaction that continues to this day. I am forever trying to figure out what pool or other body of water we can swim in next. Visits to Arizona, her visits to California and, of course, to Hawaii are always planned around time in the water. During my six months in Phoenix in 2003, we swam virtually every day. When larger bodies are not available, long baths, sometimes two a day, have to do. Eventually, Chelsey became part of the planning. She is unafraid and at home in the ocean, so our summer month-long times together on the Big Island have been filled with delightful long afternoons in the surf, watching her develop her own dolphin-like movements under water and engaging in both silent and verbal, playful interacting far more readily than on dry land. I used to play the water game of throwing her high into the air with the count of, "one, two, three!" literally for hours. Soon she became too heavy for that, but Jaquelyn and I have delighted in trips to the "Hot Pool" in the southern part of the Big Island, where Chelsey moves gracefully beneath the surface in the warm sunlit mixture of hot vulcanic and ocean water, her hair moving in slow motion, a hint of a smile on her lips. We swim past each other underwater like two dolphins, close but not touching. Anyone watching us play would never guess she had any special needs at all.

Not long after our swimming relationship had begun, Liz and I took Chelsey to see a psychologist with extensive past experience doing movement work with ASD children, Dr. Beth Kalish-Weiss.[1] After Beth observed Chelsey and Liz for more than an hour, I told her about our strong water connection, so Beth asked me to swim with Chelsey in their backyard pool. Watching us play together in the water, Beth noticed the immediate increase in Chelsey's relational capacity. When Jaquelyn and I returned a month later to receive her formal evaluation, Beth remarked how touched she had been watching us in the water. Jaquelyn took that moment to raise a question she had been incubating ever since our first extended time with Chelsey in Hawaii. "What do you think would serve Chelsey the most at this point in her life [she was then five], to live full time with Jack and me or continue on in Arizona with her family [now grown to six with the recent birth of Adam]?"

Beth hesitated only a moment. "I think the opportunity for Chelsey to spend that kind of time with you and Jack would be invaluable. She would get a lot of focused attention that would help her greatly at this age. With three other children in the family, Liz and Jim have their hands full. This is an important time in Chelsey's development. As she gets older, it will be more difficult for changes to be made." Jaquelyn gave me a look that would have awakened a statue. The following evening we went right to the edge.

"I have to go down the path with Chelsey all the way," Jaquelyn said. "There's something going on in all of this—even beyond her getting better, as important as that is to me. I don't pretend to understand the depth of my love for her, but I know I have to follow the call. I hope you can come with me, but if you can't, I still have to go."

"What do you mean, 'go,' " I said, suddenly feeling my mouth get dry.

"I don't know and I don't mean to sound threatening or dramatic. I just know that my love for Chelsey is an awakening of something as strong as our relationship has been—and I have to follow it. I want her to get better more than anything else in the world and I want to do whatever I can to help that happen. The grandmother and doctor—and yes the mother in me—all hear the call strongly. I need for you to understand. I want you to come with me because

I know you can be of great help in Chelsey's healing. I'm not sure I can do what needs to be done without you but, if I have to, I will."

The weeks that followed shook the foundations of our twenty-five years together. I knew, as did Jaquelyn, that I couldn't "go" along with her unless the healing journey with Chelsey was a profound reality for me as well. Otherwise, our relationship would veer out of balance, flounder and lose the remarkable synergy that had inspired every aspect of our life and work together.

By that time, I had already witnessed Jaquelyn's extraordinary emergence as "sleuth/physician" in her quest to find the right bio-medical treatment program for Chelsey. After the visits with Beth, it became clear that these talents would be well complemented by my way of entering Chelsey's world and finding a common language—silent and verbal—in which to express feelings. It was then that we began to see that together there was a possibility of using the power of our highly energetic relational "field" to help Chelsey emerge and heal. We saw that by working intimately together we might be able to create a conscious synergy between the biomedical treatments Chelsey was undergoing (with only limited success to that point) and the ongoing highly energized interactions we were having with her.

I had always been slightly uncomfortable with the singular focus on "getting Chelsey better." I wondered whose definition of `better' we had adopted. I wondered about this great goal of "normalcy" we were striving for. I found the temerity to ask Jaquelyn: "Why isn't Chelsey responding to the protocols you're using successfully with so many of the other kids in your practice?" Finally, I found the real questions that were stirring in me:

"What's the message in all this?"

And also, for the first time, I asked, "By what authority do we have the right to try and 'fix' her?"

For a while Jaquelyn felt the second question was irrelevant and distracting. Obviously, Chelsey needed to get better because she was ill and otherwise wouldn't have an independent and creative life—one that would not be a perpetual burden on her parents. I saw the truth of that, of course, but still the questions haunted me.

They haunted me right into realizing that I wanted to go down the path with Jaquelyn, not primarily because I didn't want to risk losing my life partner, but because *I saw that Chelsey was the next challenge in further deepening our relationship and our service to others, particularly in the realm of healing.* At the same time, I felt my life couldn't take Chelsey on full time because of all the many involvements that already filled it to overflowing. To take her on would mean giving up almost everything that I was doing, because I knew I would be the one primarily playing the interactive role in Chelsey's healing. Perhaps it was selfish; perhaps my resistance was appropriate. Looking back now, years later, I see that it was probably both. Liz and Jim were Chelsey's parents, I argued. She had entered their lives and it was their gift as well as burden to learn what they had to learn from her message of awakening. Yet, even though it appeared impossible, some part of me was tempted to say yes and release my entire life as I knew it—if only I could be sure I had something tangible to offer Chelsey.

Liz and I talked it all over. Giving up Chelsey for a while would greatly ease her over-filled parental life, but Liz agreed that she and Jim (and Andrea, Alisha—and now Adam too) had been given the gift of Chelsey's presence in their lives. They all needed to honor that, Liz felt. Our conversation that day launched a series of talks that continued regularly, mostly on the phone, until just a few months before Chelsey's ninth birthday. During that period Liz came to see Chelsey as an awakener in all of our lives. Even during the hard times dealing with the formidable parental challenges she faces (not only with Chelsey!), the major part of Liz knows that it is all perfect and part of her adventure in consciousness.

The final commitment to the path of healing Chelsey took place in a "council" between Jaquelyn and me a few months after our visit with Beth. We felt Chelsey with us, in the way she had been literally many times during our councils together, though she was actually many miles away sleeping in her bed in Phoenix. I picked up the talking piece and asked for guidance from the spirit of our relationship (which we call our "Third"): "Do we have permission to attempt to change the basic course of Chelsey's life, to completely change her biomedical status and to 'bring her into the world of relationship?" We sat quietly for several minutes, listening for a response. It came in a few moments loud and surprisingly clear. Giving it a human voice, this is what we heard:

"You have permission to find ways to alter Chelsey's body and life so you can have a fuller relationship with her, as long as you are willing to transform your lives in an equally fundamental way."

The message was so obviously right that neither of us had a moment's hesitation. Our "Yes" has never wavered over the years since then and Chelsey has held to her part of the bargain. She changes as we do, slowly, two-steps-forward-one step back, challenging us all the way.

In the fall of 2002 Jaquelyn went to Phoenix to present clinical material at an autism conference. She returned looking tired and down; as soon as we met at the airport I knew something was up about Chelsey. Jaquelyn wasted no time in letting me know what it was.

"We're losing her," she began. "None of the biomedical protocols are helping her improve right now. We've gotten all that we can from the GF/CF/SF diet, the supplements, the antivirals and chelation. As usual Chelsey is not responsive to the new treatments. She seems less verbal and relational than the last time we were with her in Hawaii—more isolated and into herself. She hardly noticed me. We're losing her and I know the only way that it's going to turn around is if she spends more time with us—with you particularly. She needs someone to reach into her world and draw her out. I am sure of it."

I was in a different state than several years earlier and heard the ring of truth in Jaquelyn's voice, a tone that I had come to associate with the authority of our relationship—the voice of our Third. This time it also carried the power of the goddess as well, that particular quality of the Divine Feminine that understands the mysteries of healing. Without any hesitation, I let what she said enter me fully.

We had three choices. We could take Chelsey to Hawaii and live there with her, bring her to our condo in Los Angeles or I could go to Phoenix and become part of her family on a daily basis. It took us only a day to see that the third possibility was the only one that made sense because of the importance of her staying connected to her family and continuing to attend the excellent school for special needs kids she was enjoying. There were no comparable schools in Los Angeles or Hawaii, as far as we knew at the time. The idea of living in Phoenix and being separated from Jaquelyn for an extended period was not exactly my dream, but she was so committed to traveling the country giving talks that we would have many separations anyway. Phoenix was clearly the right option and we set the wheels in motion right away.

After three months and many deep conversations with Liz (and the rest of the family), I had made arrangements to adjust all my professional commitments. By January I found myself living in an apartment complex just a few miles from Chelsey's home. For six months I picked up Chelsey every day after school, took her back to "2066" (my apartment number became her name for our times together), spent four or five hours with her, fed her and took her home in time for me to report on our adventures to Liz and Jim before bed time.

Our intense program included music (listening and recording Chelsey singing both familiar and original songs); daily swimming, of course; computer work, including neurofeedack; field trips to Tower Records and other places of delight; and a lot of hanging out together. Chelsey came to call our time, "Grandpa's After School Program"—GASP—which described my state on many occasions in the late evening as I attempted to catch up with my "other life." I also found the motivation and time to slowly introduce Chelsey to a range of new foods that included avocados, tomatoes, raw peas, wild rice, pears and blueberries. I used the "you-have-to-eat-these-before-you-can-have-the-hamburger-and-french-fries" technique. It worked and Chelsey entered the world of a varied diet for the first time. This feature of GASP particularly pleased Liz and Jaquelyn. I also played Jaquelyn's biomedical assistant, implementing magadoses of Vitamin A, and applying glutathione and TTFD creams daily to my squirming playmate.

I kept a daily journal of my adventures with Chelsey that, together with the multitude of other stories accumulated over the years, may end up in a collection someday that describes our family's adventure in awakening. I returned home that summer a grateful, somewhat wiser and inspired grandpa. We continued to spend a month each summer with Chelsey until she turned thirteen and entered young womanhood, in what became our permanent home in Hawaii.

During the time in Phoenix and since, I have watched Liz and the rest of the family mature in wondrous ways. Despite creating a GF/CF diet for Chelsey, implementing treatment programs and trying to find time for the other kids, Liz has been blessed with many personal realizations. Even by the end of Chelsey's third year, she began to recognize patterns in herself that were subtle versions of Chelsey ways of behaving. "Chelsey comes by her autism naturally," Liz told us one day with a mixture of chagrin and delight. "Being with her so intensely has led me to see those parts of myself that are just like her, only not so obvious. I often avoid direct eye contact and have some trouble expressing my deeper feelings to another person, even someone close to me. She does what I do but much more so." We had been aware of this connection already but hearing Liz give voice to it revealed another piece of the mystery of Chelsey's role in our family.

Besides personal revelations, Liz has reaped a nourishing harvest from raising Chelsey. The fruit includes deepening her practice of prayer, remembering wonderful dreams from which she derives guidance, learning how to search for an entirely new level of meaning in events and experiences, and the discovery of a variety of capabilities in herself that had never been tapped before. Shortly after Chelsey's seventh birthday, Liz told me on the phone one day, "I feel blessed to have Chelsey as my child. I was playing with her today when I suddenly realized that she's a very special being, a high being, probably higher than all of us. It's just hidden behind all those symptoms. I have come to see her now." I put down the phone shortly after that with tears in my eyes. I had never felt such love and admiration for Liz!

In 2007, Liz took on a new life as autism research coordinator that utilizes her two-year training as a nurse. She works with Defeat Autism Now! physicians in Phoenix directly dealing with many parents who are testing new treatment protocols with their ASD children. Being a full-time mother and now research coordinator has given Liz deeply meaningful work in the world and an even broader perspective about Chelsey's healing and her daughter's role as awakener in the family's life.

Awareness of Subtle Relationships

Parts of our story are probably familiar to most of you. Many parents and grandparents we have spoken with over the years have stories to tell of deepening insights and awakenings inspired by their ASD child. Even before starting treatment, many parents begin to expand their old notions of what it means to relate. Our culture's primary focus on cognitive and verbal development tends to undervalue and so under-nourish more subtle relationship skills. But having a child with ASD behavior—particularly in the more extreme portion of the spectrum—leaves us no choice but to learn how to relate without the support of words and familiar facial expressions. We begin to see that a lot of relating occurs beyond speech and in the silences between the few words that may be spoken. We learn to sense the nuances of expression that previously escaped our attention. Ways to "read the field" are found that almost certainly would never have been discovered were it not for facing the unique challenges of raising an ASD child.

We learn to observe in silence, watching patiently for a sign that our presence is being acknowledged. We begin to develop what might be called an *intuitive relational capacity* that expands the familiar one often ascribed to mothers who "know" their children's needs from a subtle gesture or the tone of their cry. The ability to relate intuitively grows in raising a special needs child, because *it has to* in order to get through the day in one piece.

Soon, the pleasures of little gifts become an important part of our life. "We made eye contact during his bath today and I swear I saw the beginning of a smile when I showed him how to pour water from one cup into another." "I was singing a song to myself after a disastrous lunch, probably just to cheer myself up, and she stopped stimming for a moment and sat still. It was extraordinary." "It's almost as if I can sense what he's thinking inside that complicated brain of his. I'm learning to get his transmissions. I'm learning his silent language."

As educational and biomedical treatment begins—and hopefully language, eye contact and facial gestures become more developed (even if ever so slowly)—parents have the opportunity to "calibrate" their intuitive knowledge with more ordinary means of communication. This can be a rich period of exploration and learning for everyone involved. As we explore "language" in this way and enter our child's world more fully, he or she begins to enter ours. More accurately , both adult and child enter an expanded *joint world of subtle communion* that is mysterious, compelling and at times profoundly satisfying. Soon we are launched on the journey of exploring that world together.

By the time parents and children have entered this phase of the journey, it is hard for anyone in the family to remember what life was like before autism spectrum disorder ("BASD") entered their lives. The BASD world seems two-dimensional in retrospect. On the other hand, the world after ASD ("AASD") is multidimensional, full of surprises and transformational almost on a daily basis. Priorities have shifted. What seemed important BASD now may feel quaint or distant. Life AASD usually feels more dramatic, passionate and directed by an intelligence beyond the familiar. When other children are involved, family dynamics may change dramatically.

The great amount of care required by the ASD child makes it difficult for siblings to receive what they and their parents may feel is their "fair share" of parental attention. Making this "all right" requires enormous patience, many dialogues with siblings, family meetings and special child care arrangements. Ultimately, the sibling issue also requires a major transformation in our notion of fairness, from one based primarily on each child getting "equal time" to one based on need. Reaching this level of understanding in a family with an ASD child is a major achievement and liberating for everyone involved.

The ASD child may be the source of other challenging "gifts" as well. Many parents speak of the uncanny ability of their special needs child to create exactly those demands that push everyone's creative capabilities to the limit. If Chelsey had responded in a significant way to the secretin protocol when she was four, or to anti-viral treatment at five, or chelation at six, or . . . Jaquelyn would probably never have written this book. Instead, Chelsey has continuously called her grandmother/physician back to the drawing board to expand her medical horizons. As Chelsey moved into double digits, we tried more chelation, methyl-B12, HBOT, LDN and much more. When she began to develop at eleven, we wondered if the approaching hormonal surge would unbalance her further or help in the healing. At first she seemed to regress in behavior exhibiting a lot of angry acting out and less contact. But as her twelfth birthday passed and menstruation began, Chelsey appeared to welcome her new womanhood with grace and even a touch of wisdom befitting the goddess in training that she is. Her relationship with Liz in particular has deepened and she is beginning to relate in ways that are new and encouraging. There is still a long ways to go, but in Chelsey's case, the infusion of estrogen and all that comes with it appears to be good biomedicine.

Throughout these past few years, Jaquelyn and I (and Liz, Jim and her siblings as well) have been challenged continuously to work better together as a team, integrating our diverse perspectives about healing more creatively and generally becoming more conscious in all of our relationships. The gift-list is long and impressive—and continues growing as we write these words. Most of our "failures" have led to discovering new levels of perseverance, patience and creativity that have led us to a clearer overview of the complex nature of ASD.

Final Words

I would like to end this chapter on a personal note by adding a few witness comments about Jaquelyn. The quest to heal Chelsey has transformed my life partner into a combined medical sleuth *par excellence*, a human body systems analyst, a physician quite knowledgeable about the biochemistry of that body and, I must add, an alchemist working on the edge of the mystery of healing. Her love for Chelsey has been the primary force in forging all her talents together synergistically to help her become a member of the growing group who practice the "new medicine."

We need look no further than the writing of this book to see explicitly how a single ASD child inspired her grandmother/physician to be of service to many other children (not to mention how its writing has drawn me into a level of collaboration I never dreamed possible). And there are hundreds of professionals and lay people alike who have been inspired to serve others with similar devotion and success. We can only imagine what awakenings are now taking place in the lives of those just touched by one or more of the thousands of ASD children that have appeared in recent years. As we each discover our unique path of healing with them, may we continue to nourish our hearts. That's our part of the bargain. That's the message we're being given. When we get it—really get it—then they will have done their job, our hearts will be more open and their brains will no longer need to be starving to get our attention.

References

[1] Dr. Beth Kalish-Weiss was a pioneer some thirty-five years ago in working with children in the autistic spectrum through individual and group movement therapy. She has published voluminously about her successful work, which was done quantitatively and with controls. Dr. Kalish-Weiss lives in Los Angeles where she now has a private practice for adults.

APPENDIX A

PROGRESS IN GASTROINTESTINAL RESEARCH AND ITS RELATIONSHIP TO IMMUNITY IN AUTISM

Teresa Binstock
Autism Researcher

Since 2001, various studies delineate aspects of gastrointestinal pathologies found in autistic children. Concurrently, food hypersensitivities are increasingly elucidated in both autistic and non-autistic populations, as are altered immune profiles—both intestinal and peripheral—as a result of gastrointestinal pathology. We present here not a thorough review but instead a survey of recent developments, even as they are best understood in the context of preceding studies.

D'Eufemia et al[1] excluded autistic children with clinical or laboratory indications of intestinal pathology and nonetheless found increased intestinal permeability in 43% of the remaining children (9 of 21). In 2002, Wakefield, Murch, and colleagues commented upon this finding and wrote: "reliance upon symptomatology will substantially underestimate the proportion of autistic individuals with possible gastrointestinal pathology." Furthermore, underestimates "will be compounded by the combination of raised pain threshhold... and by their restricted ability to communicate symptoms."[2]

That same year, Knivsberg et al reported improvement in a small number of autistics following a gluten-free, casein-free diet[3]. and Parent Ratings data amassed by Bernie Rimland, Ph.D., and the Autism Research Institute indicate that gluten free and/or casein-free diets are efficacious for many autistic children[4]. In 2006, Balzola et al described beneficial results of elimination diets combined with other therapies[5]. Of note, hypersensitivity to a food antigen can induce increased intestinal permeability and other pathologies[6, 7]

Circa 2007, Andrew J. Wakefield, M.D., remains controversial. In 1998, Wakefield et al published data describing intestinal pathologies in a small group of autistic children (n = 12) whose parents felt the child had regressed following the MMR vaccination[8]. For the validity of the concept "regressive autism", see—for example–Siperstein and Volkmar[9]. Subsequently, a retraction of Wakefield et al's 1998 study's speculative interpretation was published[10], even though the 1998 article's primary findings have not been retracted. Furthermore, a number of peer-reviewed studies have confirmed, nuanced, and expanded upon the original (1998) findings[11-16]. These studies demonstrate that lymphoid nodular hyperplasia (LNH) and other gastrointestinal pathologies are found in many autistic children and differ from LNH in non-autistic children and also from ulcerative colitis and from Crohn's disease1[4, 17, 18].

Let us be clear: the retraction focused upon the *speculative interpretation* of the 1998 findings. The findings themselves have not been retracted. And what was the interpretation? The abstract states "We identified associated gastrointestinal disease and developmental regression in a group of previously normal children, which was generally associated in time with possible environmental triggers." The heresy by Wakefield and colleagues lay in suggesting that there might be a subgroup of children in whom the MMR had been injurious. Subsequent studies about the MMR have been divided, with some finding "no problem" and others questioning that conclusion[19]. Importantly, challenge-rechallenge methodology has demonstrated that physiological effects of the MMR can be alleviated and then recur subsequent to reexposure[20].

Aside from the issue of whether or not the MMR can be injurious to a small percentage of toddlers, several studies have found measles virus (MV) in intestinal tissue of autistic children[2, 11,16], and in at least two of those studies, intestinal MV is consistent with the vaccine strain[11, 16], as was MV found in cerebrospinal fluid of three autistic children[21]. When reading published medical literature about gastrointestinal pathologies in autism, keep in mind that they now have various names, eg, autistic enterocolitis, ileal lymphoid hyperplasia, ileocolonic lymphonodular hyperplasia, and gastritis.

Important new developments are being offered by autism researchers who have been evaluating gastrointestinal pathologies in relation to alterations of intestinal and peripheral immunity. Many such studies present analysis of peripheral blood mononuclear cells (eg, [22-28]). Some such studies evaluate the child's immune response to dietary antigens (eg, [22-25]).

Increased appreciation of food hypersensitivities, intestinal pathologies, and their significance in non-autistic populations is reflected in major reviews[7, 29-32]. As an example, celiac disease is realized to be a spectrum wherein villous atrophy is not necessarily present[33-35]. Furthermore, various behavioral traits and nutritional deficits associated with autism are described in non-autistic celiac disease. Importantly, for subgroups of non-autistic patients with gluten hypersensitivity and with behavioral or mood problems, an elimination diet is often helpful for boosting nutritional status and for alleviating adverse traits[36-38]. Similar efficacy is true in autism[3, 5].

Reinforced by these studies about intestinal pathologies, food hypersensitivity, and immunity, a new perspective is emerging, one that links gut, immunity, and brain. Many and probably most autistic children have one or more gastrointestinal pathologies—ranging from increased intestinal permeability and/or a food hypersensitivity all the way to severe inflammation such as ileocolonic lymphoid hyperplasia. Many of these pathologies are associated with altered profiles of peripheral cytokines (prior cites, also [39]). That peripheral cytokines are altered in autism suggests yet another way for brain function to be made atypical, because cytokines affect brain function[40-43].

Furthermore—as discussed elsewhere in this text —relationships between familial autoimmunity and autism subgroups are increasingly described[44-48]; and Connolly and colleagues have continued their work, in 1999 describing endothelia-related autoantibodies in autism and other neurologic disorders; in 2006 affirming the researchers' original findings while also decribing increased levels not only of brain derived neurotrophic factor (BDNF) but also of IgG and IgM antibodies against BDNF, which itself modulates immunity[49-50]. They also describe elevated IgG and IgM against myelin basic protein (MBP;[50]), thus confirming the elevated MBP titers described by VK Singh[51].

In summary: recent studies of gastrointestinal pathologies and immune nuances in autism and in non-autistic populations are prompting acceptance of significant relationships among food hypersensitivities, intestinal pathologies, and changes in peripheral immunity—as well as alterations of nutritional status and behavior. Healing the gut remains an important focus for clinicians and parents of children with autism.

References

1   D'Eufemia P et al. Abnormal intestinal permeability in children with autism. Acta Paediatr. 1996 Sep;85(9):1076-9.

2   Uhlmann V et al. Potential viral pathogenic mechanism for new variant inflammatory bowel disease. Mol Pathol. 2002 55(2):84-90.

3   Knivsberg AM et al. A randomised, controlled study of dietary intervention in autistic syndromes. Nutr Neurosci. 2002 Sep;5(4):251-61.

4   Autism Research Institute. Parent ratings of behavioral effects of biomedical interventions. http://www.autismwebsite.com/ari/treatment/form34q.htm

5   Balzola F et al. Beneficial effects of IBD therapy and gluten/casein-free diet in an Italian cohort of patients with autistic enterocolitis followed over one year. Conference presentation 2006.

6   Heyman M, Desjeux JF. Cytokine-induced alteration of the epithelial barrier to food antigens in disease. Ann N Y Acad Sci. 2000;915:304-11.

7   Nowak-Wegrzyn A et al. Food protein-induced enterocolitis syndrome caused by solid food proteins. Pediatrics. 2003 Apr;111(4 Pt 1):829-35. http://pediatrics.aappublications.org/cgi/reprint/111/4/829

8   Wakefield AJ et al. Ileal-lymphoid-nodular hyperplasia, non-specific colitis, and pervasive developmental disorder in children. Lancet. 1998 Feb 28;351(9103):637-41.

9   Siperstein R, Volkmar F. Brief report: parental reporting of regression in children with pervasive developmental disorders. J Autism Dev Disord. 2004 34(6):731-4.

10 Murch SH et al. Retraction of an interpretation. Lancet. 2004 363(9411):750.

11   Kawashima H et al. Detection and sequencing of measles virus from peripheral mononuclear cells from patients with inflammatory bowel disease and autism. Dig Dis Sci. 2000 45(4):723-9.

12   Furlano RI et al. Colonic CD8 and gamma delta T-cell infiltration with epithelial damage in children with autism. J Pediatr. 2001 138(3):366-72.

13   Torrente F et al. Small intestinal enteropathy with epithelial IgG and complement deposition in children with regressive autism. Mol Psychiatry. 2002 7(4):375-82, 334.

14   Torrente F et al. Focal-enhanced gastritis in regressive autism with features distinct from Crohn's and Helicobacter pylori gastritis. Am J Gastroenterol. 2004 99(4):598-605.

15   Balzola F et al. Autistic enterocolitis: confirmation of a new inflammatory bowel disease in an Italian cohort. Conference presentation 2005.

16   Walker SJ et al. Persistent ileal measles virus in a large cohort of regressive autistic children with ileocolitis and lymphonodular hyperplasia: revisitation of an earlier study. IMFAR. June 1, 2006.   http://thoughtfulhouse.org/pr/053106.htm

17   Wakefield AJ et al. The significance of ileo-colonic lymphoid nodular hyperplasia in children with autistic spectrum disorder. Eur J Gastroenterol Hepatol. 2005 17(8):827-36.

18   Walker-Smith JA et al. Practical Paediatric Gastroenterology. Butterworths, 1983.

19   Goldman GS, Yazbak FE. An investigation of the association between MMR vaccination and autism in Denmark. J Am Physicians & Surgeons 2004 9(3):70-75. http://www.jpands.org/vol9no3/goldman.pdf

20   Wakefield AJ et al. Gastrointestinal comorbidity, autistic regression, and Measles-containing vaccines: positive re-challenge and biological gradient. Medical Veritas 2006 3:796-802.

21   Bradstreet JJ et al. Detection of measles virus genomic RNA in cerebrospinal fluid of children with regressive autism: a report of three cases. J Am Physicians Surgeons 2004 9(2):38-45.

22   Jyonouchi H et al. Proinflammatory and regulatory cytokine production associated with innate and adaptive immune responses in children with autism spectrum disorders and developmental regression. J Neuroimmunol. 2001 Nov 1;120(1-2):170-9.

23   Jyonouchi H et al. Innate immunity associated with inflammatory responses and cytokine production against common dietary proteins in patients with autism spectrum disorder. Neuropsychobiology. 2002;46(2):76-84.

24   Jyonouchi H et al. Dysregulated innate immune responses in young children with autism spectrum disorders: their relationship to gastrointestinal symptoms and dietary intervention. Neuropsychobiology. 2005;51(2):77-85.

25   Jyonouchi H et al. Evaluation of an association between gastrointestinal symptoms and cytokine production against common dietary proteins in children with autism spectrum disorders. J Pediatr. 2005 May;146(5):605-10.

26   Ashwood P et al. Spontaneous mucosal lymphocyte cytokine profiles in children with autism and gastrointestinal symptoms: mucosal immune activation and reduced counter regulatory interleukin-10.   J Clin Immunol. 2004 24(6):664-73.

27   Ashwood P, Wakefield AJ. Immune activation of peripheral blood and mucosal CD3+ lymphocyte cytokine profiles in children with autism and gastrointestinal symptoms. J Neuroimmunol. 2006 173(1-2):126-34.

28 Molloy CA et al. Elevated cytokine levels in children with autism spectrum disorder. J Neuroimmunol. 2006 172(1-2):198-205.

29 Mack DR et al. Peripheral blood intracellular cytokine analysis in children newly diagnosed with inflammatory bowel disease. Pediatr Res. 2002 51(3):328-32.

30 Latcham F et al. A consistent pattern of minor immunodeficiency and subtle enteropathy in children with multiple food allergy. J Pediatr. 2003 143(1):39-47.

31 Shek LP et al. Humoral and cellular responses to cow milk proteins in patients with milk-induced IgE-mediated and non-IgE-mediated disorders. Allergy. 2005 60(7):912-9.

32 Murch SH. Clinical manifestations of food allergy: the old and the new. Eur J Gastroenterol Hepatol. 2005 17(12):1287-91.

33 Murray JA. The widening spectrum of celiac disease. Am J Clin Nutr. 1999 69(3):354-65.

34 Cronin CC, Shanahan F. Exploring the iceberg--the spectrum of celiac disease. Am J Gastroenterol. 2003 Mar;98(3):518-20.

35 Esteve M et al. Spectrum of gluten sensitive enteropathy in first degree relatives of coeliac patients: clinical relevance of lymphocytic enteritis. Gut. 2006.

36 Pynnonen PA et al. Untreated celiac disease and development of mental disorders in children and adolescents. Psychosomatics. 2002 43(4):331-4.

37 Pynnonen PA et al. Mental disorders in adolescents with celiac disease. Psychosomatics. 2004 45(4):325-35.

38 Pynnonen PA et al. Gluten-free diet may alleviate depressive and behavioural symptoms in adolescents with coeliac disease: a prospective follow-up case-series study. BMC Psychiatry. 2005 Mar 17;5(1):14.

39 Burgess NK et al. Hyperserotoninemia and Altered Immunity in Autism. J Autism Dev Disord 2006.

40 Biber K et al. Chemokines in the brain: neuroimmunology and beyond. Curr Opin Pharmacol. 2002 2(1):63-8.

41 Sperner-Unterweger B. Immunological aetiology of major psychiatric disorders: evidence and therapeutic implications. Drugs. 2005;65(11):1493-520.

42 Biber K et al. Chemokines and their receptors in central nervous system disease. Curr Drug Targets. 2006 7(1):29-46.

43 Ashwood P et al. The immune response in autism: a new frontier for autism research. J Leukoc Biol. 2006 80(1):1-15.

44 Comi AM et al. Familial clustering of autoimmune disorders and evaluation of medical risk factors in autism. J Child Neurol. 1999 14(6):388-94.

45 Sweeten TL et al. Increased prevalence of familial autoimmunity in probands with pervasive developmental disorders. Pediatrics. 2003 112(5):e420.

46 Croen LA et al. Maternal autoimmune diseases, asthma and allergies, and childhood autism spectrum disorders: a case-control study. Arch Pediatr Adolesc Med. 2005 159(2):151-7.

47 Molloy CA et al. Familial autoimmune thyroid disease as a risk factor for regression in children with Autism Spectrum Disorder: a CPEA Study. J Autism Dev Disord. 2006 Apr;36(3):317-24.

48 Valicenti-McDermott M et al. Frequency of gastrointestinal symptoms in children with autistic spectrum disorders and association with family history of autoimmune disease. J Dev Behav Pediatr. 2006 Apr;27(2 Suppl):S128-36.

49 Connolly AM et al. Serum autoantibodies to brain in Landau-Kleffner variant, autism, and other neurologic disorders. J Pediatr. 1999 134(5):607-13.

50 Connolly AM et al. Brain-derived neurotrophic factor and autoantibodies to neural antigens in sera of children with autistic spectrum disorders, Landau-Kleffner syndrome, and epilepsy. Biol Psychiatry. 2006 15;59(4):354-63.

51 Singh VK, Lin SX, Newell E, Nelson C. Abnormal measles-mumps-rubella antibodies and CNS autoimmunity in children with autism. J Biomed Sci. 2002 9(4):359-64.

APPENDIX B

AUTISM, METALS, AND THE MERCURY IN VACCINES

Introduction by Teresa Binstock
Autism Researcher

In 1999, an FDA report revealed that ethylmercury was present in several vaccines mandated for infants and toddlers. That announcement caused several parents of autistic children to realize that injected ethylmercury may have caused their children's regression. That insight prompted extensive research and led to the writing of a medical paper called the "mercury/autism paper " published in a medical journal.[1]

Along the way, various individuals provided citations or other information including, but certainly not limited to, Woody McGinnis, MD, Boyd Haley, PhD, and Vas Aposhian, PhD. Thus far, this mercury/autism paper has led to a Congressional Hearing by the U.S. Government Reform Committee, to an international hearing hosted by the National Academy of Science's Institute for Medicine, and to the removal of ethylmercury from most vaccines.

An important question is why most children who were injected with ethylmercury did not become autistic? Medical literature describes individuals with increased susceptibility—whether from acquired and/or genetic reasons. Furthermore, medical history offers the lesson of acrodynia, also known as Pink Disease, a form of mercury poisoning from commercial powders used for diaper rash and teething. Acrodynia illustrates the significance of susceptibility. Approximately 1 in 400 exposed individuals developed symptoms of Pink Disease.[2]

Several CDC studies (Spring of 2000) found that early exposure to ethylmercury was indeed associated with autism-spectrum disorders including ADHD, tics, and autism. The CDC's internal documents—obtained by Freedom of Information Act filings—were more forthright than were early press releases describing those findings.[3]

Since CSB was first published, public perceptions of thimerosal's etiologic role in neurologic disorders remain shaped by politics. The CDC, AAP, and IOM would have us believe that thimerosal injections are not injurious to the developing brain, but recent studies suggest otherwise. As excellently summarized by David Kirby, a CDC study (2000) found elevated risk of various neurologic sequelae from thimerosal injections into infants. ADD, ADHD, sleep disorders, impaired language, other developmental delays, and autism were linked with thimerosal injections into infants[4]. However, as revealed by documents obtained by *freedom of information act* (FOIA), individuals who conducted this CDC study proceeded to dilute their own data[5, 6]. Subsequently (2003), after a series of deliberate dilutions which made the associations disappear, the CDC researchers—in concert with the editors of "Pediatrics "—published an article claiming that thimerosal injections had no role in the autism epidemic[7].

That "Pediatrics" published deliberately altered data[7] is part of a larger trend. In 2001, the Institute of Medicine (IOM) hosted a thimerosal hearing in which various experts and others submitted testimony. Among the IOM's conclusions was the biologic plausability of the thimerosal autism hypothesis[8]. Despite and perhaps because of this important conclusion, chicanery by the CDC and IOM continued.

A 2nd IOM hearing occurred in 2004. Thimerosal and the MMR were the primary topics. The hearing's agenda prompted Congressman Dave Weldon (R-Fla) to write that the time allocated for thimerosal concerns was "heavily biased and would not allow for a fair and balanced discussion of the [medical] literature."[9] Most importantly, additional documents obtained by FOIA delineated a contractual relationship between the CDC and the IOM and revealed that the CDC predetermined the hearing's conclusions as would be announced by the IOM at the end of its 2004 hearing[10, 11].

Despite the IOM's 2004 recommendation to direct research away from thimerosal, findings in a number of recent studies further elucidate the mechanisms by which thimerosal causes damage to developing brains.

For instance, Deth & colleagues found that mercury levels found in human infants vaccinated with a thimerosal-containing vaccine[12] were sufficient to impair function of methionine synthase, an enzyme crucial for methylation[13]. Hornig et al reported that autoimmune-related genetic susceptibility predisposes for thimerosal damage[14], whereas James et al published evidence showing that many autistic children have nutrient deficiencies that impair detoxification[15]. More recently, findings by Burbacher, Clarkson, & colleagues make clear that thimerosal's ethylmercury enters the brain more efficiently than does methylmercury, thus causing ethylmercury to deposit a higher level of inorganic mercury, prompting the conclusion, "A higher percentage of the total Hg in the brain was in the form of inorganic Hg for the thimerosal-exposed monkeys (34% vs. 7%)."[16]

A simple, clear review of important studies about thimerosal can be found on a website hosted by Generation Rescue[17], one of several autism-parent organizations increasingly influential in resisting the CDC's and IOM's demand that adverse effects from thimerosal and the MMR not be studied. If fact, websites by parents' organizations have become repositories of good information—including summaries of peer-reviewed scientific studies, presentations of FOIA documents, and calls to political action. For instance, while Safeminds remains the flagship of autism groups formed in response to thimerosal's adverse effects, other groups are making important contributions, eg:

NoMercury.org
MomsAgainstMercury.org
GenerationRescue.org
PutChildrenFirst.org
NationalAutismAssociation.org
TheAutismAutoimmunityProject (taap.info)

Dan Olmsted—science editor for United Press International—became curious about the vaccinations/autism controversy. His investigative and writing skills have resulted in a series of news columns, entitled the "The Age of Autism ", which present vaccine ironies in an understandable way[18], not the least of which are seqeulae that seem to occur when chickenpox or the chickenpox vaccination occur in temporal proximity with the MMR.

In July of 2006, "Pediatrics" published an article by Eric Fombonne et al[19]. The article and attendant publicity conveyed that neither thimerosal nor the MMR is associated with autism. However, perusal of the article suggests it is more a diatribe than a scientific publication. Consider a quote from page e141:

> "By and large, biological studies of ethylmercury exposure have also failed to support the thimerosal hypothesis. Despite the accumulation of negative studies, concerns from the public have not been entirely alleviated, and fears continue to be fueled by well-publicized media accounts of a spectacular nature."

Unlike actual scientific articles wherein peer-reviewers request that alternative findings be mentioned, Fombonne et al fail to cite peer-reviewed studies contrary to the researchers' preferred position (eg, see[17]). Furthermore, the political agenda of Fombonne et al[19] is conveyed by their phrasing "media accounts of a spectacular nature". Categorizing Kirby's book Evidence of Harm (EOH) as a spectacular media account appears to be a deliberate distortion because EOH includes a vast array of peer-reviewed citations, links to IOM testimonies, and quotes from CDC and IOM documents obtained by FOIA.

As this new edition of CSB goes to press, a bill (HR 5887) has been introduced by Dave Weldon (R-Fla) & Carolyn Maloney (D-NY). The bill's purpose is to dilute the CDC's conflict of interest inherent in the fact that rhw CDC is paid far more to promote vaccinations than to evaluate their safety. HR 5887 would take safety evaluations away from CDC and place them within the Department of Health and Human Services, while allowing the CDC to continue its role in promoting vaccines.

The controversy is far from over. The mechanisms by which thimerosal induces adverse effects in susceptible individuals is increasingly understood.

References

1   Bernard S., Enayati A., Redwood L., Roger H., Binstock T. Autism: A novel form of mercury poisoning. Med. Hypotheses. 2001 Apr;56(4): 462-71

2   Dally A. "The rise and fall of pink disease, " Soc Hist Med. 1997 Aug; 10(2): 291-304

3   "Thimerosal Linked to Autism in Confidential CDC Study. " Mothering Magazine, March/April 2002

4   p380. Kirby D. Evidence of Harm: Mercury in vaccines and the autism epidemic: a medical controversy; St. Martins Press, 2005.

5   p283-4, ibid.

6   Generation Zero Full Analysis with Charts - Safe Minds 2004 http://www.nationalautismassociation.org/library/GenerationZeroPres.pdf

7   Verstraeten T et al. Safety of thimerosal-containing vaccines: a two-phased study of computerized health maintenance organization databases. Pediatrics. 2003 112(5):1039-48. Erratum in: Pediatrics. 2004 113(1):184.

8   Stratton K et al. Immunization Safety Review: Thimerosal Containing Vaccines and Neurodevelopmental Disorders. Institute of Medicine, National Academy Press; Washington DC, 2001.

9   p305, Kirby.

10 http://putchildrenfirst.org/chapter6.html

11 http://putchildrenfirst.org/media/6.3.pdfldrenfirst.org/media/6.3.pdf

12 Pichichero ME et al. Mercury concentrations and metabolism in infants receiving vaccines containing thiomersal: a descriptive study. Lancet. 2002 30;360(9347):1737-41.

13 Waly M et al. Activation of methionine synthase by insulin-like growth factor-1 and dopamine: a target for neurodevelopmental toxins and thimerosal. Mol Psychiatry. 2004 9(4):358-70.

14 Hornig M et al. Neurotoxic effects of postnatal thimerosal are mouse strain dependent. Mol Psychiatry. 2004 Sep;9(9):833-45.

15 James SJ et al. Metabolic biomarkers of increased oxidative stress and impaired methylation capacity in children with autism. Am J Clin Nutr. 2004 80(6):1611-7. http://www.ajcn.org/cgi/content/full/80/6/1611

16 Burbacher TM et al. Comparison of blood and brain mercury levels in infant monkeys exposed to methylmercury or vaccines containing thimerosal. Environ Health Perspect. 2005 113(8):1015-21. http://www.ehponline.org/members/2005/7712/7712.html

17 Generation Rescue summaries of Top Scientific Reports: http://generationrescue.org/evidence_reports.html

18 Olmsted D. "The Age of Autism ": http://theageofautism.com

19 Fombonne E et al. Pervasive developmental disorders in Montreal, Quebec, Canada: prevalence and links with immunizations. Pediatrics. 2006 118(1):e139-50.

During the final stages of writing the ethylmercury/autism paper, two versions were prepared for publication. One version focused upon comparing traits and physiological abnormalities common in autistic children and in victims of mercury poisoning. That version was submitted and published. An alternative version called attention to technical aspects and susceptibility was also prepared; that version is here published for the first time.

Autism: Mercury Poisoning by Thimerosal Injections

Sallie Bernard[*1], Albert Enayati[1],
Heidi Roger[1], Lyn Redwood[1], Teresa Binstock[2]

*sbernard@arcresearch.com—June 27, 2000
1. parent of autistic child
2. autism researcher (diagnosed with Asperger's Syndrome)

Abstract: Autism is a syndrome characterized by impairments in social relatedness, language and communication, a need for routine and sameness, abnormal movements, and sensory dysfunction. Mercury (Hg) is a toxic metal that can exist as a pure element or in a variety of inorganic and organic forms and can cause immune, sensory, neurological, motor, and behavioral dysfunctions similar to traits defining or associated with autism; the similarities extend to neuroanatomy, neurotransmitters, immunity, and epileptiform activity. Thimerosal, a preservative frequently added to childhood vaccines, has become a major source of Hg in human infants and toddlers. According to the EPA and the American Academy of Pediatricians, fully vaccinated children, within their first two years, receive a potentially neurotoxic quantity of Hg. A review of medical literature and U.S. government data suggests that

1. Many and perhaps most cases of idiopathic autism are induced by early exposure to Hg in thimerosal.

2. This type of autism represents a unique and heretofore unrecognized mercurial syndrome.

3. Certain genetic and non-genetic factors establish a predisposition whereby thimerosal's adverse effects occur only in some children.

4. Causal mechanisms include mercurial effects upon astrocytes, microtubules, neuronal function, and synaptogenesis and gastrointestinal function.

Introduction: Originally described by Kanner (1943;1), the incidence of autism and autism-spectrum disorders (ASD) has been steadily increasing, especially during the 1980s and again during 1990s (2,3). Since the 1930s, an ethylmercury compound (thimerosal; TMS) has been used as a preservative in certain mandatory vaccines (4), and increased ASD-rates during the last several decades may represent a heretofore unrecognized form of mercurialism. Recently, the FDA reported that the total amount of ethylmercury (eHg) injected into infants and toddlers during mandatory vaccinations is worthy of concern, and the CDC has recommended that TMS be removed from vaccines (5-6). In fact, the neurotoxicity of eHg compounds has long been known (7), and profound similarities between autism and mercury poisoning (HgP) suggest that many cases of autism and related neurobehavioral disorders may be manifestions of HgP caused by TMS injections during vaccinations.

This hypothesis is supported not only by traits comparisons but also by similarities in neuroanatomy, neurotransmitters, immune profiles, and epileptiform activity. Additional support derives from Hg's neurotoxic mechanisms and the timings of exposure to injected Hg. Furthermore, HgP literature provides basis for understanding why only some children develop CNS impairment from TMS. The fact that some children experience neurobehavioral improvements after chelation therapies (8) is consistent with a causal link between HgP and ASD.

Traits similarities: HgP literature describes traits consistent

1. with ASD's defining criteria, and
2. with virtually all ASD-associations such as sensory impairments, hand-flapping, and shifted immune profiles. For instance: juvenile monkeys prenatally exposed to mercury exhibit decreased social play, increased passive behavior, and impaired face recognition (9-11). Humans exposed to mercury vapor also perform poorly on face recognition tests and may present with a "mask face " (12). Emotional instability can occur in children and adults exposed to Hg. For instance, Iraqi children poisoned by methylmercury (mHg) had a tendency "to cry, laugh, or smile without obvious provocation " (13-14), a trait seen in ASD (15)).

HgP children show difficulties with speech (16-18). Even children exposed prenatally to "safe " levels of mHg performed less well on standardized language tests than did unexposed controls (19). Iraqi babies exposed prenatally either failed to develop language or presented with severe language deficits in childhood; many exhibited "exaggerated reaction " to sudden noise; and some had reduced hearing. Iraqi children who were postnatally poisoned from bread containing either methyl- or ethyl-mercury developed articulation problems, from slow, slurred word production to an inability to generate meaningful speech. Most had impaired hearing and a few became deaf (13-14,20). Acrodynia's symptoms include noise sensitivity and hearing problems (21).

Five additional examples:

1. The amygdala are increasingly implicated in autism in regard to gaze avoidance and dysregulations in sociality, emotions, appetite, anxiety, depression (22-24). Furthermore, via bidirectional pathways with the orbitofrontal cortex, amygdaloid dysfunction is linked with motor, cognitive, and other perseverative behaviors (25-27). Organic Hg migrates into amygdaloid nuclei of primates (28-29).

2. Similar cerebellar-changes occur in autism and HgP (30-31;32-34).

3. Elevated antibodies to myelin-basic protein (MBP) are associated with autism (35) and derive from CNS neurons (VK Singh, personal communication). HgP induces elevations of antibodies against MBP (36).

4. Hand-flapping is such an unusual trait that one author has suggested it can be an early diagnostic marker for ASD in some children (37). HgP can produce flapping motions (16,17)

5. Epileptiform activity occurs in many ASD children and is often subtle and hard to detect (38-39). HgP elevates extracellular glutamate, which inclines towards epilepiform activity, and can induce seizure activity with lower threshholds and reduced amplitude (40-43).

These examples illustrate that HgP/ASD similarities exist on numerous levels. Additional parallels are presented in Tables 1-3 that follow.

TABLE 1 HgP/ASD parallels for autism's diagnostic criteria

I. Social relatedness (45):

ASD: 96, 105-108   HgP: 9-12,40,85,102

II. Communication impairments (45) including loss of
speech, failure to develop speech, dysarthria, articulation
problems, speech comprehension deficits, echolalia,
pragmatic errors, lower verbal-IQ scores; deficits in abstract
reasoning:

ASD: 96,110-111   HgP: 16-21,33,40

III. Repetitive, perseverative, or stereotyped behaviors (45):

ASD: 96,108,113-114,179   HgP: 115-117

Amygdala/orbitofrontal substrates: 25-29,46,118

TABLE 2 ASD/HgP parallels for associated traits

Anxiety:

    ASD: 118   HgP: 40,119-120

Auditory impairments:

    ASD: 96,126-127   HgP: 18,20,33.

Clumsiness, mobility and postural impairments, toe walking, rocking, choreiform movements.

    ASD: 96,179,189   HgP: 12,18,20,21,76

Depression:

    ASD: 121-123   HgP: 119,124

OCD, schizoid traits, emotional lability:

    ASD: 15,96,121-123,125   HgP: 40,85,109,119,124

Touch aversion, excessive mouthing of objects, oral and tactile hypersensitivities, insensitivities to pain:

    ASD: 96,129-130. HgP:14,17,20,90,109,128,132

Spatial orientation:

    ASD: 132,133.   HgP: 134

TABLE 3 An ASD/HgP miscellany

ASD/HgP parallels in neuroanatomy for amygdala, cerebellum, hippocampi:

> ASD: 22-24,30-31,137-139.
> HgP: 28,29,32,33,46,60,135,137-140.

ASD/HgP parallels in serotonin, dopamine, acetylcholine, glutamate:

> ASD: 141-144; 96,145-147; 148; 157-158.
> HgP: 147-152; 91,153-154; 47,155-156; 40, 159-160.

ASD/HgP parallels in sulfur, glutathione, purines, & mitochondria:

> ASD: 161-162; 80,161,164; 96,165; 140,167.
> HgP: 33,163; 33,78-79,159; 32-33; 168-169

ASD/HgP parallels in allergy, autoimmunity, asthma; Th1/Th2 shifts, and NK cells:

> ASD: 81,167; 171; 172-173.
> HgP: 42,91,174; 82,84,175-176; 177.

Additional ASD/HgP parallels can be found in numerous areas including movement and motor funtion (178;40), cognition (179;40,180), behaviors (181-182;33,109), vision (96,183;13-14,20); rashes and dermatitis (170,184;108,185-186); autonomic disturbance (15,133;76,109); gastrointestinal atypicalities (78,187-188; 33,109,186).

Causal and temporal links between Hg-injections and autism: Organic mercury's effects upon microtubules, which participate in neuronal function and synaptogenesis, are increasingly described (cites below). Timings of infant and toddler thimerosal injections correspond to major critical periods of neuronal development (eg, Harlow et al, reviewed in 22; 44). Synaptogenesis during these post-natal months subserves eye-contact, smiling, early language, and other traits central to autism's diagnostic criteria (44-45). Injected eHg that enters the infant and toddler brain would interfere with critical periods for these developmental processes. Therefore, associations among vaccination timings, injected mercury, and autistic regressions are likely to have been both causal and temporal.

Ethylmercury toxicity is similar to that of mHg, and injected Hg is especially harmful (7, 46-48). When eHg's entry route is by injection delivering a vaccine, the amount of eHg that crosses the BBB (blood brain barrier) (49) or enters gastrointestinal tissues is likely to be increased via vaccination-induced elevations of cytokines such as interferon gamma, which expands permeability of tight-junction tissues (50-52).

Mechanisms of toxicity. Gradually, circulating organic-Hg compounds localize in brain areas implicated in autism (23,28-29,31). Within the CNS, organic Hg gradually converts to an inorganic form (Hg++) (28). Inorganic Hg is unable to cross the BBB, thus tends to remain in the CNS (central nervous system), and is more likely than organic Hg-compounds to induce autoimmune responses (53-54). CNS Hg has diverse mechanisms of neurotoxicity (36,55-57).

Ethyl-Hg has an affinity for –SH (sulfhydryl) molecules and is used as a vaccine preservative because of eHg's ability to inhibit cell function, leading to cellular stasis or death (58). Organic Hg–compounds primarily affect the CNS, are most toxic to a developing brain, and are more likely to enter postnatal brains because an infant's BBB is not fully developed (59-61) and because infants under 6 months are unable to excrete Hg, probably due to an inability to produce bile, the main excretion route for organic Hg (32,62). The longer Hg remains in the CNS, the greater the neurotoxic effects (63-64).

Hg++ and and eHg affect astrocytic and neuronal function (36,65-67) and interfere with microtubules (68-69), which participate in neuronal function and synaptogenesis (70-72). Furthermore, although most cells respond to mercurial injury by modulating levels of glutathione (GSH), metallothionein, hemoxygenase, and other stress proteins, neurons tend to be "markedly deficient in these responses " and thus are less able to remove Hg and more prone to Hg-induced injury (73-74).

Why only some children? Pink Disease (acrodynia) was caused by mercury in teething powders, ear ointments, and other topical remedies, occurred in approximately 1 in 500 to 1 in 1000 exposed children, and generated a range of symptoms with much inter-individual variation (29,75-76). Studies in humans and other species have identified genetic and non-genetic factors which, as co-factors, contribute to why only some children are affected by organic Hg compounds.

For instance, a child's response to injected eHg would be shaped by his or her GSH (glutathione) status (73-74), the presence of chronic or recent infections that alter GSH levels (77), gastrointestinal problems (78), hepatic function (79); and detoxification capabilities (80); and these variables occur in a background of the child's individual and familial genetics regarding autoimmunity (33,81-84).

Large inter-individual differences exist for Hg's adverse effects; and, as evidenced by acrodynia, these differences occur in children (76,85), especially those will asthma or other allergies (76). Genetic implications of autism's high concordance rate in monozygotic twins (86) may reflect a family's Hg-response genetics.

The various factors that influence detoxification and neurotoxicity of organic Hg interact in complex ways. Nonetheless, a dose response curve reveals that at low doses, only a small percentage of HgP victims develop adverse sequelae (79). As with mercury exposures that led to acrodynia, so too injected eHg's neurotoxic effects would occur only in some children; and the phenotypic range of these effects would be modified by other exposures (eg, RhoGam; 87) in susceptible individuals.

Discussion. Vaccines are a source of Hg; the amount injected into most infants and toddlers exceeds government safety limits (4,88); and since at least 1977, TMS has been recognized as potentially dangerous (42,89-90). In July of 1999, the CDC asked manufacturers to start removing TMS from vaccines and rescheduled the hepatitis B vaccine for 6 months of age instead of at birth (6). For infants and toddlers vaccinated during the 1990s, Hg-injection amounts are 12.5 micrograms at birth, 62.5 micrograms at 2 months, 50 at 4 months, 62.5 at 6 months, and a final 50 micrograms around 15 months. In relation to infant and toddler body weights, these Hg quantities are significant. The 2-month dose of Hg is at least 30 times higher than the recommended daily maximum exposure (88).

Present EPA "safe" limit for Hg ought to be lowered. Doses not thought to be associated with adverse effects have induced damage in humans (19); infants are especially vulnerable to Hg (91); and the EPA's recently published "safe" guideline is too high (47). Two points are noteworthy: *First*: Because vaccinations induce immune reactions that include extended cytokines pulses (eg, interferon gamma; 50), vaccinal mercury is more dangerous than injected-mercury; studies suggest this is because mercury compounds and interferon gamma increase permeability of tissues such as the blood-brain barrier and gastrointestinal tract (49,51-52). Thus, when a bolus dose of ethylmercury circulates during a vaccination response, more eHg is likely to enter the CNS. *Second*: The EPA's determination was based upon the amount of ingested mercury needed to induce adverse neurologic sequelae in 10% of exposed fetuses. But vaccinal eHg is not first filtered by the maternal liver or placenta, as was the HgP incident used in the EPA calculations.

Furthermore, a 10% rate of neurologic sequelae is clearly not acceptable. To induce a 1% rate of neurologic sequelae, the necessary Hg level would be even lower than the EPA's current estimate; and to achieve a .25% rate of neurologic sequelae—which approximates the rate of autism during the 1990s—an even lower level of organic mercury would be sufficient (92-95).

For these reasons and because of Hg's dose-response curve, the EPA's current guideline for mercury toxicity is artificially high and ought be lowered. In fact, substantial evidence suggests that there is no "safe " level for injected eHg in humans and, given susceptibility factors and the distribution of organic Hg's toxic effects (93-95), the amount of vaccinal-eHg already injected into infants and toddlers is likely to have caused neurologic damage in large subgroups of susceptible children.

Sex ratio: Autism is more prevalent among boys than girls, with the ratio generally recognized as approximately 4:1 (96). Mercury studies consistently report greater effects on males than females, except for kidney damage (47). At high doses, both sexes are affected equally; at low doses only males are affected. This is true of mice as well as humans (19,33,47,97-99).

Parallel increases for thimerosal & autism: Autism's initial description and subsequent epidemiological increase mirror the introduction and use of thimerosal as a vaccine preservative. In the late 1930s, Leo Kanner, an experienced child psychologist, first began to notice the type of child he would later label "autistic. " His initial paper mentioned that this type of child had never been described previously: "Since 1938, there have come to our attention a number of children whose condition differs so markedly and uniquely from anything reported so far, that each case merits a detailed consideration of its fascinating peculiarities. " (1) All these patients were born in the 1930s. TMS was introduced as a component of vaccine solutions in the 1930s (4).

The vaccination rate and total amount of injected eHg (via TMS) have steadily increased since the 1930s, with coverage-rates in 1999 as high as 90% for some vaccines (100). Relatedly, since the syndrome was first described (1), the incidence of autism and ASD has increased dramatically. Prior to 1970, studies described an average prevalence of 1 in 2000; for studies after 1970, the average rate had doubled to 1 in 1000 (2). In 1996, the NIH estimated the autism-incidence rate to be 1 in 500 (101); and, as documented by several states' departments of education, a large increase in prevalence has been occurring since the mid-1990s (3). Thus, for several decades, these increased incidence-rates have paralleled the rising eHg-intake caused by vaccines containing eHg. In 1991, two vaccines, HIB and Hepatitis B, both of which generally include TMS as a preservative, were added to the recommended vaccine schedule (4) and may account for the increasing prevalence of autism and related neurologic diagnoses, including anorexia (102). The likelihood of a causal relationship is augmented by the fact the eHg preferentially seeks the amygdala (46; 103).

Conclusion: Based upon extensive phenotype-parallels between autism and HgP, this review establishes the likelihood that vaccinal TMS is etiologically significant in ASD, even as HgP's latency period (20) served to mask the connection. Furthermore, prior HgP epidemics have generated unique phenotypes, none of which would be classified as autism; however, the injecting of eHg when vaccinating infants and toddlers has never been studied and would induce its own unique mercurialism—which our society is experiencing as an unprecedented increase in ASD and related disorders (3,104). Safe chelation therapies ought to be considered for children who have been injected with thimerosal as infants and toddlers.

References

1. Kanner L. Autistic disturbances of affective contact. *The Nervous Child* 1942-1943;2:217-250.
2. Gillberg C, Wing L. Autism: not an extremely rare disorder. *Acta Psychiatr Scand* 1999;99:399-406.
3. Yazbak F.E. Autism `99, a national emergency. Internet publication 1999. http://www.garynull.com/documents/autism_99.htm
4. Egan W.M. Thimerosal in vaccines. presentation to the FDA, September 14 1999.
5. CDC. Thimerosal in vaccines: a joint statement of the American Academy of Pediatrics and the Public Health Service. *MMWR* 1999;48.26:563-565.
6. CDC. Recommendations regarding the use of vaccines that contain thimerosal as a preservative. *MMWR* 1999;48.43.996-998.
7. Suzuki T, Takemoto T.I., Kashiwazaki H, Miyama T. Metabolic fate of ethylmercury salts in man and animal. Ch 12, p209-233 in: Mercury, Mercurials, and Mercaptans. Miller MW, Clarkson TW, editors; Charles C. Thomas, Springfield, 1973.
8. Redwood L. Chelation case-histories http://tlredwood.home.mindspring.com/case_studies.htm

9.   Gunderson V.M., Grant K.S., Burbacher T.M., Fagan 3rd J.F., Mottet N.K. The effect of low-level prenatal methyl mercury exposure on visual recognition memory in infant crab-eating macaques. *Child Dev* 1986;57:1076-1083.

10.   Gunderson V.M., Grant K.S., Burbacher T.M., Fagan 3rd J.F., Mottet N.K. Visual recognition memory deficits in methyl mercury exposed Macaca fascicularis infants. *Neurotoxicol Teratol* 1988;10:373-379.

11.   Burbacher T.M., Sackett G.P., Mottet N.K. Methylmercury effects on the social behavior of Macaca fascicularis infants. *Neurotoxicol Teratol* 1990;12:65-71.

12.   Vroom F.Q., Greer M. Mercury vapour intoxication. *Brain* 1972;95:305-318.

13.   Amin-Zaki L, Elhassani S, Majeed M.A., Clarkson T.W., Doherty R.A., Greenwood M. Intra-uterine methylmercury poisoning in Iraq. *Pediatrics* 1974;54:587-595.

14.   Amin-Zaki L, Majeed M.A., Elhassani S.B., Clarkson T.W., Greenwood M.R., Doherty R.A. Prenatal methylmercury poisoning. *Am J Dis Child* 1979;133:172-177.

15.   Wing L, Attwood A. Syndromes of autism and atypical development. p3-19 in: Handbook of Autism and Pervasive Developmental Disorders; John Wiley & Sons, Inc., 1987.

16.   Pierce P.E., Thompson J.F., Likosky W.H., Nickey L.N., Barthel W.F., Hinman A.R. Alkyl mercury poisoning in humans. *JAMA* 1972;220:1439-1442.

17.   Snyder R.D. The involuntary movements of chronic mercury poisoning. *Arch Neurol* 1972;26:379-3381.

18.   Kark RA, Poskanzer DC, Bullock JD, Boylen G. Mercury poisoning and its treatment with N-acetyl-D, L-penicillamine. *NEJM* 1971;285:10-16.

19.   Grandjean P, Weihe P, White R.F., Debes F. Cognitive performance of children prenatally exposed to "safe " levels of methylmercury. *Environ Res* 1998;77:165-172.

20.   Amin-Zaki L, Majeed M.A., Clarkson T.W., Greenwood M.R. Methylmercury poisoning in Iraqi children: clinical observations over two years. *Br Med J* 1978; 1(6113):1613-616.

21.   Farnesworth D. Pink Disease Survey Results. Pink Disease Support Group Site, 1997 http://www.users.bigpond.com/difarnsworth

22.   Baron-Cohen S, Ring H.A., Bullmore E.T., Wheelwright S, Ashwin C, Williams S.C. The amygdala theory of autism. *Neurosci Biobehav Rev* 2000;24:355-64.

23.   Bachevalier J. Medial temporal lobe structures: a review of clinical and experimental findings. *Neuropsychologia* 1994;32:627-648.

24.   Waterhouse L, Fein D, Modahl C. Neurofunctional mechanisms in autism. *Psychol Rev* 1996;103:457-89.

25.   Rolls E.T. Memory systems in the brain. *Ann Rev Psychol* 2000;51:599-630.

26.   Bechara A, Damasio H, Damasio A.R. Emotion, decision making and the orbitofrontal cortex. *Cereb Cortex* 2000;10:295-307.

27.   Breiter H.C., Rauch S.L., Kwong et al. Functional magnetic imaging of symptom provocation in obsessive-compulsive disorder. *Arch Gen Psychiatry* 1996;53:595-606 1996.

28.   Vahter M, Mottet N.K., Friberg L, Lind B, Shen D.D., Burbacher T. Speciation of mercury in the primate blood and brain following long-term exposure to methyl mercury. *Toxicol Appl Pharmacol* 1994;124:221-229.

29. Warfvinge K, Hua J, Logdberg B. Mercury distribution in cortical areas and fiber systems of the neonatal and maternal cerebrum after exposure of pregnant squirrel monkeys to mercury vapor. *Environ Res* 1994;67:196-208.

30. Bauman M., Kemper T.L. Histoanatomic observations of the brain in early infantile autism. Neurol 1985;35:866-874.

31. Courchesne E. Brainstem, cerebellar and limbic neuroanatomical abnormalities in autism. *Curr Opin Neurobiol* 1997; 7:269-78.

32. Koos B.J., Longo L.D. Mercury toxicity in the pregnant woman, fetus, and newborn infant. *Am J Obstet Gynecol* 1976;126:390-406.

33. Clarkson T.W. Mercury: major issues in environmental health. *Environ Health Perspect* 1992;100:31-8.

34. Faro L.R.F., Nascimento J.L.M., Alfonso M, Duran R. Acute administration of methylmercury changes In vivo dopamine release from rat striatum. *Bull Environ Contam Toxicol* 1998;60:632-638.

35. Singh V.K., Warren R.P., Odell J, Warren W et al. Antibodies to myelin basic protein in children with autistic behavior. *Brain Behav Immun* 1993;7:97-103.

36. El-Fawal H.A., Waterman S.J., DeFeo A., Shamy M.Y. Neuroimmunotoxicology: humoral assessment of neurotoxicity and autoimmune mechanisms. *Environ Health Perspect* 1999;107:sl5:767-775.

37. Brasic J.R. Movements in autistic disorder. *Med Hypoth* 1999;53:48-9.

38. Lewine J.D., Andrews R., Chez M., Patil A.A. et al. Magnetoencephalographic patterns of epileptiform activity in children with regressive autism spectrum disorders. *Pediatrics* 1999;104:405-18.

39. Rapin I. Autistic regression and disintegrative disorder: how important the role of epilepsy? *Semin Pediatr Neurol* 1995;2:278-85.

40. O'Carroll R.E., Masterton G., Dougnall N., Ebmeier K.P. The neuropsychiatric sequelae of mercury poisoning: The Mad Hatter's disease revisited. *Br J Psychiatry* 1995;167:95-98 1995.

41. Scheyer R.D. Involvement of Glutamate in Human Epileptic Activities. *Prog Brain Res* 1998;116:359-69.

42. Rohyans J., Walson P.D., Wood G.A., MacDonald W.A. Mercury toxicity following merthiolate ear irrigations. *J Pediatr* 1984;104:311-313.

43. Szasz A, Barna B, Szupera Z, De Visscher G et al. Chronic low-dose maternal exposure to methylmercury enhances epileptogenicity in developing rats. *Int J Dev Neurosci* 1999;17:733-742.

44. Greenspan S., Greenspan N.T. First Feelings: milestones in the emotional development of your baby and child. Penguin Books, 1985.

45. Diagnostic and Statistical Manual of Mental Disorders, Fourth Edition, Washington D.C., American Psychiatric Association, 1994.

46. Magos L., Brown A.W., Sparrow S., Bailey E., Snowden R.T., Skipp W.R. The comparative toxicology of ethyl- and methylmercury. *Arch Toxicol* 1985;57:260-267.

47. Environmental Protection Agency (EPA); Hassett-Sipple B., Swartout J., Schoeny R., et al. Health Effects of Mercury and Mercury Compounds. Mercury Study Report to Congress, v5, December 1997.

48. Santucci B, Cannistraci C, Cristaudo A, Camera E, Picardo M. Thimerosal positivities: the role of SH groups and divalent ions. *Contact Dermatitis* 1998;39:123-6.

49. Kuwabara T, Yuasa T, Hidaka K, Igarashi H, Kaneko K, Miyatake T. [The observation of blood-brain barrier of organic mercury poisoned rat: a Gd-DTPA enhanced magnetic resonance study]. [Article in Japanese] *No To Shinkei* 1989;41:681-5.

50. Pabst H.F., Boothe P.M., Carson M.M. Kinetics of immunologic responses after primary MMR vaccination. *Vaccine* 1997;15:10-4 1997.

51. Madara J.L., Stafford J. Interferon-gamma directly affects barrier function of cultured intestinal epithelial monolayers. *J Clin Inv* 1989;83:724-7 1989.

52. Huynh H.K., Dorovini-Zis K. Effects of interferon-gamma on primary cultures of human brain microvessel endothelial cells. *Am J Pathol* 1993;142:1265-78.

53. Pedersen M.B, Hansen J.C., Mulvad G, Pedersen H.S., Gregersen M, Danscher G. Mercury accumulations in brains from populations exposed to high and low dietary levels of methyl mercury. Concentration, chemical form and distribution of mercury in brain samples from autopsies. *Int J Circumpolar Health* 1999;58:96-107.

54. Hultman P, Hansson-Georgiadis H. Methyl mercury-induced autoimmunity in mice. *Toxicol Appl Pharmacol* 1999;154:203-211.

55. Dave V, Mullaney K.J., Goderie S, Kimelberg H.K., Aschner M. Astrocytes as mediators of methylmercury neurotoxicity: effects on D-aspartate and serotonin uptake. *Dev Neurosci* 1994;16:222-231.

56. Fujiyama J, Hirayama K, Yasutake A. Mechanism of methylmercury efflux from cultured astrocytes. *Biochem Pharmacol* 1994;47:1525-1530.

57. Philbert M.A., Billingsley M.L., Reuhl K.R. Mechanisms of injury in the central nervous system. *Toxicologic Pathol* 2000;28:43-53.

58. FDA Panel Report: Mercury Containing Drug Products for Topical Antimicrobial Over-the-Counter Human Use; Establishment of a Monograph. Federal Register, January 5 1982 ;47:436-442.

59. Grandjean P, Budtz-Jorgensen E, White R.F., Jorgensen P.J. et al. Methylmercury exposure biomarkers as indicators of neurotoxicity in children aged 7 years. *Am J Epidemiol* 1999;150:301-305.

60. Davis L.E., Kornfeld M, Mooney H.S., Fiedler K.J. et al. Methylmercury poisoning: long term clinical, radiological, toxicological, and pathological studies of an affected family. *Ann Neurol* 1994;35:680-688.

61. Wild G.C., Benzel E.C., Essentials of Neurochemistry, Jones and Bartlett Publishers, Inc., 1994.

62. Clarkson,T.W. Molecular and ionic mimicry of toxic metals. *Annu Rev Pharmacol Toxicol* 1993;32:545-571.

63. Bakir F, Damluji S.F., Amin-Zaki L, Murtadha M et al. Methylmercury poisoning in Iraq. *Science* 1973;181:230-241.

64. Aschner M, Aschner J.L. Mercury Neurotoxicity: mechanisms of blood-brain barrier transport. *Neurosci Behav Rev* 1990;14:169-176.

65. Charleston J.S., Body R.L., Bolender R.P., Mottet N.K., Vahter M.E., Burbacher T.M. Changes in the number of astrocytes and microglia in the thalamus of the monkey Macaca fascicularis following long-term subclinical methlymercury exposure. *Neurotoxicol* 1996;17:127-38.

66. Huszti Z, Madarasz E, Schlett K, Joo F, Szabo A, Deli M. Mercury-stimulated histamine uptake and binding in cultured astroglial and cerebral endothelial cells. *J Neurosci Res* 1997;48:71-81.

67. Kramer K.K., Zoelle J.T., Klaassen C.D. Induction of metallothionein mRNA and protein in primary murine neuron cultures. *Toxicol Appl Pharmacol* 1996;141:1-7.

68. Miura K, Koide N, Himeno S, Nakagawa I, Imura N. The involvement of microtubular disruption in methylmercury-induced apoptosis in neuronal and nonneuronal cell lines. *Toxicol Appl Pharmacol* 1999;160:279-88.

69. Trombetta L.K., Kromidas L. A scanning electron-microscopic study of the effects of methylmercury on the neuronal cytoskeleton. *Toxicol Lett* 1992;60:329-41.

70. Roos J, Kelly R.B. Preassembly and transport of nerve terminals: a new concept of axonal transport. *Nat Neurosci* 2000;3:415-417.

71. Sanchez C, Diaz-Nido J, Avila J. Phosphorylation of microtubule-associated protein 2 (MAP2) and its relevance for the regulation of the neuronal cytoskeleton function. *Prog Neurobiol* 2000;61:133-68.

72. van den Pol A.N., Spencer D.D. Differential neurite outgrowth on astrocyte substrates: interspecies facilitation in green fluorescent protein-transfected rat and human neurons. *Neurosci* 2000;95:603-16.

73. Aschner M, Mullaney KJ, Wagoner D, Lash L.H., Kimelberg H.K. Intracellular glutathione (GSH) levels modulate mercuric chloride (MC)- and methylmercuric chloride (MgHgCl)-induced amino acid release from neonatal rat primary astrocyte cultures. *Brain Res* 1994;664:133-40.

74. Sarafian T.A., Bredesen D.E., Verity M.A. Cellular resistance to methylmercury. *Neurotoxicol* 1996;17:27-36.

75. Cheek D.B. Acrodynia. In: Brennemann's Practice of Pediatrics, Chapter 17D, as reprinted on Pink Disease website, http://www.users.bigpond.com/difarnsworth/pcheek42.htm

76. Warkany J, Hubbard D.H. Acrodynia and mercury. *J Ped* 1953;42:365-386.

77. Aukrust P, Svardal A.M., Muller F, Lunden B, Berge R.K., Froland S.S. Decreased levels of total and reduced glutathione in CD4+ lymphocytes in common variable immunodeficiency are associated with activation of the tumor necrosis factor system: possible immunopathogenic role of oxidative stress. *Blood* 1995;86:1383-1391.

78. Horvath K, Papadimitriou J.C., Rabsztyn A, Drachenberg C et al. Gastrointestinal abnormalities in children with autistic disorder. *J Ped* 1999;135:559-563.

79. Klaassen C.D., editor. Casaret & Doull's Toxicology: the Basic Science of Poisons. 5th ed; McGraw-Hill, 1996.

80. Edelson S.B., Cantor D.S. Autism: xenobiotic influences. *Toxicol Ind Health* 1998;14:553-563.

81. Comi A.M., Zimmerman A.W., Frye V.H., Law P.A. et al. Familial clustering of autoimmune disorders and evaluation of medical risk factors in autism. *J Child Neurol* 1999;14:388-394.

82. Johansson U, Hansson-Georgiadis H, Hultman P. The genotype determines the B cell response in mercury-treated mice. *Int Arch Allergy Immunol* 1998;116:295-305.

83. Hultman P, Nielsen J.B. The effect of toxicokinetics on murine mercury-induced autoimmunity. *Environ Res* 1998;77:141-148.

84. Bagenstose L.M., Salgame P, Monestier M. Murine mercury-induced autoimmunity: a model of chemically related autoimmunity in humans. *Immunol Res* 1999;20:67-78.

85. Clarkson, T.W. The toxicology of mercury. *Crit Rev Clin Lab Sci* 1997;34:369-403.

86. Bailey A, Phillips W, Rutter M. Autism: Towards an integration of clinical, genetic, neuropsychological, and neurobiological perspectives. *J Child Psychol Psychiatry* 1996;37:89-126.

87. Luka R.E., Oppenheimer J.J., Miller N, Rossi J, Bielory L. Delayed hypersensitivity to thimerosal in RhO(D) immunoglobulin. *J Allergy Clin Immunol* 1997;100:138-9.

88. Halsey N.A. Limiting infant exposure to thimerosal in vaccines and other sources of mercury. *JAMA* 1999;282:1763-6.

89. Fagan D.G., Pritchard J.S., Clarkson T.W., Greenwood M.R. Organ mercury levels in infants with omphaloceles treated with organic mercurial antiseptic. *Arch Dis Child* 1977;52:962-964.

90. Matheson D.S., Clarkson T.W., Gelfand E.W. Mercury toxicity (acrodynia) induced by long-term injection of gammaglobulin. *J Ped* 980;97:153-155.

91. Gosselin R.E., Smith R.P., Hodge H.C. Clinical toxicology of commercial products, section III, Therapeutic index (ed 5). Baltimore, Williams & Wilkins, 1984: pp262-271.

92. Gilbert S.G., Grant-Webster K.S. Neurobehavioral effects of developmental methymercury exposure. *Environ Health Perspect* 1995;103;s6:135-42.

93. Hattis D, Banati P, Goble R. Distributions of individual susceptibility among humans for toxic effects. How much protection does the traditional tenfold factor provide for what fraction of which kinds of chemicals and effects? *Ann N Y Acad Sci* 1999;895:286-316.

94. Hattis D. The challenge of mechanism-based modeling in risk assessment for neurobehavioral end points. *Environ Health Perspect* 1996;104:s2:381-90.

95. Hattis D, Glowa J, Tilson H, Ulbrich B. Risk assessment for neurobehavioral toxicity: SGOMSEC joint report. *Environ Health Perspect* 1996;104:s2:217-26.

96. Gillberg C, Coleman M. The Biology of the Autistic Syndromes; 2nd ed, Mac Keith Press, 1992.

97. Rossi A.D., Ahlbom E, Ogren SO, Nicotera P, Ceccatelli S. Prenatal exposure to methylmercury alters locomotor activity of male but not female rats. *Exp Brain Res* 1997;117:428-436.

98. Sager P.R., Aschner M, Rodier P.M. Persistent differential alteration in developing cerebellar cortex of male and female mice after methylmercury exposure. *Brain Res Dev Brain Res* 1984;12:1-11.

99. McKeown-Eyssen G.E., Ruedy J, Neims A. Methyl mercury exposure in northern Quebec: II. Neurologic findings in children. *Am J Epidemiol* 1983;118:470-479.

100. CDC press release. Record Immunization Rate, 80% of Kids Getting Vaccinated. Associated Press, September 23, 1999.

101. Bristol M, Cohen D, Costello E, Denckla M et al. State of the science in autism: report to the National Institutes of Health. *J Aut Dev Disorders* 1996;26:121-157.

102. Florentine M.J., Sanfilippo DJ 2d. Elemental mercury poisoning. Clin Pharm 1991;10:213-21.

103. Szczech J. Phosphatase and esterase activity in the amygdaloid body of rats after ethylmercury p-toluenesulfonyl poisoning. (Polish) *Neuropathol Pol* 1980;18:71-81.

104. Kelleher K.K., McInerny T.K., Gardner W.P., Childs G.E., Wasserman R.C. Increasing identification of psychosocial problems: 1979-1996. *Pediatrics* 2000;105:1313-1321.

105. Capps L, Kehres J, Sigman M. Conversational abilities among children with autism and children with developmental delays. *Autism* 1998;2:325-44.
106. Tonge B.J., Brereton A.V., Gray K.M., Einfeld S.L. Behavioural and emotional disturbance in high-functioning autism and Asperger's syndrome. *Autism* 1999;3:117-130.
107. Klin A, Sparrow S.S., de Bildt A, Cicchetti D.V., Cohen D.J., Volkmar F.R. A normed study of face recognition in autism and related disorders. *J Aut Dev Disorders* 1999;29:499-508.
108. Rapin I, Katzman R. Neurobiology of autism. *Ann Neurol* 1998;43:7-14 1998.
109. Fagala G.E.,Wigg C.L. Psychiatric manifestions of mercury poisoning. *J Am Acad Child Adolesc Psychiatry* 1992;31:306-311.
110. Bailey A, Luthert P, Dean A, Harding B et al. A clinicopathological study of autism. *Brain* 1998;121:889-905.
111. Dawson G. Brief report: neuropsychology of autism: a report on the state of the science. *J Aut Dev Disorders* 1996;26:179-184.
112. Adrien J.L., Martineau J, Barthelemy C, Bruneau N, Garreau B, Sauvage D. Disorders of regulation of cognitive activity in autistic children. *J Aut Dev Disord* 1995;25:249-63.
113. Howlin P, Asgharian A. The diagnosis of autism and Asperger syndrome: findings from a survey of 770 families. *Dev Med Child Neurol* 1999;41:834-9.
114. Turner M. Annotation: repetitive behaviour in autism: a review of psychological research. *J Child Psychol Psychiatry* 1999;40:839-49.
115. Elsner J. Testing strategies in behavioral teratology. III. Microanalysis of behavior. *Neurobehav Toxicol Teratol* 1986;8:573-84.
116. Cuomo V. Evidence that exposure to methyl mercury during gestation induces behavioral and neurochemical changes in offspring of rats. *Neurotoxicol Teratol* 1990;12:23-28.
117. White R.F., Feldman R.G., Moss M.B., Proctor S.P. Magnetic resonance imaging (MRI), neurobehavioral testing, and toxic encephalopathy: two cases. *Environ Res* 1993;61:117-23.
118. Muris P, Steerneman P, Merckelbach H, Holdrinet I, Meesters C. Comorbid anxiety symptoms in children with pervasive developmental disorders. *J Anxiety Disord*1998;12:387-393.
119. Haut M.W., Morrow L.A., Pool D, Callahan T.S., Haut J.S., Franzen MD Neurobehavioral effects of acute exposure to inorganic mercury vapor. *Appl Neuropsychol* 1999;6:193-200.
120. Uzzell B.P., Oler J. Chronic low-level mercury exposure and neuropsychological functioning. *J Clin Exp Neuropsychol* 1986;8:581-93.
121. Clarke D, Baxter M, Perry D, Prasher V. The diagnosis of affective and psychotic disorders in adults with autism: seven case reports. *Autism* 1999;3:149-164.
122. DeLong G.R. Autism: new data suggest a new hypothesis. *Neurology* 1999;52:911-916.
123. Piven J, Palmer P. Psychiatric disorder and the broad autism phenotype: evidence from a family study of multiple-incidence autism families. *Am J Psychiatry* 1999;156:557-563.
124. Hua M.S., Huang C.C., Yang Y.J. Chronic elemental mercury intoxication: neuropsychological follow up case study. *Brain Inj* 1996;10:377-84.

125. Howlin P. Outcome in adult life for more able individuals with autism or Asperger syndrome *Autism* 2000;4:63-84.

126. Rosenhall U, Johansson E, Gillberg C. Oculomotor findings in autistic children. *J Laryngol Otol* 1988;102:435-439.

127. Vostanis P, Smith B, Corbett J, Sungum-Paliwal R et al. Parental concerns of early development in children with autism and related disorders. *Autism* 1998;2:229-242.

128. Joselow M.M., Louria D.B., Browder A.A. Mercurialism: environmental and occupational aspects. *Ann Int Med* 1972;76:119-130.

129. Williams D. Autism - An Inside-Out Approach. 1996, Jessica Kingsley Publishers Ltd, London.

130. Baranek G. Autism during infancy: a retrospective video analysis of sensory-motor and social behaviors at 9-12 months of age. *J Aut Dev Disorders* 1999;29:213-224.

131. Tokuomi H, Uchino M, Imamura S, Yamanaga H, Nakanishi R, Ideta T. Minamata disease (organic mercury poisoning): neuroradiologic and electrophysiologic studies. *Neurology* 1982;32:1369-1375.

132. Grandin T. Brief report: response to National Institutes of health report. *J Aut Dev Disord* 1996;26:185-187.

133. Ornitz E.M. Neurophysiologic studies of infantile autism. p148-65 in: Handbook of Autism and Pervasive Developmental Disorders. John Wiley & Sons, Inc., 1987.

134. Dales L.D. The neurotoxicity of alkyl mercury compounds. *Am J Med* 1972;53:219-232.

135. Anuradha B, Rajeswari M, Varalakshmi P. Degree of peroxidative status in neuronal tissues by different routes of inorganic mercury administration. *Drug Chem Toxicol* 1998;21:47-55.

136. Abell F, Krams M, Ashburner J, Passingham R et al. The neuroanatomy of autism: a voxel-based whole brain analysis of structural scans. *NeuroReport* 1999;10:1647-1651.

137. Hoon A.H., Riess A.L. The mesial-temporal lobe and autism: case report and review. *Dev Med Child Neurol* 1992;34:252-265.

138. Otsuka H, Harada M, Mori K, Hisaoka S, Nishitani H. Brain metabolites in the hippocampus-amygdala region and cerebellum in autism: an 1H-MR spectroscopy study. *Neuroradiol* 1999;41:517-9.

139. Kates W.R., Mostofsky S.H., Zimmerman A.W., Mazzocco M.M. et al. Neuroanatomical and neurocognitive differences in a pair of monozygous twins discordant for strictly defined autism. *Ann Neurol* 1998;43:782-791.

140. Larkfors L, Oskarsson A, Sundberg J, Ebendal T. Methylmercury induced alterations in the nerve growth factor level in the developing brain. *Brain Res Dev Brain Res* 1991;62:287-91.

141. Chugani D.C., Muzik O, Behen M, Rothermel R et al. Developmental changes in brain serotonin synthesis capacity in autistic and nonautistic children. *Ann Neurol* 1999;45:287-95.

142. Leboyer M, Philippe A, Bouvard M, Guilloud-Bataille M. Whole blood serotonin and plasma beta-endorphin in autistic probands and their first-degree relatives. *Biol Psychiatry* 1999;45:158-63.

143. Cook E.H. Autism: review of neurochemical investigation. *Synapse* 1990;6:292-308.

144. McDougle C.J., Holmes J.P., Bronson M.R., Anderson G.M. et al. Risperidone treatment of children and adolescents with pervasive developmental disorders: a prospective open-label study. *J Am Acad Child Adolesc Psychiatry* 1997;36:685-693.

145. Ernst M, Zametkin A.J., Matochik J.A., Pascualvaca D, Cohen R.M. Low medial prefrontal dopaminergic activity in autistic children. *Lancet* 1997;350:638.

146. Gillberg C, Svennerholm L. CSF monoamines in autistic syndromes and other pervasive developmental disorders of early childhood. *Br J Psychiatry* 1987;151:89-94.

147. Rimland B, Baker S.M. Brief report: alternative approaches to the development of effective treatments for autism. *J Aut Dev Disord* 1996;26:237-241.

148. Perry E, Lee M, Court J, Perry R. Cholinergic activities in autism: nicotinic and muscarinic receptor abnormalities in the cerebral cortex. Presentation to Cure Autism Now Foundation, 2000.

149. O'Kusky J.R., Boyes B.E., McGeer E.G. Methylmercury-induced movement and postural disorders in developing rat: regional analysis of brain catecholamines and indoleamines. *Brain Res* 1988;439:138-146.

150. Thrower E.C., Duclohier H, Lea E.J., Molle G, Dawson A.P. The inositol 1,4,5-trisphosphate-gated Ca2+ channel: effect of the protein thiol reagent thimerosal in channel activity. *Biochem J* 1996;318:61-66.

151. Sayers L.G., Brown G.R., Michell R.H., Michelangeli F. The effects of thimerosal on calcium uptake and inositol 1,4,5-triosphate-induced calcium release in cerebellar microsomes. *Biochem J* 1993;289:883-887.

152. Atchison W.D., Joshi U, Thornburg J.E. Irreversible suppression of calcium entry into nerve terminals by methylmercury. *J Pharmacol Exp Ther* 1986;238:618-624.

153. Bartolome J, Whitmore W.L., Seidler F.J., Slotkin T.A. Exposure to methylmercury in utero: effects on biochemical development of catecholamine neurotransmitter systems. *Life Sci* 1984;35:657-670.

154. McKay S.J., Reynolds J.N., Racz W.J. Effects of mercury compounds on the spontaneous and potassium-evoked release of [3H]dopamine from mouse striatal slices. *Can J Physiol Pharmacol* 1986;64:1507-1514.

155. Hrdina P.D., Peters D.A., Singhal R.L. Effects of chronic exposure to cadmium, lead and mercury of brain biogenic amines in the rat. *Res Comm Chem Pathol Pharmacol* 1976;5:483-493.

156. Kung M.P., Kostyniak P.J., Olson J.R., Sansone F.M. et al. Cell specific enzyme markers as indicators of neurotoxicity: effects of acute exposure to methylmercury. *Neurotoxicol* 1989;###:41-52

157. Carlsson M.L. Hypothesis: is infantile autism a hypoglutamatergic disorder? Relevance of glutamate-serotonin interactions for pharmacotherapy. *J Neural Trans* 1998;###:525-535.

158. Moreno-Fuenmayor H, Borjas L, Arrieta A, Valera V, Socorro-Candanoza L. Plasma excitatory amino acids in autism. (Spanish) *Invest Clin* 1996;7:113-128.

159. Volterra A, Trotti D, Cassutti P, Tromba C et al. High sensitivity of glutamate uptake to extracellular free arachidonic acid levels in rat cortical synaptosomes and astrocytes. *J Neurochem* 1992;9:600-6.

160. Aschner M, Yao C.P., Allen J.W., Tan K.H. Methylmercury alters glutamate transport in astrocytes. *Neurochem Int* 2000;37:199-206.

161. O'Reilly B.A., Waring R. Enzyme and sulfur oxidation deficiencies in autistic children with known food/chemical intolerances. *J Orthomol Med* 1993;4:198-200.

162. Alberti A, Pirrone P, Elia M, Waring RH, Romano C. Sulphation deficit in "low-functioning " autistic children: a pilot study. *Biol Psychiatry* 1999;46:420-424.

163. Markovich D, Knight D. Renal Na-Si Cotransporter NaSi-1 is inhibited by heavy metals. *Am J Renal Physiol* 1998;274:283-289.

164. Golse B, Debray-Ritzen P, Durosay P, Puget K, Michelson A.M. Alterations in two enzymes: superoxide dismutase and glutathione peroxidase in developmental infantile psychosis. *Revue Neurologic* (Paris) 1978;134:699-705.

165. Fuchs J, Packer L, Zimmer G. Lipoic Acid in Health and Disease. Marcel Dekker, Inc., 1997.

166. Page T, Coleman M. Purine metabolism abnormalities in a hyperuricosuric subclass of autism. *Biochim Biophys Acta* 2000;1500:291-296

167. Lombard J. Autism: a mitochondrial disorder? *Med Hypoth* 1998;50:497-500.

168. Atchison W.D., Hare M.F. Mechanisms of methylmercury-induced neurotoxicity. *FASEB J* 1994;8:622-629.

169. Rajanna B, Hobson M. Influence of mercury on uptake of [3H]dopamine and [3H]norepinephrine by rat brain synaptosomes. *Toxicol Let* 1985;27:7-14.

170. Whiteley P, Rogers J, Shattock P. Clinical features associated with autism: observations of symptoms outside the diagnostic boundaries of autistic spectrum disorders. *Autism* 1998;2:415-422.

171. Gupta S, Aggarwal S, Rashanravan B, Lee T. Th1- and Th2-like cytokines in CD4+ and CD8+ T cells in autism. *J Neuroimmunol* 1998;85:106-109.

172. Plioplys A.V., Greaves A., Kazemi K., Silverman E. Lymphocyte function in autism and Rett Syndrome. *Neuropsychobiol* 1994;29:12-6.

173. Warren R.P., Margaretten N.C., Foster A. Reduced natural killer cell activity in autism. *J Am Acad Child Adolesc Psychiatry* 1987;26:333-335.

174. Nielsen J.B., Hultman P. Experimental Studies on genetically determined susceptibility to mercury-induced autoimmune response. *Ren Fail* 1999;21:343-348.

175. Peterson J.D., Herzenberg L.A., Vasquez K, Waltenbaugh C. Glutathione levels in antigen-presenting cells modulate Th1 versus Th2 response patterns. *Proc Nat Acad Sci USA* 1998;95:3071-6.

176. Hu H, Moller G, Abedi-Valugerdi M. Mechanism of mercury-induced autoimmunity: both T helper 1- and T helper 2-type responses are involved. *Immunol* 1999;96:348-357.

177. Ilback N.G. Effects of methyl mercury exposure on spleen and blood natural-killer (NK) cell-activity in the mouse. *Toxicol* 1991;67:117-124.

178. Kugler B. The differentiation between autism and Asperger syndrome. *Autism* 1998;2:11-32.

179. Filipek P, Accardo P, Baranek G, Cook E et al. The screening and diagnosis of autistic spectrum disorders. *J Aut Dev Disord* 1999;29:439-484.

180. Myers G.J., Davidson P.W. Prenatal methylmercury exposure and children: neurologic, developmental, and behavior research. *Environ Health Perspect* 1998;106;s3:841-847.

181. Richdale A.L. Sleep problems in autism: prevalence, cause, and intervention. *Dev Med Child Neurol* 1999;41:60-6.

182. Gedye A. Anatomy of self-injurious, stereotypic, and aggressive movements: evidence for involuntary explanation. *J Clin Psychol* 1992;48:766-778.

183. O'Neill M, Jones R.S. Sensory-perceptual abnormalities in autism: a case for more research? *J Aut Dev Disord* 1997;27:283-293.

184. O'Neill J.L. Through the Eyes of Aliens. Jessica Kingsley Publishers Ltd., 1999.

185. Pfab R, Muckter H, Roider G, Zilker T. Clinical course of severe poisoning with thiomersal. *Clin Toxicol* 1996;34:453-460.

186. Florentine M.J., Sanfilippo II D.J. Grand Rounds: elemental mercury poisoning. *Clin Pharm* 1991;10:213-221.

187. D'Eufemia P, Celli M, Finocchiaro R, Pacifico L. Abnormal intestinal permeability in children with autism. *Acta Paediatr* 1996:85:1076-1079.

188. Shattock P, Savery D, Autism as a Metabolic Disorder, Autism Research Unit, University of Sunderland, Sunderland, UK, 1997.

189. Kugler B. The differentiation between autism and Asperger syndrome. *Autism* 1998;2:11-32

190. Teitelbaum P, Teitelbaum O, Nye J, Fryman J et al. Movement analysis in infancy may be useful for early diagnosis of autism. *Proc Nat Acad Sci USA* 1998; 95:13982-13987.

INTRA-BODY TOXINS

Toxins in the Human Body:
Nutrient-Depletion Increases Susceptibility

Teresa Binstock
Autism Researcher

Although the word "toxin" originally referred to an organic molecule produced by organisms, contemporary use in peer-reviewed journals such as Toxicology, Neurotoxicology and Environmental Health Perspectives establishes that "toxin" can refer to molecules such as PCBs, arsenic, phthalates, etc.

In recent years, studies have documented large numbers of toxins within the human body[1-19]. Some of these toxins are linked with pathologies in humans, including effects upon cognition and behavior (eg,[20-21]). Other studies document a spectrum of inter-human variance in the ability to detoxify human-made toxins, with an adult range of 64 to 164 times for at least one organophosphate pesticide, with newborns generally more likely to be affected[22]. When considered together, findings about intra-body toxins and interpersonal variations in susceptibility have relevance to etiologies and treatments of autism.

A recent finding associates autism with an organophosphate insecticide, with autism more likely if a weak allele of the paraoxonase

1 (PON1) gene is present[23]. A subsequent study documented high levels of homocysteine and low PON1 arylesterase in 12 children with autism[24]. Additional research is needed because geographic differences are important[23]; because ethnicity is linked with rates of weak alleles[25], and because PON1 gene expression is associated with different levels of enzymatic activity in pregnant women and neonates[26]. Furthermore, lead and other toxic metals reduce expression of the PON1 gene[27-29].

Since peer-reviewed evidence now documents an etiologic relationship among autism, a specific gene's weak alleles, and a common class of pesticides, the fact that numerous toxins are present in the human body merits concern of physicians, researchers, and people with a child or grandchild on the autism spectrum. But autism is not unique in regard to toxic molecules. Additional findings link various"low dose" intra-body toxins with non-autism pathologies in humans, including cancer, asthma, and allergies[30-36].

Phthalates are small molecules used in many products and have become ubiquitous in modern society. They are found in the human body and can affect reproductive tissues and gender behaviors[20-21, 37] as well as cognitive processes[38-41]. Similar sequelae of PCB exposure are documented[42-47], and the effects of flame retardants (PBDEs) are beginning to be studied (eg,[48-49]).

For the forseeable future, escape from toxic molecules is impossible. They are found in the placenta, amniotic fluid, cord blood, and breast milk of humans[51-54], and adverse effects are more likely in children who had higher toxin levels as infants[55]. Furthermore, there is an inverse relationship between immunity and levels of intra-body toxins[38], thus enabling toxins to augment effects of weak alleles for genes whose protein products are involved in detoxification and immunity (eg,[57-59]). Despite these findings, industry continues to fund disparagements of the idea that toxins cause damage to humans and other species (see Figure 1).

Increased oxidative stress has become a common finding in autism[60-62] and may provide an indirect measure of intra-body toxins & damaged tissue:

> "*Environmental stimuli such as hypoxia, toxins, or heavy metals,
> increase production of reactive oxygen species and lower energy*

reserves. Chronic exposure to oxidative radicals can adversely affect gene expression and proteolysis."[63]

Studying one toxin at a time can be misleading, because effects of multiple toxins may be additive, cumulative, or synergistic. Furthermore, toxin-induced pathologies may be exacerbated by infections and—via impaired nutritional status—by gastrointestinal difficulties[64-68]. In 1997 Claudia S. Miller published "Toxicant-induced Loss of Tolerance"[69]. Her hypothesis is relevant to various epidemics. Although more studies about additive and synergistic effects are needed, there is another mechanism whereby multiple intra-body toxins increase the likelihood of adverse sequelae. A hypothesis is here offered. It may already have been published in scientific literature. If so, please let us know by providing the citation.

Hypothesis: The large number of toxins in the fetus, infant, or toddler deplete glutathione and other detoxification nutrients, thereby increasing the likelihood of adverse effects from one or more of the toxicants, even if each toxin's level is supposedly "safe". The likelihood of adverse effects is increased by concurrent illnesses, by encounters with bolus doses, and by various genetic and/or acquired reasons whereby an individual has suboptimal, intra-body nutritional status and thus has impaired detoxification. There is an inverse correlation between the number of intra-body toxins and the level of nutrients needed for detoxification.

In other words, the higher the number of intra-body toxins, the likelier that nutrients necessary for detoxification will become depleted. If and as this occurs in a pregnant woman, embryo, fetus, infant or toddler, developing one or more toxin-related pathologies may ensure lifelong challenges.

Inter-child variance among autistic children has long been a challenge. As toxin-related environmental factors are researched, the interplay of etiologic factors needs be kept in mind. For instance, whether or not an infant or toddler is sick at the time of exposure may affect the intra-body distribution of toxins (eg,[64, 66, 68]).

Reducing the toxic load in autistic children is important. A first example came from chelation of toxic metals (eg,[70-74]). An increased body burden of toxic metals will decrease activity of PON1, thereby increasing risk from organophosphate insecticides[22-23, 27-29]. Moreover, various toxins are detoxified by processes which utilize certain nutrients (eg, glutathione;[75-81]). The fact that most lab tests do not measure non-metal toxins in feces or urine does not demonstrate such toxins aren't being excreted. Instead, we ought consider the possibility that children who improve in response to detoxification procedures are reducing their load of intra-body metal and/or non-metal toxins.

Lastly, the liver is a major participant in detoxification[82-83]. Having an adequate hepatic supply of Phase 1 and Phase 2 nutrients is crucial. Supoptimal intra-body nutritional status is a risk factor for adverse effects from toxins including but not limited to heavy metals [84-85]. Minimizing a child's and the family's contact with toxins is recommended (eg,[86]). The sequence Heal the gut, Optimize nutritional status, and Detoxify remains important for many and perhaps most autistic children.

FIGURE 1

Spinning Science to Manufacture Uncertainty

These sources delineate how scientific findings of adverse effects are misconstrued to create doubt about scientific findings of adverse effects described in peer-reviewed articles.

Toxic Sludge Is Good for You:
Lies, Damn Lies and the Public Relations Industry.
Sheldon Rampton, John Stauber; Common Courage Press, 1995

Science Under Siege:
The Politicians' War on Nature and Truth.
Todd Wilkinson; Johnson Books, 1998.

Global Spin: The Corporate Assault on Environmentalism.
Sharon Beder; Chelsea Green Publishing Company, 1998.
Wargo, John. 1998.

Our Children's Toxic Legacy:
How Science and Law Fail to Protect Us from Pesticides.
Yale University Press.

Trust Us We're Experts:
How Industry Manipulates Science
and Gambles with Your Future.
Sheldon Rampton, John Stauber; J P Tarcher,
Los Angeles, California, USA; 2000.

What the Chemical Industry Fears.
Rachel's Environment and Health News. 30 October 2003.
http://www.rachel.org/bulletin/index.cfm?issue_ID=2392

Bisphenol A
Analysis of the politics of commercial "science":
An OurStolenFuture analysis of:
vom Saal, F and W Welshons. 2006.
Large effects from small exposures.
II. The importance of positive controls in low-dose research
on bisphenol A. Environmental Research 100: 50-76.
http://www.ourstolenfuture.org/NewScience/oncompounds/
bisphenola/2006/2006-0101vomsaalandwelshons/
2006-0101vomsaalandwelshons.html

References

[1] Toxic chemicals and children's health in North America. North American Commission for Environmental Cooperation. 26 May 2006. http://www.cec.org/news/details/index.cfm?varlan=english&ID=2704

[2] Pollution In People. Toxic-Free Legacy Coalition. 24 May 2006. http://pollutionin-people.org/results

[3] Across Generations: Mothers and Daughters. Environmental Working Group. 10 May 2006. http://www.ewg.org/reports/generations/execsumm.php

[4] An Investigation of Factors Related to Levels of Mercury in Human Hair. Greenpeace International. 9 February 2006.http://www.greenpeace.org/usa/press/reports/mercury-report

5 Children's health and the environment in North America. North American Commission for Environmental Cooperation. 4 February 2006. http://wec.org/pubs_docs/documents/index.cfm?varlan=english&ID=1917

6 Toxic Nation. Pollution, It's in You! Environmental Defence Canada. 19 January 2006.http://www.environmentaldefence.ca/toxicnation/home.php

7 Teflon chemicals in food packaging. Ohio Citizen Action. 18 January 2006. http://www.ohiocitizen.org/campaigns/dupont_c8/consumer.htm

8 LDDI analysis – CDC biomonitoring. The Learning and Developmental Disabilities Initiative. 11 November 2005.http://www.iceh.org/LDDISummaryCDC.html

9 Generations X. World Wildlife Fund - UK. 6 October 2005.http://www.panda.org/campaign/detox/news_publications/news.cfm?uNewsID=23635

10 A present for life: Hazardous chemicals in cord blood. Greenpeace International, World Wildlife Fund - UK. 8 September 2005. http://www.wwfuk.org/news/n_0000001830.asp

11 The Pollution in Newborns. Environmental Working Group. 14 July 2005. http://www.ewg.org/reports/bodyburden2/newsrelease.php

12 Contaminated: the next generation. World Wildlife Fund - UK. 10 October 2004. http://www.wwf-uk.org/news/n_0000001830.asp

13 Chemical Trespass. Pesticide Action Network. 11 May 2004.http://www.panna.org/campaigns/docsTrespass/chemicalTrespass2004.dv.html

14 Chemical Check Up. World Wildlife Fund - UK. 21 April 2004. http://www.panda.org/campaign/detox/news_publications/news.cfm?uNewsID=12622

15 Body Of Evidence: New Science In The Debate Over Toxic Flame Retardants And Our Health. US Public Interest Research Group. 15 February 2004. http://uspirg.org/uspirg.asp?id2=12225

16 ContamiNATION, the results of the WWF's Biomonitoring survey. World Wildlife Fund - UK. 24 November 2003.http://www.wwf.org.uk/News/n_0000001055.asp

17 Confronting Toxic Contamination in Our Communities: Women's Health and California's Future. Women's Foundation of California. 10 October 2003. http://www.womensfoundca.org/fullreport10_7.pdf

18 Environmental Exposures and Racial Disparities. Environmental Justice and Health Union. 1 August 2003. http://www.ejhu.org/disparities.html

19 Body burden: the pollution in people. Environmental Working Group. 31 January 2003. http://www.ewg.org/reports/bodyburden/es.php

20 Vreugdenhil HJ et al.Effects of perinatal exposure to PCBs and dioxins on play behavior in Dutch children at school age. Environ Health Perspect. 2002 110(10):A593-8.

21 Weiss B. Sexually dimorphic nonreproductive behaviors as indicators of endocrine disruption. Environ Health Perspect. 2002 110 Suppl 3:387-91.

22 Furlong CE et al.PON1 status of farmworker mothers and children as a predictor of organophosphate sensitivity.Pharmacogenet Genomics. 2006 16(3):183-90.

23 D'Amelio M et al.Paraoxonase gene variants are associated with autism in North America, but not in Italy: possible regional specificity in gene-environment interactions. Mol Psychiatry. 2005 10(11):1006-16.

[24] Pasca SP et al. High levels of homocysteine and low serum paraoxonase 1 arylesterase activity in children with autism. Life Sci. 2006 78(19):2244-8.

[25] Chen J et al. Haplotype-phenotype relationships of paraoxonase-1. Cancer Epidemiol Biomarkers Prev. 2005 14(3):731-4.

[26] Chen J et al. Increased influence of genetic variation on PON1 activity in neonates. Environ Health Perspect. 2003 111(11):1403-9.

[27] Cole TB et al. 2002. Inhibition of paraoxonase (PON1) by heavy metals [Abstract]. Toxicol Sci 66(1-S):312.

[28] Debord J et al. 2003 Inhibition of human serum arylesterase by metal chlorides. J Inorg Biochem 94(1–2):1–4.

[29] Wan-Fen Li et al. 2006. Lead Exposure Is Associated with Decreased Serum Paraoxonase 1 (PON1) Activity and Genotypes. Environ Health Perspect 114:1233–1236. http://www.ehponline.org/members/2006/9163/9163.html

[30] Birnbaum LS, Fenton SE. Cancer and developmental exposure to endocrine disruptors. Environ Health Perspect. 2003 111(4):389-94.

[31] McDuffie HH. Host factors and genetic susceptibility: a paradigm of the conundrum of pesticide exposure and cancer associations. Rev Environ Health. 2005 20(2):77-101.

[32] Vineis P, Husgafvel-Pursiainen K.Air pollution and cancer: biomarker studies in human populations. Carcinogenesis. 2005 26(11):1846-55.

[33] Kortenkamp A.Breast cancer, oestrogens and environmental pollutants: a re-evaluation from a mixture perspective. Int J Androl. 2006 29(1):193-8.

[34] Reichrtova E et al.Cord serum immunoglobulin E related to the environmental contamination of human placentas with organochlorine compounds. Environ Health Perspect. 1999 107(11):895-9.

[35] Bornehag CG et al.The association between asthma and allergic symptoms in children and phthalates in house dust: a nested case-control study. Environ Health Perspect. 2004 112(14):1393-7.

[36] Sunyer J et al. Prenatal dichlorodiphenyldichloroethylene (DDE) and asthma in children. Environ Health Perspect. 2005 113(12):1787-90.

[37] Lottrup G et al. Possible impact of phthalates on infant reproductive health. International Journal of Andrology 2006: 29:172.

[38] Perera FP et al. A summary of recent findings on birth outcomes and developmental effects of prenatal ETS, PAH, and pesticide exposures. Neurotoxicology. 2005 26(4):573-87.

[39] Rohlman DS et al. Neurobehavioral performance in preschool children from agricultural and non-agricultural communities in Oregon and North Carolina. Neurotoxicology. 2005 26(4):589-98.

[40] Young JG et al. Association between in utero organophosphate pesticide exposure and abnormal reflexes in neonates. Neurotoxicology. 2005 26(2):199-209.

[41] Kofman O et al. Motor inhibition and learning impairments in school-aged children following exposure to organophosphate pesticides in infancy. Pediatr Res. 2006 60(1):88-92.

[42] Colborn T.Neurodevelopment and endocrine disruption. Environ Health Perspect. 2004 112(9):944-9. http://www.ehponline.org/members/2003/6601/6601.html

[43] Nguon K et al. Perinatal exposure to polychlorinated biphenyls differentially affects cerebellar development and motor functions in male and female rat neonates. Cerebellum. 2005;4(2):112-22.

[44] Saito K et al. Systematic analysis and overall toxicity evaluation of dioxins and hexachlorobenzene in human milk. Chemosphere. 2005 61(9):1215-20.

[45] Newman J et al. PCBs and cognitive functioning of Mohawk adolescents. Neurotoxicol Teratol. 2006 Jun 27; [Epub ahead of print]

[46] Carpenter DO. Polychlorinated biphenyls (PCBs): routes of exposure and effects on human health. Rev Environ Health. 2006 21(1):1-23.

[47] Sharlin DS et al. Polychlorinated biphenyls exert selective effects on cellular composition of white matter in a manner inconsistent with thyroid hormone insufficiency. Endocrinology. 2006 147(2):846-58.

[48] Fonnum F et al. Molecular mechanisms involved in the toxic effects of polychlorinated biphenyls(PCBs) and brominated flame retardants (BFRs). J Toxicol Environ Health A. 2006 8;69(1-2):21-35.

[49] Lilienthal H et al. Effects of developmental exposure to 2,2 ,4,4 ,5-pentabromodiphenyl ether (PBDE-99) on sex steroids, sexual development, and sexually dimorphic behavior in rats. Environ Health Perspect. 2006 114(2):194-201.

[50] Lackmann GM et al. Organochlorine compounds in breast-fed vs. bottle-fed infants: preliminary results at six weeks of age. Sci Total Environ. 2004 Aug 15;329(1-3):289-93.

[51] Foster W et al. Detection of endocrine disrupting chemicals in samples of second trimester human amniotic fluid. J Clin Endocrinol Metab. 2000 85(8):2954-7.

[52] Hamel A et al. Effects of low concentrations of organochlorine compounds in women on calcium transfer in human placental syncytiotrophoblast. Toxicol Sci. 2003 76(1):182-9.

[53] Suzuki G et al. Distribution of PCDDs/PCDFs and Co-PCBs in human maternal blood, cord blood, placenta, milk, and adipose tissue: dioxins showing high toxic equivalency factor accumulate in the placenta. Biosci Biotechnol Biochem. 2005 69(10):1836-47.

[54] Bradman A et al. Measurement of pesticides and other toxicants in amniotic fluid as a potential biomarker of prenatal exposure: a validation study. Environ Health Perspect. 2003 111(14):1779-82.

[55] Jacobson JL, Jacobson SW. Breast-feeding and gender as moderators of teratogenic effects on cognitive development. Neurotoxicol Teratol. 2002 24(3):349-58.

[56] de Swart RL et al. Impaired immunity in harbour seals (Phoca vitulina) exposed to bioaccumulated environmental contaminants: review of a long-term feeding study. Environ Health Perspect. 1996 104 Suppl 4:823-8.

[57] Torres AR et al. The association of MHC genes with autism. Front Biosci. 2001 6: D936-43.

[58] Latcham F et al. A consistent pattern of minor immunodeficiency and subtle enteropathy in children with multiple food allergy. J Pediatr. 2003 143(1):39-47.

[59] Warren RP et al. Increased frequency of the null allele at the complement C4b locus in autism. Clin Exp Immunol. 1991 83(3):438-40.

[60] James SJ et al. Metabolic biomarkers of increased oxidative stress and impaired methylation capacity in children with autism. Am J Clin Nutr. 2004 80(6):1611-7. http://www.ajcn.org/cgi/content/full/80/6/1611

[61] McGinnis WR. Oxidative stress in autism. Altern Ther Health Med. 2004 10(6):22-36.

[62] Chauhan A, Chauhan V.Oxidative stress in autism. Pathophysiology. 2006

[63] Potashkin JA, Meredith GE. The role of oxidative stress in the dysregulation of gene expression and protein metabolism in neurodegenerative disease. Antioxid Redox Signal. 2006 8(1-2):144-51.

[64] Scrimshaw NS.Historical concepts of interactions, synergism and antagonism between nutrition and infection. J Nutr. 2003 133(1):316S-321S. http://jn.nutrition.org/cgi/reprint/133/1/316S

[65] Madsen C. Prevalence of food additive intolerance. Hum Exp Toxicol. 1994 13(6):393-9.

[66] Nowak-Wegrzyn A et al.Food protein-induced enterocolitis syndrome caused by solid food proteins. Pediatrics. 2003 111(4 Pt 1):829-35. http://pediatrics.aappublications.org/cgi/reprint/111/4/829

[67] Lau K et al.Synergistic interactions between commonly used food additives in a developmental neurotoxicity test. Toxicol Sci. 2006 90(1):178-87.

[68] Darnerud PO et al.Common viral infection affects pentabrominated diphenyl ether (PBDE) distribution and metabolic and hormonal activities in mice. Toxicology. 2005 210(2-3):159-67.

[70] Miller CS. Toxicant-induced Loss of Tolerance--An Emerging Theory of Disease? Environ Health Perspect 105(Suppl 2):445-453 (1997) http://www.ehponline.org/members/1997/Suppl-2/miller-full.html

[71] Lonsdale D et al.Treatment of autism spectrum children with thiamine tetrahydrofurfuryl disulfide: a pilot study. Neuro Endocrinol Lett. 2002 Aug;23(4):303-8.

[72] Bradstreet J et al. A Case-Control Study of Mercury Burden in Children with Autistic Spectrum Disorders, J. Am. Phys. Surg 8(3) 2003 76-79.

[73] Autism Research Institute. Treatment Options for Mercury/Metal Toxicity in Autism and Related Developmental Disabilities: Consensus Position Paper. February 2005. http://www.autismwebsite.com/ARI/vaccine/heavymetals.pdf

[74] Bradstreet et al. Biological Evidence of Significant Vaccine Related Side-effects Resulting in Neurodevelopmental Disorders. http://www.aapsonline.org//iom/bradstreet-slides.pdf

[75] Hansen LG. Biotransformation of organophosphorus compounds relative to delayed neurotoxicity. Neurotoxicology. 1983 4(1):97-111.

[76] Hathway DE. Toxic action/toxicity. Biol Rev Camb Philos Soc. 2000 75(1):95-127.

[77] Slim R et al. Cellular glutathione status modulates polychlorinated biphenyl-induced stress response and apoptosis in vascular endothelial cells. Toxicol Appl Pharmacol. 2000 166(1):36-42.

[78] Ludewig G et al.Mechanisms of toxicity of PCB metabolites: generation of reactive oxygen species and glutathione depletion. Cent Eur J Public Health. 2000 8 Suppl:15-7.

[79] Abel EL et al.Biotransformation of methyl parathion by glutathione S-transferases. Toxicol Sci. 2004 79(2):224-32.

80   Shen D et al. Glutathione redox state regulates mitochondrial reactive oxygen production. J Biol Chem. 2005 280(27):25305-12.

81   Cho HJ et al.Enhanced expression of plasma glutathione peroxidase in the thymus of mice treated with TCDD [dioxin] and its implication for TCDD-induced thymic atrophy. Mol Cells. 2006 30;21(2):276-83.

82   Diehl-Jones WL, Askin DF. The neonatal liver, Part 1: embryology, anatomy, and physiology. Neonatal Netw. 2002 21(2):5-12.

83   Pineiro-Carrero VM, Pineiro EO.Liver. Pediatrics. 2004 113(4 Suppl):1097-106. http://pediatrics.aappublications.org/cgi/content/full/113/4/S1/1097

84   Liska DJ. The detoxification enzyme systems. Altern Med Rev. 1998 3(3):187-98.

85   Quig D. CysteineMetabolism and metal toxicity. Altern Med Rev. 1998 3(4):262-70.

86   Lu C et al.Organic diets significantly lower children's dietary exposure to organophosphorus pesticides. Environ Health Perspect. 2006 114(2):260-3.

MITOCHONDRIAL CONCERNS

Background and New Definition

Teresa Binstock, Researcher

Mitochondria are the powerhouses of our cells. They are responsible for generating energy as an adenosine triphosphate (ATP) and heat and are involved in the apoptosis-signaling pathway. (Pieczenik & Neustadt 2007) (1A)

MtD: Mitochondrial dysfunction
ASD: autism-spectrum disorder
ATP: adenosine triphosphate
ETC: Electron-chain transport
MRC: Mitochondrial respiratory chain
mtDNA: mitochondrial DNA
nDNA: nuclear DNA

Background: Autism and Mitochondria

In early 2008, Hannah Poling, a young autistic child, renewed interest in a possible link between vaccinations and autism. "On Nov. 9, 2007, HHS medical experts conceded through the Department of Justice that Hannah's autism was triggered by nine childhood vaccinations administered when she was 19 months of age." That such a lovely child was induced to regress into autism brought forth a potpourri of issues including but not limited to: multiple vaccinations per incident, the politics of vaccination science in America, and mitochondria.

In an op-ed column in the Atlanta Journal-Constitution, her father - who is a M.D., Ph.D. neurologist - set forth a major ramification: "To understand Hannah's case, it is important to understand mitochondria, which act like batteries in our cells to produce energy critical for normal function. Because the government's concession hinged on the presence of Hannah's underlying medical condition, mitochondrial dysfunction, some claim the decision is relevant to very few other children with autism. As a neurologist, scientist and father, I disagree." (1B) As we shall see, the meaning of "mitochondrial dysfunction" is changing, expanding to include a spectrum of signs and symptoms.

In recent years, various research groups have focused upon mitochondria in autism. For instance, in 2005, Oliveira at al reported that among 69 autistic children, 14 had hyperlactacidemia (2), and when 11 were tested further, 9 of 11 had an elevated lactate/pyruvate ratio. In 2006, Poling et al found aspartate aminotransferase significantly elevated in autistics versus controls (3); and Correia et al described a "high frequency of biochemical markers of mitochondrial dysfunction, namely hyperlactacidemia and increased lactate/pyruvate ratio, in a significant fraction of 210 autistic patients." (4) These studies explored rates of mitochondrial dysfunction in large groups of autistic children. In contrast and more recently, Weissman and colleagues focused upon "25 patients with ASD [autism and PDD/NOS] who had unequivocal evidence of a disorder of oxidative phosphorylation." (5) Although the study provides important insights, we need make clear that the group studied by Weissman et al was preselected and did not represent subjects with idiopathic autism. Nonetheless, Weissman group's observations are important. "Even a clear-cut deficiency of one or more ETC activities in vitro does not prove a genetic defect of oxidative phosphorylation because ETC deficiencies can be secondary to other conditions." (5) "For most individuals with defects of oxidative phosphorylation, the diagnosis is made through ETC determination but an underlying nuclear or mitochondrial mutation usually cannot be identified..." (5)

Hui et al summarize similarly: "It is... very difficult to establish normal reference ranges for MRC activities that can reliably distinguish patients with a primary MRC enzyme defect from those with a secondary defect due to other pathology..." (6)

Preliminary summary: A number of studies have presented mitochondria-related findings in autism. Here, we mention only some of those studies. Trends emerge: there is a range of signs and symptoms which suggest one degree or another of dysfunction in pathways related to mitochondria. As presented in the second part of this chapter, whether or not a mutation in mtDNA or nDNA has been identified, **various treatments are known to improve mitochondria function.**

A New Definition of Mitochondria Dysfunction

The classic definition of mitochondrial disease is being refined. Mitochondria dysfunction can occur even in the absence of an identified genetic mutation in mtDNA, even in the absence of a complete set of symptoms associated with classic mitochondria disease. In an important review available free online, Rossignol and Bradstreet summarize a number of autism studies that focused upon mitochondria (7). As other researchers wrote, "The broad clinical spectrum is one of the hallmarks of mitochondrial disease... Signs and symptoms that were not present early in the course of disease may appear as the disease progresses. The absence of a specific sign is not evidence of the absence of mitochondrial disease." (8) Furthermore, "Classical mitochondrial diseases occur in a subset of individuals with autism and are usually caused by genetic anomalies or mitochondrial respiratory pathway deficits. However, in many cases of autism, there is evidence of mitochondrial dysfunction (MtD) without the classic features associated with mitochondrial disease... In comparison to classical mitochondrial disease, MtD occurs more commonly in autism..., is not as severe in symptomatology, and is not associated with any discernable mitochondrial abnormality upon muscle biopsy. It is, however, associated with laboratory evidence of lowered mitochondrial functioning." (7)

The review by physicians Rossignol and Bradstreet calls attention to signs and symptoms associated with mitochondrial dysfunction *even in cases wherein not all markers of classic mitochondrial disease are present* in a specific child. As recently as 2004, a prominent researcher wrote, "A comprehensive classification system for mitochondrial diseases has not yet been developed." (9) Nonetheless, researchers continue to elaborate mitochondria's many functions in health and disease (e.g., 10).

Significant Issues

1. What percentage of autistic children, other ASD children, or pre-ASD children have signs and/or symptoms suggesting mitochondrial dysfunction?

2. If such signs and symptoms are present, are safe treatments described in peer-reviewed medical literature?

3. Should screening for signs of mitochondria dysfunction occur prior to infant and toddler vaccinations?

In this still developing field, terminology is important. Scientific papers generally categorize mitochondrial pathologies as disorders, diseases, and dysfunction. These categories are not necessarily distinct. Furthermore, some diseases not categorized as a "mitochondrial disease" are associated with signs or symptoms of mitochondrial dysfunction (6). Moreover, not all researchers use mitochondria-related terms identically. For instance, an emphasis upon "genetic" is traditional: Gabriele Siciliano and colleagues recently offered, "Mitochondrial diseases... with respiratory chain defects are caused by genetic mutations that determine an impairment of the electron transport chain functioning." (11) In stark contrast, Rossignol and Bradstreet emphasize that non-classical, milder forms of mitochondrial dysfunction (MtD) merit attention, thus we reiterate: **"Classical mitochondrial diseases occur in a subset of individuals with autism and are usually caused by genetic anomalies or mitochondrial respiratory pathway deficits. However, in many cases of autism, there is evidence of mitochondrial dysfunction (MtD) without the classic features associated with mitochondrial disease."** (7)

In other words, signs of MtD may be important even if a classically defined mito-disorder is not fully present.

Poling et al comment similarly, "It is unclear whether mitochondrial dysfunction results from a primary genetic abnormality, atypical development of essential metabolic pathways, or secondary inhibition of oxidative phosphorylation by other factors. If such dysfunction is present at the time of infections and immunizations in young children, the added oxidative stresses from immune activation on cellular energy metabolism are likely to be especially critical for the central nervous system, which is highly dependent on mitochondrial function." (3) Given the discordance in meanings of "mitochondrial dysfunction", autistic children, parents, and physicians confront a dilemma. Should diagnosis and treatment of mitochondria disease be based entirely upon signs and symptoms reinforced by the finding of a mutation in mtDNA or in mito-related nDNA? We think not. A wider definition of mitochondria dysfunction (and related treatments) has become justified in clinical settings. Recent findings in celiac disease offer a parallel.

The Expanding Spectrum of Celiac Disease

In celiac disease, the definition and diagnostic criteria are increasingly perceived as a *spectrum* ranging from classical presentations to milder, even seemingly silent forms. A 1997 article stated, "The widespread use of sensitive diagnostic tools, such as the serum antigliadin and the anti-endomysial antibodies, has shown not only that coeliac disease is one of the commonest disorders in Western countries but also that this condition is characterized by a higher degree of clinical variability than previously thought (typical, atypical and silent forms)." (12) In 1999, "The classic sprue syndrome of steatorrhea and malnutrition coupled with multiple deficiency states may be less common than more subtle and often monosymptomatic presentations of the disease." (13). In other words, by the late-1990s, celiac disease was becoming appreciated as having a wider range of signs and symptoms than had originally been postulated.

Similarly circa 2008, genetically documented mitochondrial disorders and associated diseases are becoming realized to be one endpoint on a larger continuum whose other endpoint is comprised of signs and symptoms summarized by Rossignol and Bradstreet and labeled as MtD (7).

IMPORTANT POINTS:

a) Within individuals, mutations in mtDNA can increase across time, and "Mitochondrial DNA undergoes a higher rate of spontaneous mutation than nuclear DNA." (8).

b) Individuals can be mosaic for mutations of mtDNA (14).

c) Pollutants and oxidative stress are associated with mtDNA mutations (15-16).

d) Elevated oxidative stress is associated with autism (17-19).

e) Mutations in mtDNA or in mito-related nDNA are often not found (5).

f) Pollutants, antibiotics, thimerosal, and aluminum can impair mitochondrial function (see below). Indeed, Rossignol and Bradstreet write, "Exposure to environmental toxins is the likely etiology for MtD in autism." (6)

Respectfully, we note that Richard H. Hass and colleagues have come to their expertise from the classical position wherein mutations in mtDNA or nDNA confirm a diagnosis of mitochondria disease. But we reiterate: Haas et al (10) specify a meaning of "mitochondrial dysfuntion" quite different from that set forth by Rossignol and Bradstreet, who offer: "MtD appears to be more common in autism and presents with less severe signs and symptoms. It is not associated with discernable mitochondrial pathology in muscle biopsy specimens despite objective evidence of lowered mitochondrial functioning." (7)

Pollutants, Oxidative Stress, Mitochondria, and Autism

Pregnancies occur in a polluted world, infants develop in a polluted environment. Peer-reviewed studies about pollution, oxidative stress, and mitochondria suggest a likelihood of suboptimal mitochondria function in all of us. Indeed, mito-related reference ranges are probably biased downwards from what ought to be signs of healthful mitochondria function in non-polluted environments (wherever they might be). Here is a summary:

- Pollutants, antibiotics, thimerosal, and aluminum can impair mitochondrial function (e.g., 20-23)
- Pollutants exacerbate oxidative stress (24)
- Elevated oxidative stress is associated with autism (25)
- Excessive oxidative stress impairs mitochondria function (e.g., 26-29)

Additional Relationships Linking Autism and Mitochondria

Adequate glutathione is important for mitochondria including brain mitochondria (30-35). Estrogen is protective against mitochondrial dysfunction (e.g., 36). Thus mitochondria in the context of pollutants may contribute to the male/female ratio in autism.

Vascular anomalies related to oxidative stress have been described in autism (37-38).

Vascular pathologies are related to mitochondrial dysfunction. Mitochondria participate in endothelial processes. MtD may negatively alter vascular function, consistent with vascular findings in autism. (39-40)

Air pollution is common in numerous locales worldwide. Airborne pollutants can "induce oxidative stress and mitochondrial damage" and are associated with autism (41-43). Note: these findings are based upon human data (e.g., 44-45). We should we concerned.

Studies describe mitochondrial dysfunction in relation to neurogeneneration. Since a large subgroup of autistic children has non-classical MtD, does MtD contribute to impairments of neuronal function in autistic children? To long-term neurodegeneration? (e.g., 46-47)

Mitochondria, Immunity, and Autism

Immune atypicalities have long been described in autism (e.g. 48-51). Mitochondria participate in immunity (e.g., 52-56). Thus, mitochondrial dysfunction may be a factor in autism-associated immune weakness. Brain-imaging techniques can identify mitochondria problems. As mitochondria disease and dysfunction become appreciated as a spectrum, imaging specialists may be able to document non-classical mitochondrial dysfunction in autistic children, even as results seem likely to differ from brain-imaging of individuals with classic mitochondrial disease (e.g., 57-60).

The Politics of Science

Hannah and her mother share a specific mtDNA mutation not categorized as pathologic. Her mother is a nurse and lawyer and thus —if affected at all by her mtDNA mutation—she is clearly not autistic. Nor was Hannah until after she was injected with 9 vaccinal antigens, related adjuvants, preservatives, etc (1).

Scientists and news reporters wanting to deflect criticism of vaccinations often claim that Hannah's mtDNA variant was crucial to her developing autism symptoms. However, this rationale avoids the reality of her mother's achievements and lack of autism despite (presumably) having the same mtDNA mutation. Furthermore, such scientists and reporters often present interpretations rooted in classical, must-be-genetic definitions of mitochondria disease, thereby ignoring clinical data indicating that MtD is not as rare as is classic mitochondrial disease.

VACCINATIONS AND MITOCHONDRIA

A comment in Weissman et al is profoundly important: "For one of our 25 patients, the child's autism/neurodevelopmental deterioration appeared to follow vaccination... Although there may have been a temporal relationship of the events in this case, such timing does not prove causation. That said, there might be no difference between the inflammatory or catabolic stress of vaccinations and that of common childhood diseases, which are known precipitants of mitochondrial regression... Large, population-based studies will be needed to identify a possible relationship of vaccination with autistic regression in persons with mitochondrial cytopathies." (5)

Jon Poling & colleagues made a similar observation: "It is unclear whether mitochondrial dysfunction results from a primary genetic abnormality, atypical development of essential metabolic pathways, or secondary inhibition of oxidative phosphorylation by other factors. If such dysfunction is present at the time of infections and immunizations in young children, the added oxidative stresses from immune activation on cellular energy metabolism are likely to be especially critical for the central nervous system, which is highly dependent on mitochondrial function. Young children who have dysfunctional cellular energy metabolism therefore might be more prone to undergo autistic regression between 18 and 30 months of age if they also have infections or immunizations at the same time." (3)

Furthermore, Edmonds et al 2002 describe how mitochondrial disease and infection can interact to induce neurodegeneration and offer a summary relevant to autism and the expanding spectrum of MtD: "We found no disease-specific presenting symptoms or characteristic age of presentation of mitochondrial disease..., although developmental delay was observed in 40%... **The broad clinical spectrum is one of the hallmarks of mitochondrial disease...** Signs and symptoms that were not present early in the course of disease may appear as the disease progresses. The absence of a specific sign is not evidence of the absence of mitochondrial disease." (8)

Poling et al elaborate the risk in a subgroup: "Young children who have dysfunctional cellular energy metabolism therefore might be more prone to undergo autistic regression between 18 and 30 months of age if they also have infections or immunizations at the same time. Although patterns of regression can be genetically and prenatally determined... it is possible that underlying mitochondrial dysfunction can either exacerbate or affect the severity of regression. Abnormalities of oxidative phosphorylation can be developmental and age related and can normalize with time..." (3)

What Does All This Mean?

The findings summarily reviewed hereinabove suggest several ramifications.

1. Pre-vaccination screening for MtD would minimize adverse reactions and life-long impairments.
2. Vaccination-guidelines could be improved by precluding sick or recently sick children.
3. As is presented in the rest of this chapter, according to peer-reviewed studies, elevated oxidative stress and/or mitochondrial dysfunction may respond to therapeutic protocols.

Circa 2008, "Biomarkers for mitochondrial dysfunction have been identified, but seem widely under-utilized despite available therapeutic interventions." (7)

References

1A Pieczenik SR, Neustadt J. Mitochondrial dysfunction and molecular pathways of disease. Exp Mol Pathol. 2007 83(1):84-92.

1B Pohling, Jon S, Father: Child's case shifts autism debate. Atlanta Journal-Constitution 4/11/08 http://www.ajc.com/opinion/content/opinion/stories/2008/04/11/polinged0411.html

2 Oliveira G et al. Mitochondrial dysfunction in autism spectrum disorders: a population-based study. Dev Med Child Neurol 2005 47(3):185-9.

3 Poling JS, Frye RE, Shoffner J, Zimmerman AW. Developmental regression and mitochondrial dysfunction in a child with autism. J Child Neurol 2006 21(2):170-2.

4 Correia C et al. Brief report: High frequency of biochemical markers for mitochondrial dysfunction in autism: no association with the mitochondrial aspartate/glutamate carrier SLC25A12 gene. J Autism Dev Disord 2006 36(8):1137-40.

5 Weissman JR, Kelley RI, Bauman ML et al. Mitochondrial disease in autism spectrum disorder patients: a cohort analysis. PLoS ONE. 2008;3(11):e3815. Epub 2008 Nov 26. http://www.plosone.org/article/info:doi/10.1371/journal.pone.0003815

6 Hui J, Kirby DM, Thorburn DR, Boneh A. Decreased activities of mitochondrial respiratory chain complexes in non-mitochondrial respiratory chain diseases. Dev Med Child Neurol 2006 48(2):132-6.

7 Rossignol DA, Bradstreet JJ. Evidence of Mitochondrial Dysfunction in Autism and Implications for Treatment. Am J Biochem Biotech 2008 4(2):208-17.

8 Edmonds JL et al. The otolaryngological manifestations of mitochondrial disease and the risk of neurodegeneration with infection. Arch Otolaryngol Head Neck Surg 2002 128(4):355-62.

9 Naviaux RK. Developing a systemic approach to the diagnosis and classification of mitochodrial disease. Mitochondrion 2004 4:351-61.

10 Haas RH et al. The in-depth evaluation of suspected mitochondrial disease. Mol Gen Metab 2008 94:16-37.

11 Siciliano G et al. Functional diagnostics in mitochondrial diseases. Biosci Rep 2007 27:53-67.s

12 Catassi C, Fabiani E. The spectrum of coeliac disease in children. Baillieres Clin Gastroenterol 1997 11(3):485-507.

13 Murray JA. The widening spectrum of celiac disease. Am J Clin Nutr 1999 69(3):354-65. http://www.ajcn.org/cgi/content/full/69/3/354

14 Bendall KE et al. Variable levels of a heteroplasmic point mutation in individual hair roots. Am J Hum Genet 1997 61(6):1303-8.

15 Simon DK et al. Low mutational burden of individual acquired mitochondrial DNA mutations in brain. [oxidative stress] Genomics 2001 73(1):113-6.

16 Nomiyama T et al. Accumulation of somatic mutation in mitochondrial DNA extracted from peripheral blood cells in diabetic patients. [oxidative stress] Diabetologia 2002 45(11):1577-83.

17 James SJ et al. Metabolic endophenotype and related genotypes are associated with oxidative stress in children with autism. Am J Med Genet B Neuropsychiatr Genet. 2006 141B(8):947-56.

18 Chauhan A, Chauhan V. Oxidative stress in autism. Pathophysiology. 2006 13(3):171-81.

19 Kern JK, Jones AM. Evidence of toxicity, oxidative stress, and neuronal insult in autism. J Toxicol Environ Health B Crit Rev. 2006 9(6):485-99.

20 Li N, Sioutas C, Cho A et al. Ultrafine particulate pollutants induce oxidative stress and mitochondrial damage. Environ Health Perspect. 2003 Apr;111(4):455-60.

21 Antibiotics and Mitochondria http://www.autism.com/medical/research/advances/autism-mitoantibiotics.htm

22 Yel L et al. Thimerosal induces neuronal cell apoptosis by causing cytochrome c and apoptosis-inducing factor release from mitochondria. Int J Mol Med 2005 16(6):971-7.

23 Murakami K, Yoshino M. Aluminum decreases the glutathione regeneration by the inhibition of NADP-isocitrate dehydrogenase in mitochondria. J Cell Biochem 2004 93(6):1267-71.

24 Pollutants and oxidative stress http://www.autism.com/medical/research/advances/autism-polloxi.htm

25 Oxidative stress and autism http://www.autism.com/medical/research/advances/autism-oxidative.htm

26 Chinopoulos C, Adam-Vizi V. Calcium, mitochondria and oxidative stress in neuronal pathology. Novel aspects of an enduring theme. FEBS J 2006 273(3):433-50. "The interplay among reactive oxygen species (ROS) formation, elevated intracellular calcium concentration and mitochondrial demise is a recurring theme in research focusing on brain pathology, both for acute and chronic neurodegenerative states."

27 Sas K et al. Mitochondria, metabolic disturbances, oxidative stress and the kynurenine system, with focus on neurodegenerative disorders. J Neurol Sci 2007 257(1-2):221-39.

28 Somayajulu M et al. Role of mitochondria in neuronal cell death induced by oxidative stress; neuroprotection by Coenzyme Q10. Neurobiol Dis 2005 18(3):618-27.

29 Patel M. Mitochondrial dysfunction and oxidative stress: cause and consequence of epileptic seizures. Free Radic Biol Med 2004 37(12):1951-62.

30 Fernández-Checa JC et al. Oxidative stress: role of mitochondria and protection by glutathione. Biofactors 1998 8(1-2):7-11.

31 Fernández-Checa JC et al. Mitochondrial glutathione: importance and transport. Semin Liver Dis 1998 18(4):389-401.

32 Heales SJ, Bolaños JP. Impairment of brain mitochondrial function by reactive nitrogen species: the role of glutathione in dictating susceptibility. Neurochem Int 2002 40(6):469-74.

33 Fernandez-Checa JC, Kaplowitz N. Hepatic mitochondrial glutathione: transport and role in disease and toxicity. Toxicol Appl Pharmacol 2005 204(3):263-73.

34 Lash LH. Mitochondrial glutathione transport: physiological, pathological and toxicological implications. Chem Biol Interact 2006 163(1-2):54-67. http://www.pubmedcentral.nih.gov/picrender.fcgi?artid=1621086&blobtype=pdf

35 Sims NR et al. Mitochondrial glutathione: a modulator of brain cell death. J Bioenerg Biomembr 2004 36(4):329-33.

36 Duckles SP et al. Estrogen and mitochondria: a new paradigm for vascular protection? Mol Interv 2006 6(1):26-35. http://molinterv.aspetjournals.org/cgi/content/full/6/1/26

37 Cohen DJ, Johnson WT. Cardiovascular correlates of attention in normal and psychiatrically disturbed children. Blood pressure, peripheral blood flow, and peripheral vascular resistance. Arch Gen Psychiatry 1977 34(5):561-7.

38 Yao Y et al. Altered vascular phenotype in autism: correlation with oxidative stress. Arch Neurol 2006 63(8):1161-4. http://archneur.ama-assn.org/cgi/content/full/63/8/1161

39 Davidson SM, Duchen MR. Endothelial mitochondria: contributing to vascular function and disease. Circ Res 2007 100(8):1128-41.

40 Zhang DX, Gutterman DD. Mitochondrial reactive oxygen species-mediated signaling in endothelial cells. Am J Physiol Heart Circ Physiol 2007 292(5):H2023-31. http://ajpheart.physiology.org/cgi/reprint/292/5/H2023

41. Palmer RF et al. Environmental mercury release, special education rates, and autism disorder: an ecological study of Texas. Health Place. 2006 Jun;12(2):203-9.

42 Windham GC et al. Autism spectrum disorders in relation to distribution of hazardous air pollutants in the san francisco bay area. Environ Health Perspect. 2006 114(9):1438-44.

43 Palmer RF et al. Proximity to point sources of environmental mercury release as a predictor of autism prevalence. Health Place 2009 15(1):18-24.

44 Törnqvist H, Mills NL, Gonzalez M et al. Persistent endothelial dysfunction in humans after diesel exhaust inhalation. Am J Respir Crit Care Med. 2007 Aug 15;176(4):395-400.

45 Crüts B, van Etten L, Törnqvist H et al. Exposure to diesel exhaust induces changes in EEG in human volunteers. Part Fibre Toxicol 2008 5:4.

46 Mancuso M, Coppede F, Migliore L, Siciliano G, Murri L. Mitochondrial dysfunction, oxidative stress and neurodegeneration. J Alzheimers Dis 2006 10(1):59-73.

47 Keating DJ. Mitochondrial dysfunction, oxidative stress, regulation of exocytosis and their relevance to neurodegenerative diseases. J Neurochem 2008 104(2):298-305.

48 Pardo CA, Vargas DL, Zimmerman AW. Immunity, neuroglia and neuroinflammation in autism. Int Rev Psychiatry 2005 17(6):485-95.

49 Cohly HH, Panja A. Immunological findings in autism. Int Rev Neurobiol 2005 71:317-41

50 Ashwood P, Wills S, Van de Water J. The immune response in autism: a new frontier for autism research. J Leukoc Biol 2006 80(1):1-15.

51 Jyonouchi H et al. Dysregulated innate immune responses in young children with autism spectrum disorders: their relationship to gastrointestinal symptoms and dietary intervention. Neuropsychobiology 2005 51(2):77-85.

52 McWhirter SM et al. Connecting mitochondria and innate immunity. Cell 2005 122(5):645-7.

53 Nagy G et al. Nitric oxide, mitochondrial hyperpolarization, and T cell activation. Free Radic Biol Med 2007 42(11):1625-31.

54 Deming PB, Rathmell JC. Mitochondria, cell death, and B cell tolerance. Curr Dir Autoimmun 2006 9:95-119.

55 Grimaldi M et al. Mitochondria-dependent apoptosis in T-cell homeostasis. Curr Opin Investig Drugs 2005 6(11):1095-102.

56 Perl A et al. Mitochondrial hyperpolarization: a checkpoint of T-cell life, death and autoimmunity. Trends Immunol 2004 25(7):360-7.

57 Finsterer J. Cognitive decline as a manifestation of mitochondrial disorders (mitochondrial dementia). J Neurol Sci. 2008 Sep 15;272(1-2):20-33. Epub 2008 Jun 24.

58 Kim J et al. Neuroradiologic findings in children with mitochondrial disorder: correlation with mitochondrial respiratory chain defects. Eur Radiol. 2008 Aug;18(8):1741-8. Epub 2008 Apr 4.

59 Lee YM, Kang HC, Lee JS et al. Mitochondrial respiratory chain defects: underlying etiology in various epileptic conditions. Epilepsia. 2008 Apr;49(4):685-90. Epub 2008 Feb 5.

60 Ramaekers VT et al. Mitochondrial complex I encephalomyopathy and cerebral 5-methyltetrahydrofolate deficiency. Neuropediatrics. 2007 Aug;38(4):184-7.

IMPLICATIONS FOR MEDICINE, EDUCATION AND THE ENVIRONMENT

By Jack Zimmerman, PhD

A Paradigm Change in Medicine

Perhaps the ASD children's most direct message to the culture is the necessity to change some of the ways many of us view medicine and the way we relate to physicians. Searching for ASD treatment protocols not only brings researchers and physicians to the edge of their knowledge about the human body but also questions our basic allopathic perspective and practices. ASD is not the only arena in which these beliefs and practices are being challenged. Others include the challenges surrounding the growing epidemic of Alzheimer's Disease, the increasing and inevitable ineffectiveness of anti-pathogens in the face of viral adaptability and diversity, the apparent degeneration of the human immune system, the rapid rise of auto-immune illnesses, and the dilemmas surrounding whether and how to prolong the end of life through medical means—to mention just a few.

We suggest that the roots of the impending and inevitable transformation in allopathic medicine lie in the essential distinction between "healing" and "curing." The special children are virtually driving us to transform our contemporary obsession with curing symptoms and embrace the larger interactive process that deserves to be called healing. Our time with Chelsey forced us to make this distinction, not without the benefit of countless dialogues between Jaquelyn and me that were not always calm and objective.

In simple terms, I have come to see curing as a process in which one or more knowledgeable and (hopefully) compassionate individuals attempt to change the physiological and/or the psychological condition of another. The definitions of normal and healthy are set primarily by the individuals implementing the cure, again hopefully in dialogue with the one(s) requesting it—and all generally in the context of our existing cultural consensus of what it means to be healthy. In curing, the major change is to take place in the one being cured. Unless something goes wrong in pursuing the cure, those "practicing the medicine" rarely go through a transformation as profound as that of the one being cured. Setting broken bones, hip replacement surgery, heart bypass surgery and many of the new laser surgeries for the eyes are examples of "curings" that are remarkable and clearly beneficial. In these more mechanical arenas allopathic medicine shines brightly.

Healing is a more reciprocal process in which the practitioner-healer(s) and patient are both transformed in a similarly profound, although possibly quite different ways. Because it is fundamentally relational in nature, the exchange in the healing process is analogously altering to all parties involved and usually produces more surprises than arise during the curing process. It is not uncommon for physician and patient (including the patient's loved ones) to enter a situation thinking that curing is what is called for only to discover that they are drawn inexorably (and sometimes kicking and screaming) into the more demanding, multilevel experience of healing. No matter how physiological the "disease," healing always involves the human psyche as well as the body. Full healing is not possible unless the body/psyche is treated as an inseparable continuum. Examples of illnesses that call us into healing include asthma, fibromyalgia and many other autoimmune diseases, allergies, clinical depression, cancer—and ASD.

Chelsey has been quite clear that she will not be cured. As we have indicated, her impairment is still at a level that spurs us on to try new treatments, despite the fact that she has not responded dramatically as have many other children in Jaquelyn's practice. On the other hand, it is unquestionably clear that Chelsey is more responsive, more emotionally active, initiates relationally more frequently and is increasingly capable in regard to such skills as reading, writing, arithmetic, swimming, trampolining, computer games, singing, and now even helping with household chores. Affective communication remains her biggest challenge, though she loves being with other children increasingly in recent years.

What is equally and undeniably clear is that Chelsey has changed the lives of many people directly and indirectly—her parents and siblings, of course, her grandparents, the many clients that Jaquelyn has worked with, those of us who have helped her with this book and (hopefully) the people who read it. Virtually every family with a special needs child can identify with this kind of statement. Chelsey is typical in regard to the impact she has had on all of us, perhaps more recalcitrant when it comes to "getting better," but typical as a transformer nevertheless.

Chelsey has and still is delivering the message that curing will not do. "Nothing less than healing, thank you," is what I hear from her all the time. It is a message we have resisted at times of overwhelm and confusion but, after almost ten years, have come to embrace, particularly in those moments when she spontaneously blossoms into greater relationship with us. I believe that we have entered into a healing process with Chelsey that is mutually and profoundly transformative, no less for all of us as for her. As readers of this book must surely now be convinced:

ASD is unbelievably complex—too complex to cure. It can only be healed and that is why these children are an imposing force for change in our medical culture.

What else are the ASD children teaching us about medicine?

• *A Systemic approach is essential.*

ASD involves almost every aspect of the child's non-skeletal physiology: the gut, the endocrine system, literally every aspect of the brain, the body as viral host, the immune system and so on. Treatment protocols need to be applied with systemic awareness, even if only a part of the system is being treated at a given time. That is exactly what led Jaquelyn to the broad-spectrum approach that is described in this book. The reductionistic direction of allopathic medicine over the past fifty years, fueled by established medicine's embrace of "specialists" and the explosion of technology, needs a significant mid-course correction if ASD is to be eventually contained. Every physician/healer will have to develop her or his own way of working "broad spectrum" if we are to successfully heal the onslaught of ASD (as well as many other illnesses).

- ***The patient (in this case, usually the parents) must take back responsibility for being a partner in the healing process.***

This is not a new challenge, of course. Many have spoken and written about the need for patients to take more responsibility. But now it's time to walk our talk. Having an ASD child provides a powerful daily reminder to take that walk. Largely with the assistance of local support groups and a variety of closely bonded ASD Internet groups, parents have become a powerful force in the "Healing ASD Movement." Not only parents, but physicians, researchers and clinicians who have ASD children often participate at the frontier of this movement, which is another reason for its growing influence both medically and politically. As a result of the active role parents are playing, the projections of power and authority onto medical professionals that have so dominated contemporary medicine are diminishing and even disappearing in the healing of ASD children.

It is often parents who inform their pediatricians about the latest protocols and even begin their doctor's education in the mysteries of ASD. Moreover, parents are the primary clinicians in treating ASD. They are the ones trying to get the pills down, holding tightly to squirming bodies for EEG's, injections or blood sampling, and getting up in the middle of the night to follow through a chelation protocol. There are too many ASD children for physicians to treat without significant participation of parents, even when the doctors are willing to take on the enormously time-consuming challenges involved. The few who are have become swamped. As she has made clear, Jaquelyn wrote this book in part with the hope it would find its way to pediatricians and other physicians through the passionately involved parents of their ASD patients.

- ***Strengthening the immune system is an inescapable and primary component of healing.***

Prior to the increased incidence of autoimmune illnesses over the past twenty-five years, the primary thrust of establishment medicine has been to contain the symptoms of an illness and, perhaps, even remove its root cause without any significant interruption of the patient's life style. That has empowered our present medication mystique to the point that the general public expects that every disease will soon be curable through the taking of pills or other simple treatment. As a result, we consume a massive number of pills and live with the illusion that we are a healthy culture because of modern medicine's ability to generate the vast array of easily taken medications.

With the growing onslaught of autoimmune illnesses, this illusion is getting frayed around the edges. Having lost the ability to distinguish friend from foe, our bodies are turning on themselves to a greater and greater degree, crippling the functions of our digestive, hormonal and neurological systems as they kill off supposed enemies. The ASD children exemplify this situation to such a heart rendering degree that we can no longer avoid getting the message behind this exponential rise of autoimmune madness.

Humans have behaved as if there were little or no connection between their personal health and the "collective health" of the planet. We have polluted virtually every aspect of the environment and devoured natural resources voraciously, not understanding that we are literally part of this "Large Body." It seems clear to me that this disrespect for the Large Body is reflected in the epidemic of human autoimmune illnesses. It is as if unconsciousness about how we affect the environment has decimated the Large Body's immune system (the environment's ability to stay healthy) in a way that is now being reflected in the degeneration of human immune systems. We have objectified and "attacked" the environment just as an immune system can destroy its host body, no longer being able to differentiate friend from foe. Healing this planetary autoimmune disease is the single most important challenge we face as a culture—physician and non-physician alike—during the next cycle.

The diseases of the Large Body will not be cured. They must be healed. The ultimate survival of both our personal bodies and the Planetary Body depends on our ability to better understand the combined mystery of our interdependent immune systems. Human medicine must direct a greater proportion of its resources towards strengthening and reeducating our immune systems, rather than continuing our present, almost missionary, emphasis on destroying pathogens.

In the long run, the treatment of ASD will surely have to move in this direction. As indicated in Chapter Eight, for example, there is strong evidence that the myelin sheath in the brains of some autistic children is being destroyed by the child's immune system. How can this insidious "mistake" be stopped? No more important question faces medicine than how to reprogram a malfunctioning immune system. This is the primary reason for the recent excitement about Low Dose Naltrexone (LDN), which offers a way to modulate impaired immune systems. Finding out how to do this effectively will help us to understand what compromises the immune systems of the children who were adversely affected by the normal vaccination sequence, and so continue to improve the safety of such procedures.

At best the present environmental disaster will be reversed slowly over a period of many years. A few generations of children cannot wait for this to happen. Might it be possible to find ways to test a child's immune system for efficacy in utero and supplement-based remedies developed (much as can be done now with Down Syndrome children)? We can dream of the time when no child need be born with autism or with increased susceptibility to toxins.

In the meantime our present allopathic model needs to be transformed into a new medical paradigm in which the health of the immune system plays a central role. It will be medically and financially more efficient to do so.

For ASD is only one of a long list of critical autoimmune illnesses that is growing longer all the time: diabetes, MS, ALS, fibromyalgia, chronic fatigue syndrome, rheumatoid arthritis, Crohn's Disease—and, of course, AIDS and many others. The enormous number of people touched by these illnesses suggests that the "Large Body" is trying to give us the message more loudly and clearly, despite our resistance and denial: *Our collective immune system is on the ropes; focus on the immune system, not just on battling symptoms; find out more about what affects our immune systems so that you can make them stronger.* These challenges inevitably will expand medicine to include the way we eat, live our daily lives, deal with stress, conduct our relationships and set our cultural priorities.

Perhaps the most dramatic example of the need for an integrated immune system approach is the AIDS pandemic in developing countries. More than 26 million people in Africa are infected with the AIDS virus, over 6 million have active AIDS and 11 million have already died from the consequences of the devastating illness. In nine African countries life expectancy has dropped below 40 years and now 55%-60% of those infected are girls or women, many with children who are also infected. In an increasing number of villages there are few women left alive between the ages of 20 and 40. Thousands of babies are born HIV-positive and most of them die helplessly before the age of two. In sub-Saharan Africa there are 14 million AIDS orphans 50% of whom are estimated to be HIV positive.

It is widely accepted by international experts that gender inequality and men's predatory entitlement in much of Africa are primary factors in creating the AIDS pandemic catastrophe that has no historical precedent. The majority of women who are HIV-positive were infected by their husbands and, with few exceptions, do not have the capacity to refuse sex, cannot insist on condoms, and, therefore, cannot protect their own lives. The disease is threatening the very existence of women in some African countries. This social inequity between the genders in Africa is acknowledged to be a strong factor in the HIV/AIDS epidemic. The head of the U.N. along with other experts have stated that this epidemic will not abate until women are empowered to protect their own health and the health of their children.

Although the standard HAART medications are being used more widely in Africa, it is estimated that they are available to less than 25% of the people who need them, including most of the infected children. Even where they are available, these drugs are still expensive, have significant side effects for many people and require strict regular medical management and testing to be used safely.

Rebuilding the deeply injured African immune system will require mounting a large scale integrated, multi-dimensional approach that begins with improved nutrition, includes immune system enhancer/modulators (such as LDN) and includes a rebalancing of the complex gender mores that so dominate many African cultures. Bringing about radical changes through education and processes such as council among circles of men, circles of women and couples can be an essential part of strengthening the immune system of those involved—both literally through preventing infection in the first place and in creating healthier immune systems through stress reduction and the establishment of compassion as a cultural priority. Unless women begin to feel valued, respected, cherished—and empowered, the AIDS epidemic will continue, no matter how effective medical treatments become. The same is true, of course, in other parts of the developing world and, to some extent, in developed countries as well.

Jaquelyn and I are presently pursuing such an initiative with the staff of the University Hospital in Bamako, Mali, which is preparing to conduct a research study on LDN soon. We see this as a significant step along the path that leads to the New Medicine.

Education

One can learn a lot by deeply relating to just one child. My experience with Chelsey is a prime example. As I spent time with her during our extended "retreats," my six months in Phoenix and other times during the last ten years, I began to fantasize about what it would take to create a school in which she would really flourish. During this same period, I had the opportunity to speak with educators and health professionals who work with special needs students in both public and private school settings. When I was in Phoenix, I frequently visited "The High-Star Center for Children," the excellent school that Chelsey has attended for several years, and talked with their faculty. The extent and depth of the work of the many talented people devoted to the education of special needs children was astounding to me. I barely scratched the surface of the enormous body of writings and research that has been accomplished in this field over the past seventy years—particularly in the last fifteen.

Before long, my mind was spinning with educational possibilities for all the Chelseys in the world. These ideas began to flesh themselves out, first into a basic "meta-curriculum" and then into a more detailed description of how such a community of children and adults might actually function. By a meta-curriculum I mean the (hopefully conscious) agreements and principles that shape both the course content and environment of a school.

THE META-CURRICULUM

The meta-curriculum of my ideal, fantasy school for Chelsey was based on five foundation principles.

- *Inclusiveness.*

Inclusive means that ASD students and neurologically typical (NT) students co-mingle to a great extent within an integrated school environment. Many of the arts, physical and social activities are shared by all the children, along with certain portions of the academic program. The ASD children receive special academic support in very small groups (as do some of the NT children). As appropriate, older NT children are trained to tutor the ASD kids individually in academic skills. Quite a few schools in the US are now following this approach.

- *Learning takes place in a relational environment or "field" that resembles that of a well-functioning clan.*

Whatever else a "school" should be for an ASD child, it must create an environment that stimulates safe and fulfilling relationships among adults and children. Whether it's called "floor time," "stimulating interaction," "relationship development" or just plain being with children, the inclusive school's curriculum should grow out of a fabric of trust and connectedness that resembles the extended clans in traditional peaceful cultures.[1] All three generations—children, parents and grandparents (the latter as elders)—are fully present in the school and the educational program includes the exchange of life experiences, knowledge and wisdom among all the generations in the community--including the special children.

- ### *Honoring the Undirected Mind.*

Effective learning (healing too!) requires fluidity of academic structure (classes, curriculum content, schedules, etc.). Having room to breathe helps create a learning community in which spontaneous or "undirected" creative interactions—as well as academics—are encouraged.[2] To achieve such open and spacious interactions authentically requires a level of acceptance that all the children, ASD and NT alike, can participate in all school activities in their own unique way. (Of course, this does not mean acceptance of unproductive or destructive behaviors that any child, NT or ASD, may exhibit). Chelsey has taught us again and again that when we hold tightly to an agenda of changing her, she resists our expectations by becoming less relational and then regressing. She feels that we want her to be different than she is—and she reacts, sometimes strongly but usually subtly, by becoming less present. Of course, all children do this to some extent, at least until they learn to "play the game." It is just more noticeable with an ASD child.

We speak here of acceptance as an active, not passive, state of openheartedness that lies beyond patience and in which the child has room to move. It is a truism of good teaching that to effectively support growth in children requires accepting them where they are in the learning process at that particular time. Real growth is from the inside out, encouraged first by acceptance of what is and then challenging the child to extend their capabilities, knowledge and talents. The simultaneous acceptance of the being of a child and challenging her or him to grow is not a paradox but rather the basic gift of a good teacher.

- ### *Curiosity replaces quantitative goals as the primary source of motivation.*

Having goals for each child's "improvement" are inevitable, but in a clan-like relational environment these goals are held compassionately without attachment to the outcome. Thus the process is open to the possibility that student, teacher and the goals themselves can evolve and even transform significantly. What takes the place of the present philosophy of strongly held quantitative goals (grades, standardized test scores, etc) is passionate curiosity, a feeling of "what will the next moment of learning bring?" This level of curiosity brings with it at least a temporary suspension of fear-based judgment and the embracing of "Yes/And" (rather than "Yes/But" or "No/But") ways of relating among teachers and students.

• *Silence and Contemplation*

Most schools are noisy places and many children seem to both generate and thrive on a full menu of sound. Young people's music is often deafening, many sporting events are loud and urban schools are boisterous at best. It is debatable how well NT students handle all this input and what effects it has on their bodies and minds. What isn't debatable is that many ASD children are extremely sensitive to sudden and loud noises, even those that most children and adults find non-invasive. The fact that silence is becoming a rare commodity in our lives is a serious challenge for many special needs children and continuous awareness of their sensitivity to sound on everyone's part is important. Intervals of relative quiet and even silence are important for integration, reflection and release of the tensions that arise from relating. Quiet times are an essential manifestation of spaciousness. I have heard more than a few NT high school students yearn for the "good old days" (Primary School) when taking naps was part of the curriculum. ASD children yearn for this even more so, often silently.

When adults join with the kids in undirected play and quiet time, the wordless dimension of their relationships is given an opportunity to develop. This contemplative connection is essential in learning to listen deeply to ASD children and thus being able to enter their world in order to come up with ideas for productive ways of engaging them. Strong nonverbal connections often feel spontaneous and touched by grace. Such moments are obviously important in creating a strong relational field for the ASD children—and, of course for all children.

In brief then, the ideal school I imagined for Chelsey is:

An educational community—a "clan" for children, families and teachers-- that honors the undirected (as well as the academic) mind, practices acceptance, incorporates time for contemplation and honors curiosity as a primary motivation for learning.

I knew a few of the specific activities that had to be included in my fantasy school. Certainly there would be frequent councils of the ASD and NT kids all together. There would also be time for movement and music. Movement helps the ASD child to develop "I-ness"—that is, a sense of ego identity—by connecting rhythmic patterns with gross and fine motor movements. The experienced dance therapist begins by watching the child move, either in silence or with musical accompaniment, and then imitating his or her movements. This "imitation dance" sets the relational field necessary to build trust and serves as the basis for subsequent movement dialogues that include call and response, spontaneous interaction and, ultimately a developing sense of that kind of "relational movement" we call dancing. A mixed group of special needs and NT children learning to move together is an inspiring sight to behold.

Even in the early years when Chelsey's restlessness dominated her behavior, music always helped to focus her attention in a remarkable way. She would sit and listen to a favorite CD (over and over again!) all the while sitting quietly in a chair. At first she was still, except for a steady tapping of the CD case with her forefinger, the rhythm of her stimming bearing no relationship to the music's beat. As we explored and expanded her musical tastes (which have included a broad spectrum from popular Latino guitar, Bob Marley and Kenny Loggins to traditional Hawaiian music, Kitaro, Bach, Mozart and now rock and roll), she would intersperse the quiet, almost reverent, periods with dancing. She is quite clear—actually willful —about what music she wants to hear at any given time and likes to dress for the occasion. Traditional Hawaiian music can precipitate a quick change into a sarong and the Latino guitar brings out a long skirt and blouse.

One of Jaquelyn's most joyous experiences with Chelsey involved teaching her all the words to "Silent Night" and "Joy to the World" when she was six. It took writing out all the words and hours of practice but listening to their angelic duets, "there wasn't a dry eye in the house." Our musical experiences with Chelsey are shared by other families gifted with an ASD child. Many of these children seem to possess considerable latent musical talent. (Chelsey has perfect pitch, a sweet voice with a natural vibrato and a "photogenic musical memory"—talents that are not rare among ASD children, as we have discovered.)

Why does music have such a significant effect on these children? Observing Chelsey and other ASD children over the years suggests that the melodic, harmonic and rhythmic elements of music offer them a structure for the "uncoordinated" neurological activity going on in their brains. While they are listening and moving they are brought into better balance and self-awareness. It is as if the music provides a scaffold that increases the coherence of their neurological activity. Regular exposure to music and movement as part of school would strengthen coordination of neurological development with auditory capability, as well as both gross and fine motor skills. And, needless to say, Chelsey's school would have to have ready access to lots of water. A small natural looking pool would do. But if the school happened to be near a warm ocean, river or lake that would be sublime!

CAN A SCHOOL LIKE THIS REALLY BE CREATED?

I have been describing a fantasy school, based on values and ideals--however desirable--that are obviously difficult to manifest in our current critical educational scene. But perhaps continuing to try and make the present educational paradigm work is even more unreal. A well-populated generation of ASD children are becoming teenagers. The thousands of susceptible children who regressed into ASD in the late 1980's and early 1990's from viral and environmental triggers have become or are becoming adolescents. Where and how will those among them who still need a lot of daily support live meaningful lives that includes continuing their education?

I suggest that many of these ASD kids would thrive in cohesive communities, possibly together with their biological families, that are a mix of special needs and neurologically typical children and adults--communities much like my fantasy school for Chelsey. Our existing family and educational institutions will be strained to the breaking point by this surge of ASD children until they both transform themselves in radical ways. Visionary Karl Konig, MD, saw the potential of a community setting for special needs children many years ago when he started the Camp Hill Movement in Scotland. There are now more than 90 Camp Hill Communities around the world, seven in the US alone.[3] In any event we are going to have to do something quite radical with that portion of the now half-million US autistic children and the untold millions of ADHD and ADD children that still may be impaired enough after biomedical treatment to need special attention. So why not set our intentions high, apply the wisdom gained from past experience without maintaining the forms and familiar patterns of the past and see what happens?

We conducted two such "ASD in Community" experiences during the summers of 2004 and 2005, the first for four days and the second for a full week. Both autism camps were held at the Ojai Foundation's semi-wilderness setting in Ojai, California and were inspired by a vision similar to the one described in this chapter. One of our intentions was to create a temporary community of families raising ASD children that would continue to support parents, siblings and the ASD children themselves throughout the year.

Although we faced a host of challenges in organizing, planning and carrying out our vision for these autism camps, both summers exceeded our expectations in many respects. New friendships were established and old ones deepened. Families continued to assist each other in a variety of ways after camp, including the sharing of biomedical and other treatment protocols. This has helped to break down the familiar sense of isolation ASD families often experience. Particularly during the weeklong camp session, we tapped into the almost magical power of community living to support the healing of the ASD children—as well as helping parents and siblings to cope with their many challenges.

We experimented with a variety of activities to stimulate the children's self esteem and social awareness, including drumming, swimming, work projects, arts, akido, food preparation and, of course, council. The second summer we added interns to the program (both adult and youth) in order to provide more individual support for the children and to offer the parents some respite from their 24/7 "on duty" lives. The Ojai Foundation staff and both Jaquelyn and I hope to continue exploring the potential of such healing communities in the future.

Wanting to take my fantasy for the year-around education of ASD children a little further, I decided to share my vision of Chelsey's ideal school with some of my educator colleagues. I expected that many of them would feel I was being quite unrealistic. I have come to anticipate honest and strong reactions from my colleagues mixed with a certain amount of playful curiosity about what I might be coming up with next. Another reason I sought their council had to do with exploring what I call the principle of "Marginal Group Innovation" a little further.

One of the most important catalysts for educational change has always been the inadequacy of the established approach to be effective with a particular group of unusual students. Often it's the marginal elements of the student population that stimulate out-of-the-box educational thinking. Reading methods developed to work with dyslexic children have proven useful for helping "normal" children to learn to read more effectively.[4] To assist certain atypical students learn arithmetic and deaf students geometry, visual and kinesthetic methods were developed that now have found use with students possessing normal cognitive and hearing capabilities.[5]

The population of special needs children, in general, and ASD children, in particular, has reached a level that has finally received wide attention from the mainstream educational community. It is increasingly clear that supporting these students requires significant revision of a large portion of the standard curriculum, changes in the methods of training teachers and a substantial rethinking of the kind of school environments we have often created in the past. When I explored Chelsey's ideal school with my colleagues in the light of all these realities we all became quite clear—and excited—with the possibility that the ASD kids are creating a major opportunity to transform the way we educate *all* children. After going into greater detail than I have done here, the consensus seemed to be, "Why not make the kind of meta-curriculum you're suggesting the foundation for any school?"

Indeed! Why not?

In 2005 one in five middle school classrooms in the Los Angeles Unified School District (LAUSD) was devoted to special needs students—and this substantial percentage doesn't include many ASD children who were not able to be served within the school system at all. Just the economics of this situation were sufficient to create a crisis in the District.

The familiar model of segregating special needs children within regular schools or sending them to special schools was inadequate to handle the explosion of ASD population that began more than seven years ago. Many educators faced the challenge—actually the unusual opportunity—of educating all children within an inclusive school environment. The handwriting was on the wall. In 2001 LAUSD's Division of Special Education published their long-awaited report, "Schools for All Children: A Strategic Plan for Achieving Measurable Results for All Students Including Those with Disabilities" and the District set the goal to be 90% inclusive by 2005. In this plan, inclusion meant mainstreaming ASD children whenever possible. The report established 80% as the fraction of classes children with "disabilities" were to share with their NT cohorts with the remaining 20% to be special classes geared to those children that learn in ways that are different than normal children.

This decision was a bold and necessary step—and, as it turned out, a very difficult one to achieve. In particular, the retraining of teachers to incorporate ASD and other special needs children into their classrooms has turned out to be a daunting task. Curricula had to be significantly revised, teaching methods radically changed and entirely new approaches taken to structuring schools in implementing the inclusive vision. Many educators experienced overwhelm, most of the schools for special needs children had to be kept open because of parent concerns and the reality of what could be done in a short period of time. This critical situation is a familiar one in many school districts all over the country. The past few years have clearly shown that we are at the beginning of a long journey of educational transformation that will have many tumultuous turns in the road.

This is not the place to explore these complex educational issues further. What is important for those of us on the starving brains/ starving hearts journey is that many of our kids are already or soon going to be in the middle—not the fringes—of the mainstream educational scene. Those of us who spend a lot of time with ASD kids inevitably will be drawn into the coming educational revolution.

Those who have "taught" special needs children are already developing methodologies which will eventually be essential in rethinking the way we educate *all* our children. This transformation of education will be supported by embracing the principle of inclusion in schools, a principle we believe is and will be of great benefit to both the special and neurologically typical children. The changes will not come easily. Familiar educational ideas hold on tenaciously and die tumultuously. For many reasons besides the challenge of incorporating special needs children, we have entered a chaotic time in public education that undoubtedly will continue for some years to come.

A Final Word on the Environment

As we have emphasized, the present ecological crisis is inseparable from the challenges parents face in healing their ASD children. Miners in the coalfields of Pennsylvania and West Virginia often brought a canary down into the mines with them as a way to detect the presence of methane gas. As long as the canaries survived the miners were safe. When the birds stopped singing and began to die, the miners packed up their tools and headed for the surface in a hurry.

It is clear that ASD children have been cast in the role of canaries in the "mines of our culture," not only in regard to education, medicine and the need for more conscious family relationships, but also directly in regard to our relationship with the environment. Whatever the causes, their impaired immune systems cannot handle the toxins that other children and most adults are able to tolerate. They are letting us know already that the food we eat, the way in which we dispose of our industrial waste and some of the materials we have used in agriculture, dentistry and vaccines are not safe. But we are slow to get the message and continue to use many of these or similar materials, as well as support policies that are leading to an increasingly toxic environment. It is time to pack up our tools, get to the "surface" (that is, wake up) and take care of these situations in a hurry!

It has been made quite clear that the presence of mercury in fish (Chapter 4), the excessive amounts of gluten in prepared foods, as well as in breads and pasta, and the over-abundance of dairy products in our diets are intolerable for a large number of children (Chapter 5). The majority of us seem to be able to handle the unbalanced diets that are typical of children and adults today, but at what cost? Most of us may not show dramatic symptoms, as do the ASD children. But is it just a matter of time? If our immune systems become further compromised by stress, overuse of antibiotics, a toxic environment and the cumulative effect of unbalanced diets, will more and more of our children "stop singing?"

The effluents of pesticides used since the beginning of the last century and long standing industrial waste disposal practices have already had a serious contaminating effect on our fresh water supplies and the oceans. Some think it is already at or beyond the critical level. (The mercury in fish is just one direct result of failed water practices). We have only an educated guess of what effect the storage of nuclear wastes will have on our long-term health. Certain consumer products have altered the ozone layer, led to the dangers of the greenhouse effect, left a legacy of lead-poisoning and caused the destruction of much of the native rain forests that contain the vast majority of the earth's medicinal plant species. Finally, after many years of ignoring scientists' concerns about global warming, decision-makers and the mainstream of the culture are beginning to listen and debate the possibility of averting disaster.

We are making small inroads in solving some of these problems, but has the pace and magnitude of the improvements been sufficient to stem the tide? Most environmentalists say, "No!" Those in denial respond that the vast majority of people seem to be surviving, despite all the dire warnings. Besides, they say, economic factors must also be taken into consideration. But if the ASD children are seen as our advanced messengers of ill tidings, then we are already in a dangerous transition that will soon affect the health of a larger portion of the population. We feel this is the prudent hypothesis to pursue. There is a good chance that if the frightening symptoms already exhibited by the ASD children are not treated very seriously, many more children—and adults—will soon become seriously ill as well.

We believe the link between environmental toxicity and the growing number of ASD children is sufficiently "causal" to embrace new dietary patterns and a radical rethinking of all of our policies concerning industrial waste disposal, agricultural practices, the preparation and use of vaccines, the use of dental materials, the manufacture of consumer products—and much more. If we hear the message the children are bringing, we are more likely to heal the messengers. At the very least, we may be able to reduce the need for further generations of young messengers.

References

1   The Pre-Tahitian Hawaiian Culture is a good example of what I'm talking about. This clan-based culture flourished in the Islands before the more hierarchical and war-like Tahitian culture arrived. Clans were as large as 400-500, children were educated primarily by grandparents, aunts and uncles, as well as parents, and all the clans share a council-like practice called "ho'o pono pono."

2   In his seminal book, "Letters to the Schools," Krishnamurti makes the strong statement that there is no true learning without leisure. By "leisure" he means an environment which encourages students and teachers to interact in a state of undirected mind.

3   See "The Camp Hill Movement," Karl Konig, TWT Publications Ltd. 1993 (2nd edition).

4   For example, the Gillingham reading method, developed more than seventy years ago in part at the Ethical Culture Schools in New York City, was inspired by the special needs of dyslexic students.

5   I refer here to the now familiar "Cuisenaire Rods" for teaching arithmetic and Gattegno's invention of the "Geo-Board" for teaching geometry to deaf students.

POETIC VERSION OF OUR JOURNEY WITH CHELSEY

TO JAQUELYN: GODDESSES ON THE MOVE
FEBRUARY 2002

I am disappearing—white hot fire burning in a far away belly a
    lifetime below my heart—
Into this forever new moment of discovering what you call
    "Love's Body"

Disappearing—beaten by wind-chopped swells vanishing into
    union with the shore—
Into the image of your face, breast, smooth back-swell, thigh,
    sacred sea flower

Disappearance, I trust, leaves me transparent, so nothing comes
    between who you are
And what I see with these seventy year-old fading friends of mine

With that heartsight I relish my woman, fire-eyes blazing, riding a
    creature of Diana's
That surely knows the way and will not stop until she arrives
    home, done, finished

Through fresh ears, not numbed by years of listening to secular
    chatter,
I hear the hundreds of children you will touch celebrating,
    "Mommy, Daddy, we are free"

In this hoary heart, fired, shaped and tempered by our
    otherworldly blacksmith
I know they are preparing to shake off the curse of confused
    immunity

I am with you, slightly behind on your left, my hands reaching
    across our differences
To rub a back that aches with the consuming labor of your sixth
    love child

I am with you to learn how to serve a goddess sworn to devote her
   life
Completing a mission of redemption for her next embodiment as
   Chelsey

I have no choice for I am disappearing into loving both these
   goddesses
—Or are they One? I am losing the patterns of my mind…and
   finding my heart

That discovery will guide me to where you live in love's wildest
   imagination
And, so inspired, we will do our part to bring the children home,
   clear and re-awakened

After the celebrations, we bower buddies are free to see what two
   Love's Bodies become
As they slowly vanish into boundary-less knowing of the Other

Meanwhile, I still wonder about this goddess who always defines
   my love
I will likely keep on asking and you two, surely, will keep on
   moving

I am disappearing…Take a good last look…Who will be saying,
   "I love you?"
Will you remind "me" who he used to be when we make the
   crossing?

TO CHELSEY: ALMOST A YEAR LATER
JANUARY 2003

Seduced by our impassioned vision of healing, we moved ahead of
  the medicine
Already anticipating celebrations of reawakened immune systems
And parents' tearful joy on hearing: "Mommy, Daddy, I love you"
  for the first time.

In fact, the journey grows longer than expected—and steeper—
  and perplexing
How many times have you, now almost nine, sent us back to our
  lovers' laboratory
Dark with dashed expectations, challenging us to let go and try
  again?

We fear losing ground to your hormonal budding, burgeoning
  strength
And a will that shouts "Wake up! You still haven't seen clearly who
  I am behind the
Veils of seeming indifference, wild destructiveness and insatiable
  orality."

"I take no prisoners; nothing short of complete surrender—
  of who you think you are
What your life is about, and all that you know about healing and
  love—will do.
Nothing less than a heart completely devoted to *seeing* me will
  open mine."

There is no alternative…The past has been shaken up, uprooting
  patterns of a life
Devoted to getting ready to take the leap, always preparing, always
  on the brink
Of learning the secret to turning just one child's life around.

"Don't you see? There is no one child to heal, no secret curriculum
   for healing
No great knowledge to acquire, no success or end to the dance
Just show up a little more every day without expectations and
   be with me."

"Touch me softly, treat me roughly; Gramma, don't hold back the
   grief and frustration
Wooing is too one sided to entice me into a world wild with fear
And whipped into insanity by leaders falsely claiming fearlessness."

"Maybe I will woo you instead, away from the advancing darkness
Mirroring what I see until you all feel the great cry of danger from
   the world's shared
Immunity now rapidly reaching a state of irreversible pollution."

"Listen! It is not too late. Come be with me, Grampa—no drama,
   just day-to-day
Fulfill your assignment, stop stalling with that which you have
   already accomplished
Just look out the windows of your heart and write and swim and
   play with me."

"I assure you every seduction will meet its match as I fulfill my
   mission—
Not exactly chosen—birthed in me by the mystery that you two
   will also encounter
When love finally disappears you and there is no one left to write
   about it."

INVITATION
FEBRUARY 2004

Come, take my hand
So I can find you in the eye of the whirlwind
Calling medicine back to its spirit home
And welcoming the lost tribe of children
Our little adept among them
As you keep reminding me, we need to work from another level
Which means creating an entire heartscape, nothing less
Chelsey is waiting—I see the message in her big browns
"Only full surrender satisfies my mission."

Take my hand—again
As at our birth when you led me out
Of a flat world into the delights and shadows of Eros
Now, our toes curled around the edges of the past
We hesitate, seeking a still greater revelation of Love
Are we too heavy with treasured wounds and attachments to fly
Or is it fear of the demons at the doorway to ecstasy?
No matter, our courage will soon rise to the new occasion
Since it always starts with, "Gramma—Grampa will you
    dance with me?"

And so leaps of faith and healing are merging movements
Connecting you and Chelsey inside the Mystery
That we touch as well when our trust is great enough
To fall more wildly into Love's uncharted forests
And then to guide us into the clearing of our hearts
We can create similar shamanic celebrations
To re-awaken our unrelenting messenger
And so embrace her healing with enough persistent passion
To wholly feed that starving brain

This enlightening of our aim to cure
Will see through the harvest of impaired immunities
Into the innate wholeness of each ancient soul

So too our little Buddha, our Christ Child, asks for recognition
I heard the call again the night I phoned to celebrate her tenth
She said, "Hi, Grampa" in that soft and rounded voice
That opens my heart and wild eyes to smiling
She waits for us to leap and doesn't need fixing
As much as being met half way with laughter

"Here, take my hand"
Excites the biggest grin of all
Since she's been longing for our commitment
To meet in Rumi's field together
That consummation meets her challenge
To claim our fullest lives while still embodied
"But words don't matter," she says, "The joke's on you
You jumped a long time ago and have been falling forever
There's nothing else to do."

EPILOGUE: A TURN IN THE STORY
JANUARY 2005

I first noticed the change last summer walking along our favorite
    beach
When, looking up from the sand and squinting into the sun, I saw
    her hips
Outline the shape of a woman who would soon need Jaquelyn's
    guidance
I wondered whether premature waves of womanhood
Would leave her floundering, unable to speak of it.

A little later, at our Island's summer camp for special children
A pair of brothers fell wildly in love with her by the second day
One, as articulate as a troubadour, said to us, "She is so beautiful"
As the children cuddled on the resting mat between making pizza
    and computer time
For days his brother worshipped her wordlessly without response.

Soon her body called for exploration with an uninhibited curiosity
That most "normal" ten year olds have already hidden for future
    intimacy
Only nipples appeared that summer with just a hint of the swell to
    come
When she finally took notice, innocent fingers went walking to see
If Grampa might be manifesting a similar secret.

Six months later, just after Christmas, she sat on our bed in
    California
Nightshirt in hand, entranced by a favorite photo of herself at six
(Topless, feral eyes befitting a nymph, near the giant eucalyptus
    swing)
We watched unnoticed, wondering what cascade of feelings filled
    this dolphin child
As she gently touched one budding breast and then the other.

Oh, Chelsey, when the moon moves the tides in you—too soon
    perhaps
Will you understand or be confused by parental words of wisdom?
Either way, might these new stirrings feed your starving brain
Past all our medication and call your Isis in to play amongst a
    cautious culture
That has forgotten how to celebrate so powerful a Goddess.

We hope the legacy of protocols and passages we have shared
Allow us to discover the story of your emergence from childhood
    and isolation
A tale that honors your history—and births a vision for
    transcending it
A vision that your Gramma and I will draw
From the wellspring of our inexplicable love.

In the story you say to Grampa, "I'm sad I will not see you for a
    while"
And later ask Gramma, "What is it like when Grampa holds you in
    his arms?"
All real, for once in Phoenix you looked up at me in the midst of
    learning a song
On a day of my rare discouragement to ask, wide-eyed, "Grampa
    sad?"
I nodded and for the first time imagined you a woman on the path
    of intimacy.

I see you and this "Damian"—grown from a boy at summer camp
    or school
Getting to know each other beyond the residue of immune
    impairment
We will write this story with enough wisdom and transforming
    heart
To meet the karmic challenge you made silently through big
    browns afire
"The changes for both of you will have to be as deep as those you
    want for me."

May our story work the ground of your future
Leaving it fertile for you and your Damian to discover
The delights of Love's synaptic synergies
And so, through intimacy's medicine, build the far greater
    immunity
Desperately needed to transcend the poisons of our withering
    world.

Preparing you for this healing journey has already taken us
Beyond the borders of what we used to call Unbounded Love
Into new territory where spirit gardeners prune the old wood
From our cluttered hearts so that you and all the children blossom
With the blessings of a healing Spring.

Is it time to release you, charismatic catalyst
And write this story of our love with prayers of gratitude?
We must learn to heal even when deserts or oceans divide us
A story can be held anywhere
And prayers know no boundaries.

Then someday
We will become
Your spirit guides
And so come to know
The story that never ends.

(On Jaquelyn's Birthday, January 24, 2005)

HEALING FOOLISHLY
OCTOBER 2006

What is this foolishness bubbling up when I play with Chelsey?
Where does it reside when I'm not with my goddess in training
Who, in truth, is training me to find the way to her heart
So she can awaken to the path of love
In preparation for meeting Damian.

Our diversion started years ago in a California store
Where Gameboys filled the shelves
Promising a passionate path to high-tech stimming
Thereafter, she would look at me and ask with a sly smile
"Walking to the game store, yes!"

My part of the dance was to answer, "No"
Bringing my mouth close to her ear
And stretching out the "o" until she laughed
Or to say many "No's" in a row bringing about the same result
Until even a grampa's patience became threadbare.

After many months we added a wrinkle to the game
That opened a door to deeper delights
"Walking to the game store, yes," Chelsey would say
"No," I answer, "Life is not a game store; life is a game "
"Yes, life is a game," she echoes while we laugh.

Why this amused her left me wondering
Whether she understood this crude version
Of Shakespeare's great insight
But I never found out all the many months
We repeated our dialogue endlessly.

This summer the silliness shifted as we all
Did our best to stop her from picking
At her cuts, scratches and blemishes—
The latter a consequence of the hormones demanding entrance
Into the body of this unsuspecting twelve year-old.

"Stop picking," became our mantra—literally
Gramma and I must have said it a hundred times each day
And written it out for her in big letters
That she was asked to copy many times
To imprint the message…all to no avail.

Then in the tank one day she discovered that my thinning hair
Hid a few of the barnacles that come with age
And many years in the garden or swimming in the sea
Encrustations that seduced her irrepressible fingers
That are never still until she finally falls asleep, exhausted.

After I parried her pickings for a few more days
She upped the ante on this wacky way we have
Of connecting through her soggy synaptic veils
"Walking to picking grampa's head, yes," she said gaily one day
"Noooooooo," I whispered into her ear in self-defense.

We played out this version in our capsule, and in the car
And the sea, each time changing the tone, pitch and length
Of the "No," until her delight knew no bounds
And I was as foolish as a grown man can be
When love for a child goes beyond his comprehension.

The next wrinkle came a week before the flight home to Phoenix
To family, school, church and a long history of healing
I begin with "Nnnnnn," very softly, letting the tone build
Until finally the "o" pounces on her like a predatory panther
Leaving her big browns round as moons and a Cheshire smile on
    her lips.

The final twist came in the last dive of the summer
During a break from watching Pocahontas
When, after numerous "nnnnooo's," I said (thinking of Damian)
"Enough of this silly game we've been playing
We need to play a new one called the Game of Love."
"Noooooo," she answered in true terror, reversing roles.
"Yes, you are soon to enter the path of love!"

"Nooooo," she repeated with such fiery fierceness
That I knew she understood exactly what I meant
And was loath to leave her haven of impairment.

Tickling is another way we touch the mystery of Love...
During one of our dives after Jaquelyn had tucked us in the tank
I was invited to provide an armpit tickle—right armpit to be exact
And, as I did my duty, a current connected between the lymph
    node
And that mysterious network of neurons that is Chelsey's brain.

I asked her, "Is there a connection between what my fingers
Are doing under your arm and what happens here in your brain?"
I tickled her head ever so gently with my other hand...
Wanting so to feel all the years of tickling had some higher purpose
And when she nodded I played the fool in still another way.

"It must be dendritic stimulation," I said with mock awe
She understood somehow and asked for more: "Tickle—left arm
    pit!"
"I don't know what `tickling' is," I whispered, playing my part
"Dendritic stimulation," she managed to get out before we both
Dissolved in laughter ten feet down in the wondrous world of
    HBOT.*

*Special thanks to Jim Neubrander for gifting us the use of an HBOT chamber
 for our annual summer month with Chelsey in Hawaii.

RECONCILIATION: AFTER AFRICA
JANUARY 2007

Reading all the poems in sequence reveals the story
Brings out the larger meanings that are lost
When life is lived in short spasms of attention
One secret to living a life of verse when raising a special child
Is to see they are closer to poetry than most of us.

A theme emerges from all the years of reflecting
On what these special children mean to us…"Reconciliation"
Just a word, no more the true essence of these ten years with
    Chelsey
Than the map is the territory
Yet the word resounds in the chambers of my heart

And once through the door and acknowledged
More words follow their leader
Like the echoes in a deep canyon when children shout their names
Into the silent beauty, testing whether Nature knows who they are
Reconciliation…reconciliation…

Of everything…of everything?
Yes, of everything…
Of heart and mind…
Of man and woman…
Of people and planet…
Yes, and I dare to say even of illness and health
And war and peace

It is time for medicine to shift its attack on illness
To understanding sickness as part of health's way
To rebalance the eternal distortions in the Large Body
Holding that vision we become allies of the children
And, incidentally, the old ways of healing as well

Sangomas, like Mama Evalina, say they know
How to keep HIV from becoming full-blown AIDS
The herb they call (in Zulu) *inkomfe* moderates the immune
    system
Just like low dose naltrexone
Remarkable coincidence?

No, there are white sangomas there too, like Jo
Ministering the marriage of the old and new
Bringing the traditional ways into medical schools
She even brought Mama to speak to two hundred students
Just gave her the mike and Mama took over like a rock star

Using her mudra inspired hands to help transmit
The mysterious cluckings of her native tongue
(As if she were signing for herself)
Mama wowed the black and colored students
The white ones need a little pruning to prepare for the marriage

Although the land washed by oceans from East and West
Gave birth to Mandela's journey of reconciliation
And its astounding many-colored councils
There is still a generation's journey ahead
Before we can paint our lives with a full palette

Mama told Jaquelyn, "You are a sangoma who sees with spirit eyes"
And called her "Mama" to be sure the blessing wasn't missed
She challenged me to heal my ailing eyes
And gave me helichrysum to burn before dreaming
To let spirits part the veil and guide my healing hands

All her words came through Lukholo, Mama's grandson
As we sat together on the old sofa in her home in the township
That we wandered in for more than an hour to find her
Among the dirt streets, children and barking dogs
Already at twenty-four he is a sangoma-in-training

A clear light leads him to sit with circles of men
To help them redefine the meaning of masculinity
One gentle young man of magic serving the slums of Cape Town
Offering an alternative to the nightmare of male insanity
Strangling his nation by killing its women and children

The UN says containing the deadly pandemic
Demands the full empowerment of women
Finally, men must face their fear of women
As part of international policy!
The leaders of Mali say the same…How about ours?

No longer can we tolerate betraying health with politics
Nor separating environment from the climate of our souls
Global warming stems from the chilling of our hearts
In the longest of all human relationships
And pandemic autism from those in control failing to look into the
    eyes
Of a single child and actually *feeling* the message

These and the orphaned multitudes from every dark continent
Are demanding an end to denial…
"Heart of Darkness," indeed, Conrad had it right about the river…
I watched the Niger wind through the Land of our common
    Mother Ma
Until time and race disappeared in marshy banks and fishermen

The Large Body has spoken loud and clear
"Heal the ancient rift; embrace the mystery of man and woman
Or you will surely die in even greater numbers…"
Lover, what can we do with what we've learned
Trudging our path and digging foxholes of gender grief?

Have we not been bridging the primal rift between men and
    women
Since that day we met when you looked me up and down
To see if I would make a worthy opponent?
Haven't we shed some light on what Miriam and Yeshua
Were really all about?

Haven't you, Isis-like finally helped me find my manhood
So the Goddess can have a playmate worthy of her
Mystery and beauty, her fire and wisdom?
Have we not claimed the Third's realm as our home ground
And even the way to journey through the veil?

Yes, but there is still more to disappear…
When fear calls the patriarch, I become the Jack
You knew in childhood and, seen as father enemy,
You lash out at your lover of the night before
Though he held you for hours in sweet embrace

When you surrender so to impulse I think of Chelsey
But now inside a sangoma with encyclopedic knowledge
And if I follow old father gods and blame you for our separation
We repeat the story of the Garden
And once again are exiled from the Heart of Light

But if I don't and disciple myself to the emerging Goddess,
Then the wisdom of the Third grows exponentially
As in the places we touch when our bodies no longer
Need to remember even the roots of duality…
Making love in a healing way surpasses scripture

Although we are just a single wave striking a suffering shore
We bring the joys and devotion of that unique moment when
The curl offers the wind it edges for spray
In simple terms--
We can only do what we can do

Have we digested a morsel of the ancient struggle?
Has our love been enzymatic enough to
Break down those peptides of ancient fear into nourishment?
Have our practices cleared the gluten and casein from the
Diet of misunderstandings?

I dare to say, yes, a resounding YES!

We add a drop of reconciliation
To the flask of the Thirsty Healer
Each time we turn into the shadows once again
Seeking transparency—pulling ourselves
Out of the old patterns that track us from the womb

Take heart! There are many on the reconciliation path
Multitudes brought to life by the calls from darkness
Thus the flask is filling and the trek across the desert
Will be made in Lukholo's lifetime
He will show his tribe how to love a woman like a sangoma can.

A HYMN TO THE MIGHTY MITOCHONDRION
JANUARY 2009

Holding each other sharing dreams one morning long ago
You felt Our Third--our relationship—as a palpable entity
Surrounding us in a mantle of new consciousness
We honored the moment by calling our cuddling
The Embrace Meditation

Heart over heart, our different rhythms find a common beat
Our warm bodies greet each other, then forget their boundaries
And if I manage to still them long enough
My arms around you dissolve into what is left of our illusion
Of individuality

In this state our Third becomes a healer, an ancient shaman
In relational mode, ready to connect our connection
To those we are called to reach at a distance
When intimacy serves healing even the largest oceans
Are spanned by strong intentions

One regular recipient, of course, is Chelsey
Now in the torrent of the teens, almost a woman
A devoted disciple of the Goddess
But still in a body housing toxic tenants and struggling with
Mitochondrial mishaps

The mitochondrion's fertile folds cease their magic
When looted by mercury and other irresponsible intrusions
Creating a cascade of suffering
That leaves the host in misery, mourning the loss of its
Central source of energy

Yes, soiling of our sentient nest is poisoning our mitochondria
The special children are only an A in the growing list of diseases
A through Z that threaten evolution
How long can we deny the mitochondrion's mortality before we
     sweep
Ourselves to obscurity?

So a cry goes out to revive the ailing Mitochondria
Creating a broad spectrum of treatments in a new wisdom way
--Ancient alchemy, modern medicine
Recharging tiny batteries to jump-start brains weary from
Wanting a full human life

What is the link joining the Third and the mitochondrial mystery
That will empower our love to span the sea and embrace
The charismatic Chelsey as she sleeps
An astonishing adept who still has only an inkling's insight
Of her real identity?

A billion years ago the primal priestess tired of the pace of
    evolution
Brought together simple cells and our eukaryotic elders
Knowing that eons later
For humans to come to know Her we would need cells sexier
Than basic bacteria.

We were only a remote twinkle in the Goddess' eye
But that spark finally produced the mighty Mitochondrion
The original Little Engine that Could
And what it "could," produced enough power to give
Cells a prophetic life

The alchemy inside the labyrinthine laboratory
Transforms protein into ATP just by breathing and so
Evolution had a new vision
That led the way for most cells becoming tiny beings
Made up of many organs

The cells started forming families and the families created clans
And the clans went tribal until finally the Goddess
Got her wish and we appeared
--Her curiosity's creation--*in the image of a cell* as a
Multi-organ Large Body

The link is relationship, for the mitochondria made
Possible an evolution that bacteria couldn't dream of
And each cell emerged an entity
Just as our Third has materialized magically to give us
A glimmer of the Goddess

We can stop the bleeding and much more with collaborations
 Between mitochondrial alchemy and awakening Thirds
That start an evolution in healing
 And create a New Medicine to replace the old
Allopathic alliance

For when we hold each other now, merging moves beyond
Our wildest imagination and our Third becomes a source
Of power--a meta-mitochondrion
That helps each love-making conceive a new link in the
Evolutionary chain

This is the healing state, this native land of union
Holding Light and Dark, man and woman, death and life
Oppressed and dominant
Lo, we are awakening from the diseases of individuality
With the healing heart of love

To my Goddess-Healer-Lover for her 77th Birthday,
from   JZ: January 2009

INDEX

NOTES

NOTES

NOTES

NOTES

NOTES